T0203388

Extremely Preterm Birth and its Consequences

Clinics in Developmental Medicine

Extremely Preterm Birth and its Consequences: The ELGAN Study

Edited by

Olaf Dammann

Professor and Vice-Chair Department of Public Health & Community Medicine,
Tufts University School of Medicine,
Boston, MA, USA

University-Professor, Dept. of Gynecology and Obstetrics,
Hannover Medical School,
Hannover, Germany

Alan Leviton

Professor of Neurology, Harvard Medical School,
Emeritus Head of the Neuro-epidemiology Unit, Boston Children's Hospital,
Boston, MA, USA

T Michael O'Shea

C Richard Morris Distinguished Professor of Pediatrics and Division Chief for
Neonatal-Perinatal Medicine at the University of North Carolina,
Chapel Hill, NC, USA

Nigel Paneth

University Distinguished Professor, Departments of Epidemiology & Biostatistics and
Pediatrics & Human Development, Michigan State University,
East Lansing, MI, USA

2021

Mac Keith Press

© 2021 Mac Keith Press

Managing Director: Ann-Marie Halligan
Senior Publishing Manager: Sally Wilkinson
Publishing Co-ordinator: Lucy White
Project Management: Riverside Publishing Solutions Ltd

First published in this edition in 2021 by Mac Keith Press
2nd Floor, Rankin Building, 139–143 Bermondsey Street, London, SE1 3UW

British Library Cataloguing-in-Publication data
A catalogue record for this book is available from the British Library

Cover: The images depict stages of the early life journey of one individual born extremely preterm at 22 weeks.
Cover designer: Marten Sealby

ISBN: 978-1-911488-96-5

Typeset by Riverside Publishing Solutions Ltd
Printed co-ordinated by Jellyfish Solutions Ltd

Dedication

In memory of our colleagues and ELGAN co-investigators

Francis 'Frank' Bednarek (1944–2013).
Frank was the principal co-investigator at the University of Massachusetts at Memorial Health Care, Worcester, MA.

Richard 'Rich' Ehrenkranz (1946–2018).
Rich was the principal co-investigator at Yale University School of Medicine, New Haven, CT.

Contents

Author Appointments ix

Foreword xi

Preface xiii

Acknowledgements xv

1. **Introduction** 1
   Alan Leviton, Olaf Dammann, T Michael O'Shea, and Nigel Paneth

PART I Placenta and Perinatal Risk Factors 15

2. **Placental Microorganisms in ELGAN with Correlation to
   Pregnancy Outcomes, Intrauterine Inflammation, and
   Postnatal and Later-life Outcomes** 17
   Martha Scott Tomlinson and Rebecca C Fry

3. **Correlations of Placental Histology in ELGANS with Delivery
   Indications, Placental Microbiology, and Childhood
   Morbidity** 27
   Jonathan L Hecht

4. **Signal Initiators of Early Preterm Birth** 35
   Asha N Talati and Tracy A Manuck

5. **Maternal Adiposity** 43
   Jelske W van der Burg and Elizabeth T Jensen

PART II Neonatal Exposures and Outcomes 55

6. **Illness-Severity and Outcomes among Children Born
   Extremely Preterm** 57
   J Wells Logan and Olaf Dammann

7. **Bacteremia**   73
   H Reeve Bright and Kikelomo Babata

8. **Retinopathy of Prematurity**   81
   Mari Holm, Deborah VanderVeen, and Olaf Dammann

9. **Bronchopulmonary Dysplasia**   89
   Wesley M Jackson and Matthew M Laughon

PART III   Structural Brain Disorders   103

10. **Ultrasound**   105
    Genevieve Taylor and T Michael O'Shea

11. **Multispectral Quantitative MRI: Techniques and Preliminary Results**   115
    Hernán Jara and T Michael O'Shea

PART IV   Functional Brain Disorders   129

12. **Cerebral Palsy among Children Born Extremely Preterm: The ELGAN Study**   131
    Stephanie Watkins and T Michael O'Shea

13. **Cognitive and Behavioral Functioning**   145
    Lauren Bush, Megan N Scott, and Scott J Hunter

14. **Autism, Social Impairment, and Social Communication Deficits in Children Born Prior to the 28th Week of Gestation**   157
    Steven J Korzeniewski

15. **Psychiatric and Behavioral Outcomes at Age 2 and 10 Years in Individuals Born Extremely Preterm**   171
    Jean A Frazier, Hannah Zamore, and Stephen R Hooper

16. **Concluding Chapter: Please Draw Your Own Conclusions**   195
    Alan Leviton, Olaf Dammann, T Michael O'Shea, and Nigel Paneth

Glossary   219

Index   225

Author Appointments

Kikelomo Babata Assistant Professor, UT Southwestern, Department of Pediatrics, Division of Neonatal-Perinatal Medicine, Dallas, Texas, USA

H Reeve Bright Family Medicine Resident, Montefiore Medical Center, Bronx, NY, USA

Lauren Bush Clinical Psychology Doctoral Candidate and Predoctoral Intern, Northwestern University Feinberg School of Medicine & The University of Chicago, Chicago, IL, USA

Olaf Dammann Professor and Vice-Chair, Department of Public Health & Community Medicine, Tufts University School of Medicine, Boston, MA, USA

University-Professor, Department of Gynecology and Obstetrics, Hannover Medical School, Hannover, Germany

Jean A Frazier Executive Director, Eunice Kennedy Shriver Center; Professor of Psychiatry and Pediatrics, UMASS Medical School/UMMHC, Worcester, MA, USA

Rebecca C Fry Carol Remmer Angle Distinguished Professor and Associate Chair, Department of Environmental Sciences and Engineering, Gillings School of Global Public Health, UNC-Chapel Hill, Chapel Hill, NC, USA

Jonathan L Hecht Associate Professor of Pathology, Beth-Israel Deaconess Medical Center, Boston, MA, USA

Mari Holm MD, PhD and Resident, Department of Radiology and Nuclear Medicine, St. Olaus Hospital, Trondheim, Norway

Stephen R Hooper Professor; Associate Dean of Medicine; Chair, Department of Allied Health Sciences, School of Medicine, University of North Carolina-Chapel Hill, NC, USA

Scott J Hunter Professor of Psychiatry & Behavioral Neuroscience, and Pediatrics, The University of Chicago, Chicago, IL, USA

Wesley M Jackson Assistant Professor of Pediatrics, University of North Carolina at Chapel Hill, Chapel Hill, NC, USA

Hernán Jara Professor of Radiology, Boston University School of Medicine, Boston, MA, USA

Elizabeth T Jensen Associate Professor, Department of Epidemiology and Prevention, Wake Forest School of Medicine, Winston-Salem, NC, USA

Steven J Korzeniewski Associate Professor, Department of Family Medicine and Public Health Sciences, Wayne State University School of Medicine, Detroit, Michigan, USA

Matthew M Laughon Professor of Pediatrics, University of North Carolina at Chapel Hill, Chapel Hill, NC, USA

Alan Leviton Professor of Neurology, Harvard Medical School, Emeritus Head of the Neuro-epidemiology Unit, Boston Children's Hospital, Boston, MA, USA

J Wells Logan   Associate Professor of Pediatrics, The Ohio State University; Associate Director, Critical Care, Transport, Nationwide Children's Hospital, Columbus, OH, USA

Tracy A Manuck   Associate Professor, Department of Obstetrics and Gynecology, Division of Maternal Fetal Medicine, University of North Carolina-Chapel Hill, Chapel Hill, NC, USA

T Michael O'Shea   C Richard Morris Distinguished Professor of Pediatrics and Division Chief for Neonatal-Perinatal Medicine at the University of North Carolina, Chapel Hill, NC, USA

Nigel Paneth   University Distinguished Professor, Departments of Epidemiology & Biostatistics and Pediatrics & Human Development, Michigan State University, East Lansing, MI, USA

Megan N Scott   Associate Professor, Department of Psychiatry and Behavioral Neuroscience, University of Chicago, Chicago, IL, USA

Asha N Talati   Clinical Instructor, Fellow, Division of Maternal Fetal Medicine, Department of Obstetrics & Gynecology, University of North Carolina at Chapel Hill, NC, USA

Genevieve Taylor   Assistant Professor in Neonatal-Perinatal Medicine, University of North Carolina, Chapel Hill, NC, USA

Martha Scott Tomlinson   Department of Environmental Sciences and Engineering, Gillings School of Global Public Health, UNC-Chapel Hill, Chapel Hill, NC, USA

Jelske W van der Burg   Assistant Professor, Department of Environmental and Health, Vrije Universiteit, Amsterdam, The Netherlands

Deborah VanderVeen   Associate Professor, Department of Ophthalmology, Harvard Medical School, Boston Children's Hospital, Boston MA, USA

Stephanie Watkins   The University of North Carolina at Chapel Hill, Chapel Hill, North Carolina, USA

Hannah Zamore   Summer Intern at UMass Medical School; Senior, Bryn Mawr College, Bryn Mawr, PA, USA

Foreword

When you read widely in the scientific literature on neonatology, it sometimes feels as if life begins at birth and that we are all born as a blank canvas on which our neonatal teams and parents can write the future. It is clear, however, that the processes and events which lead up to preterm birth are critically important in shaping both the neonatal period and after. Something has gone awry in gestation that leads to early delivery and these events both compromise and sensitize the rapidly developing fetus. In setting out to study this interface, the ELGAN (Extremely Low Gestational Age Newborns) study has proven highly effective in unravelling some of the complex processes that lead to extremely preterm birth and its sequelae. The longitudinal nature of these studies and incorporation of important executive processing and behavioural measures at school age makes it a unique study, one that raises more questions.

Do we need a book about it? In seeking to summarize their studies and provide such an overview, Dammann et al. set their work in much broader context than was previously possible and provide insight into how all the observations they have made fit together. *Extremely Preterm Birth and its Consequences: The ELGAN Study* is an important contribution and not only clarifies, but also signposts their work and future research directions. In doing so they provide important insight into the antecedents and associates of the four major preterm neonatal morbidities: sepsis, retinopathy, bronchopulmonary dysplasia, and brain injury. These are supplemented by long-term outcomes studies that both identify important paediatric outcomes and help to connect the longitudinal impact that extremely preterm birth has on the developing child and, eventually, adult.

When the ELGAN study was conceived, the thought of trying to cross the perinatal divide had rarely successfully been achieved in longitudinal studies and certainly less so in modern times with its funding constraints and the huge cost of such projects. Other famous longitudinal studies (such as the National Collaborative Perinatal Project and the British Birth Surveys/the Avon Longitudinal Study of Parents and Children) have gone some way to doing so but concentrated on a whole birth cohort, with few children born extremely preterm. The concept of focussing not on the whole population but on inflammation as an indicator of active pathology in this focussed group, a tenet the investigators have held to throughout the study, has made this most valuable. The multiple insults or 'hits' experienced by an infant born at extremely low gestational age have been uniquely been characterized and shown to influence outcomes through to middle childhood

Studying the small proportion of preterm births who are born at extremely low gestational ages brings with it challenges. Not the least of these is to find sufficient births with which to study this critical area. Despite their small number, this group consume much of the resources allocated to prematurity and have high levels of morbidity.

One of the huge achievements made by this team is in the bringing together of a large number of institutions to contribute to this study in order to achieve the size of investigation that would provide robust and confident answers. Not only to bring them together but to commit to continue the work into childhood with excellent retention. This makes the ELGAN study one of the most important large detailed and prospective longitudinal studies in our field.

The study is not over yet. Recently there has been developing interest in the implications of preterm birth for adult life. Several groups around the world are charting adult and middle-age outcomes for cohorts who have been in intensive care and demonstrating the pervasive effect of extremely preterm birth on social, neurocognitive, psychiatric, and somatic outcomes, with implications for ageing.

The robust perinatal investigations carried out at the inception of the ELGAN study means that this is a unique opportunity to relate the longitudinal trajectories of development described in the study to the perinatal period. I predict this will be a highly fruitful series of investigations that expand our knowledge even further. This volume sets the scene for these studies.

I very much enjoyed reading this book which effectively broadens our concept of preterm birth. I found more information contained in this one volume than in much of the scientific literature I had read previously. Most importantly it shows potential routes through which we can move, from observing the biology to improving the lives of the children we care for, by understanding the interplay of pathologies on the developing human organism. The authors are to be congratulated and this relatively short volume will become an important reference book for both new and experienced investigators seeking information and background. The ELGAN study will continue to inspire researchers and clinicians for many years to come.

Neil Marlow
University College London
September 2020

Preface

This book summarizes the results of the ELGAN (Extremely Low Gestational Age Newborn) Study. Although we have published all the details in more than 150 original journal articles, we also wanted to provide a convenient and concise distillation of the main findings in one volume. You hold the result in your hands.

When we designed this book, we wanted to cast a wide net with regard to its readership. We hope that it will provide a unique epidemiological perspective about extremely preterm birth and its consequences that perinatal/neonatal clinicians and researchers, as well as practicing developmentalists and developmental scientists will find interesting and helpful.

The story of our project begins to take shape in the early 1990s, when etiological explanations of perinatal brain damage were still simple and relatively straightforward. Cerebral abnormalities in newborn infants born preterm were limited to intraventricular hemorrhage and periventricular leukomalacia, both purportedly due to some sort of disturbance of cerebral circulation. If only the purported main culprit, hypoxia-ischemia, could be prevented by improving ventilation and oxygenation, we should expect a drastic reduction in perinatal brain injury with a subsequently reduced incidence of developmental disabilities such as cerebral palsy and intellectual disability.

The development of pulmonary surfactant administration was well underway at that time. The general thinking among neonatologists and neonatal neurologists can be summarized in the following syllogism. Difficulties ventilating newborn infants leads to hypoxia-ischemia; hypoxia-ischemia leads to brain injury and developmental disabilities; therefore improving neonatal ventilation by exogenous surfactant application will help prevent brain injury and developmental disabilities.

This idea may have had its origin in a 1962 report of an uncontrolled neuropathology case series of newborn infants who died at least a decade before the modern era of neonatology and who would probably now be classified as term and near term. Betty Q. Banker and Jeanne Claudie Larroche named the entity they studied, 'Periventricular leukomalacia of infancy. A form of neonatal anoxic encephalopathy.' Yes, anoxic encephalopathy.

In those early years of the final decade before the new millennium, two major neuroepidemiological studies in very low birthweight infants born preterm were underway in the United States. The Central New Jersey Neonatal Brain Hemorrhage Study enrolled 1105 newborn infants between 501 g and 2000 g birthweight and prospectively collected neonatal data including cerebral ultrasound scans as well as brain pathology and histology data from infants who did not survive. The main results of this landmark study were published in *Brain Damage in the Preterm Infant* by Paneth et al. (1994), part of the Clinics in Developmental Medicine series. The other study, the Developmental Epidemiological Network Study, was spearheaded by Alan Leviton, Nigel Paneth, and Mervyn Susser (1921–2014). A total of 1605 infants weighing 500g to 1500g at birth, born between January 1991 and December 1993, underwent standardized cranial ultrasound studies which were analyzed vis-à-vis meticulously collected placenta histology and microbiology data. Both studies together resulted in a whole host of new knowledge about risk factors, clinical manifestations, and consequences of perinatal brain damage and laid the foundation for a sea change in our understanding of its etiology and pathogenesis in the infant born preterm.

While the New Jersey Study revolutionized our understanding of microscopic pathological abnormalities in the preterm brain, the Developmental Epidemiology Network investigators were the first to document the strong association between maternal chorioamnionitis, fetal vasculitis, and brain abnormalities. The findings of both studies confirmed the earlier proposal by Alan Leviton and Floyd Gilles, who had suggested, based on data from the same institution as Banker and Larroche, that early histological indicators of neonatal brain damage (including abnormalities of myelination) might be attributable, in part, to a circulating product of infection/inflammation.

By the late 1990s, it had become clear that a new, large prospective neonatal neuroepidemiological cohort study was needed with a focus on: (1) newborn infants defined by gestational age, not birth-weight; (2) improved placenta histology and microbiology; (3) the measurement of circulating products of inflammation (cytokines, chemokines, growth factors); and (4) long-term developmental follow-up. The decision to seek funding for what is now known as the ELGAN Study was made by the original team of co-investigators (Alan Leviton, Liz Allred, Karl Kuban, T. Michael O'Shea, Linda Van Marter, Nigel Paneth, and Olaf Dammann with invaluable support from Deborah Hirtz) at around the time of the Y2K scare (who remembers?). The rest is history.

Very many individuals have made substantial contributions to the design, implementation, and analysis of study results. These 154 individuals are listed in the Acknowledgements.

The editors of this book wish to express special gratitude to Liz Allred, for her superb biostatistical guidance and for preparing thousands of data tables that form the analytical backbone of the ELGAN Study. Deborah Hirtz, our colleague and project officer at the National Institute for Neurological Disorders and Stroke, for her continued trust and unwavering support. Linda Van Marter and Karl Kuban, for their contributions to the design and implementation of the study, and for accepting various leadership roles over the years. Beth Kring, Madeleine Lenski, Julie Rollins, and Janice Wereszczak for their unrelenting commitment to the successful implementation of study protocols and the well-being of study participants. Bernard Dan, for planting the seed for this book (and occasional watering); and Sally Wilkinson and Lucy White of Mac Keith Press, for their guidance and apparently endless patience.

At the personal level, the editors would like to thank Christiane, Lina, and Laura Dammann (OD), Roberta Leviton (AL), Lou Detty O'Shea (TMO), and Ellen Pollak (NP). Without their loving support over the past two decades, the novel insights resulting from the ELGAN Study might not exist in their current form.

Olaf Dammann, Boston
Alan Leviton, Boston
T Michael O'Shea, Chapel Hill
Nigel Paneth, East Lansing
June 2020

Acknowledgements

None of the authors has relevant financial interests, activities, relationships, or affiliations.

This study was supported by the National Institute of Neurological Disorders and Stroke (grants 5U01NS040069-05 and 2R01NS040069-09), the National Eye Institute (5R21EY019253 and 5R01EY021820) and the Office of the Director of the National Institutes of Health ((1UG3OD023348-01). The authors also gratefully acknowledge the contributions of their subjects, and their subjects' families, as well as those of their colleagues listed below.

Project Lead for ELGAN-2: Julie V. Rollins, MA

Site Principal Investigators

Baystate Medical Center, Springfield, MA: Bhahvesh Shah, MD; Rachana Singh, MD, MS. Boston Children's Hospital, Boston, MA: Linda Van Marter, MD, MPH and Camilla Martin, MD, MPH; Janice Ware, PhD. Tufts Medical Center, Boston, MA: Cynthia Cole, MD; Ellen Perrin, MD. University of Massachusetts Medical School, Worcester, MA: Frank Bednarek, MD; Jean Frazier, MD. Yale University School of Medicine, New Haven, CT: Richard Ehrenkranz, MD; Jennifer Benjamin, MD. Wake Forest University, Winston-Salem, NC: T. Michael O'Shea, MD, MPH. University of North Carolina, Chapel Hill, NC: Carl Bose, MD; Diane Warner, MD, MPH. East Carolina University, Greenville, NC: Steve Engelke, MD. Helen DeVos Children's Hospital, Grand Rapids, MI: Mariel Poortenga, MD; Steve Pastyrnak, PhD. Sparrow Hospital, East Lansing, MI: Padu Karna, MD; Nigel Paneth, MD, MPH; Madeleine Lenski, MPH. University of Chicago Medical Center, Chicago, IL: Michael Schreiber, MD; Scott Hunter, PhD; Michael Msall, MC. William Beaumont Hospital, Royal Oak, MI: Danny Batton, MD; Judith Klarr, MD.

Site Study Coordinators

Baystate Medical Center, Springfield, MA: Karen Christianson, RN; Deborah Klein, BSM, RN. Boston Children's Hospital, Boston MA: Maureen Pimental, BA; Collen Hallisey, BA; Taryn Coster, BA. Tufts Medical Center, Boston, MA: Ellen Nylen, RN; Emily Neger, MA; Kathryn Mattern, BA. University of Massachusetts Medical School, Worcester, MA: Lauren Venuti, BA; Beth Powers, RN; Ann Foley, EdM. Yale University School of Medicine, New Haven, CT: Joanne Williams, RN; Elaine Romano, APRN. Wake Forest University, Winston-Salem, NC: Debbie Hiatt, BSN (deceased); Nancy Peters, RN; Patricia Brown, RN; Emily Ansusinha, BA. University of North Carolina, Chapel Hill, NC: Gennie Bose, RN; Janice Wereszczak, MSN; Janice Bernhardt, MS, RN. East Carolina University, Greenville, NC: Joan Adams (deceased); Donna Wilson, BA, BSW; Nancy Darden-Saad, BS, RN. Helen DeVos Children's Hospital, Grand Rapids, MI: Dinah Sutton, RN; Julie Rathbun, BSW, BSN. Sparrow Hospital, East Lansing, MI: Karen Miras, RN, BSN; Deborah Weiland, MSN. University of Chicago Medical Center, Chicago, IL: Grace Yoon, RN; Rugile Ramoskaite, BA; Suzanne Wiggins, MA; Krissy Washington, MA; Ryan Martin, MA; Barbara Prendergast, BSN, RN. William Beaumont Hospital, Royal Oak, MI: Beth Kring, RN.

Psychologists

Baystate Medical Center, Springfield, MA: Anne Smith, PhD; Susan McQuiston, PhD. Boston Children's Hospital, Boston, MA: Samantha Butler, PhD; Rachel Wilson, PhD; Kirsten McGhee, PhD; Patricia

Lee, PhD; Aimee Asgarian, PhD; Anjali Sadhwani, PhD; Brandi Henson, PsyD. Tufts Medical Center, Boston, MA: Cecelia Keller, PT, MHA; Jenifer Walkowiak, PhD; Susan Barron, PhD. University of Massachusetts Medical School, Worcester MA: Alice Miller, PT, MS; Brian Dessureau, PhD; Molly Wood, PhD; Jill Damon-Minow, PhD. Yale University School of Medicine , New Haven, CT: Elaine Romano, MSN; Linda Mayes, PhD; Kathy Tsatsanis, PhD; Katarzyna Chawarska, PhD; Sophy Kim, PhD; Susan Dieterich, PhD; Karen Bearrs, PhD. Wake Forest University Baptist Medical Center, Winston-Salem NC: Ellen Waldrep, MA; Jackie Friedman, PhD; Gail Hounshell, PhD; Debbie Allred, PhD. University Health Systems of Eastern Carolina, Greenville, NC: Rebecca Helms, PhD; Lynn Whitley, PhD Gary Stainback, PhD. University of North Carolina at Chapel Hill, NC: Lisa Bostic, OTR/L; Amanda Jacobson, PT; Joni McKeeman, PhD; Echo Meyer, PhD. Helen DeVos Children's Hospital, Grand Rapids, MI: Steve Pastyrnak, PhD. Sparrow Hospital, Lansing, MI: Joan Price, EdS; Megan Lloyd, MA, EdS. University of Chicago Medical Center, Chicago, IL: Susan Plesha-Troyke, OT; Megan Scott, PhD. William Beaumont Hospital, Royal Oak, MI: Katherine M. Solomon, PhD; Kara Brooklier, PhD; Kelly Vogt, PhD.

Ophthalmologists

Ahmed Abdelsalam, University of Chicago; Antonio Capone, William Beaumont Hospital; Anthony Fraioli, Massachusetts General Hospital; Pat Droste, DeVos; Jay Duker, New England Medical Center; Robert Gise, UmassMemrl; Robert Petersen, Deborah VanderVeen – Beth Israel Deaconess Medical Center/Brigham and Women's Hospital; Michael Trese, William Beaumont Hospital, Royal Oak, Michigan; William Seefeld, Baystate; Kathleeen Stoessel, Yale; David K Wallace, Duke Eye Center; Grey Weaver, Wake Forest.

Pathologists

Karen Strehloh, University of Massachusetts Medical Center; Jonathan Hecht, Beth Israel Deaconess Medical Center; Harvey Kliman, Yale University; Solveg Pflueger, Baystate Medical Center; Chung-Ho Chang, William Beaumont Hospital; Gabriel Chamyan, Sparrow Hospital; Barbara Doss, Spectrum Health; Drucilla Roberts, Massachusetts General Hospital; Chad Livasy, University of North Carolina; Ina Bhan, New England Medical Center; Vinita Parkash, Yale University; Dennis Ross, Wake Forest University School of Medicine; Patricia Senagore, Michigan State University; Aliya Husain,University of Chicago; John Christie, East Carolina University.

Radiologists

Roy McCauley, New England Medical Center; Sara Durfee, Brigham & Women's Hospital; Kirsten Ecklund, Boston Children's Hospital; Sjirk Westra, Massachusetts General Hospital; Jane Share, Beth Israel Deaconess Medical Center; Frederick Hampf, Stanley Polansky, Baystate Medical Center; Jacqueline Wellman,University of Massachusetts Medical Center; Cindy Miller, Yale University School of Medicine; Steven Bezinque, Joseph Junewick, Bradford W. Betz, DeVos Children's Hospital; Dan Batton, William Beaumont Hospital; Ellen Cavenagh, Sparrow Hospital; Kate Feinstein, David Yousefzadeh, University of Chicago; Lynn Ansley Fordham, University of North Carolina; Barbara Specter, Wake Forest University; Ira Adler, East Carolina University; Joanna Seibert, MD – provided second readings of ultrasounds; Robert Lorenzo, MD – provided second readings of ultrasounds.

Chapter 15

This work was supported by The National Institute of Neurological Disorders and Stroke (5U01NS040069-05; 2R01NS040069-06A2) and the National Institute of Child Health and Human

Development (5P30HD018655-34). Dr Frazier has the following disclosures: she has received research support from Fulcrum Therapeutics, F Hoffmann-LaRoche Limited, Janssen Pharmaceuticals, Neuren, and SyneuRX International. No funds from these entities supported this work, and none of these entities reviewed/commented on this work. All other authors declare no financial or ethical conflicts of interest. The authors gratefully acknowledge the contributions of the research participants and their families, and of their colleagues.

Introduction

Alan Leviton, Olaf Dammann, T Michael O'Shea, and Nigel Paneth

The World Health Organization (WHO) defines extremely preterm as birth before the 28th week of gestation (WHO 2019). This book is about one longitudinal study of such children.

Most previous studies equated very low birthweight (i.e. <1500 grams) with extremely preterm birth. Such studies are potentially biased to include gestationally older newborns with fetal growth restriction (Arnold et al. 1991). To avoid this bias, and to have the opportunity to study fetal growth restriction in an unbiased way, we decided to enroll only infants who were born before the 28th week of gestation. All infants recruited for this study were extremely low gestational age newborns (ELGANs). To emphasize this entry criterion, we identified our study as the ELGAN study.

The information provided in the following chapters is about antecedents, correlates, and consequences of being born extremely preterm. One main focus of the book, and indeed the main research focus of the ELGAN study, is on exposures and outcomes related to the developing brain. Another focus is on inflammation as a major risk factor for developmental adversity.

This introduction has three parts. The first is mainly about ideas, specifically the ideas that prompted and shaped the ELGAN study. The second part is about the planning, designing, and implementation of the ELGAN study. The third, and shortest part introduces the chapters in this book.

THE IDEAS THAT PROMPTED AND SHAPED THE ELGAN STUDY

The ELGAN study had its origins about 50 years ago. Floyd Gilles had recently described four histologic features he considered the earliest visible expressions of white matter damage in the newborn brain (Gilles and Murphy 1969). Three of these histologic features appeared to precede the appearance of necrosis that is characteristic of periventricular leukomalacia (Banker and Larroche 1962), a disorder then thought to result in severe developmental limitations.

Two of these features, hypertrophic astrocytes and perivascular amphophilic globules, occurred more commonly together than would be expected by chance (Leviton and Gilles 1971). In addition, this combination occurred more frequently than expected with foci of necrosis, another of the four features of early white matter damage, especially if the interval between birth and death was ≥9 days. These two findings together strengthened the view that the combination of hypertrophic astrocytes and perivascular amphophilic globules had biologic importance, and that the occurrence of this combination preceded the onset of visually evident necrosis.

The search for antecedents/early correlates of this combination included an evaluation of all the findings usually reported for every autopsy (Leviton and Gilles 1973; Leviton et al. 1976). A routine part of the autopsy examination was, and still is, bacteriologic culture of blood aspirated from the heart.

Babies who died with hypertrophic astrocytes and perivascular amphophilic globules in their brain were much more likely than others to have bacteria recovered from their blood.

Endodotoxin Hypothesis – Postnatal

Because 85% of infants with both the combination of hypertrophic astrocytes and perivascular amphophilic globules and post-mortem bacteremia had Gram-negative organisms recovered from their blood, but none were seen in the brain, it was considered possible that a circulating product of these organisms, such as endotoxin, might have adverse effects 'on myelinogenesis or some other maturational process unique to infant white matter' (Leviton and Gilles 1973). This prompted an experiment to assess the brain-effects of endotoxin given to newborn mammals. A single intra-peritoneal injection of endotoxin (i.e. purified *E. coli* lipopolysaccharide, LPS) given to the newborn cat, rat, rabbit, and monkey resulted in diffuse astrogliosis, focal necroses, and/or enhanced karyorrhexis of glial nuclei in the telencephalic white matter (Gilles et al. 1976, 1977). These findings established that a non-infectious promoter of inflammation (such as LPS) given to mammalian newborns can contribute to histologic characteristics of cerebral white matter damage.

Endodotoxin Hypothesis – Antenatal

Among infants who died in the National Collaborative Perinatal Project (NCPP), the risk of amphophilic globules was modestly increased if the infant's mother had a urinary tract infection during the pregnancy, while the risk of the combination of hypertrophic astrocytes and amphophilic globules was prominently increased if the mother had a urinary tract infection accompanied by fever during the pregnancy (Gilles et al. 1983; Leviton and Gilles 1984). These findings suggest that the mother was likely the source of one or more substances that can cross the placenta, gain access to the fetus, and disturb normal myelinogenesis in the fetus/newborn.

More than 30 years ago, endotoxin was invoked as the link between maternal infection and brain damage in the fetus (Ornoy and Altshuler 1976). Since then, cytokines, such as those whose synthesis is stimulated by endotoxin, have been shown to be able to gain access to the central nervous system where they, in turn, stimulate fever (Prajitha et al. 2018). Thus, maternal fever might be a surrogate for information about the potential abundance of inflammation-related molecules in the fetal circulation. The ELGAN study has since shown that ELGANs whose mother had a urinary tract infection during pregnancy (regardless of whether or not fever accompanied the infection) were more likely than others to have elevated concentrations of biomarkers of inflammation, such as MPO, IL-6R, TNF-R1, TNF-R2, and RANTES on postnatal day 7 (Fichorova et al. 2015).

Prior to the ELGAN study, maternal gestational urinary tract infection had also been associated with increased risk of very low intelligence (Broman 1987), strengthening our view that antenatal inflammation is likely to damage the developing brain. Since then, maternal gestational urinary tract infection has been associated with increased risk of cognitive and language impairments (Lee 2014), and cerebral palsy (Neufeld 2005; Mann 2009; Miller 2013; Bear and Wu 2016).

Fetal Inflammation

Prior to the widespread availability of neonatal intensive care units (Philip 2005), the literature dealing with the topic of fetal inflammation was most often the purview of pathologists responsible for examination of still births and very early neonatal deaths (Davies 1971). Attention to fetal inflammation was renewed when evidence began to accrue that intra-uterine infection (Romero 1991) and inflammation

(Romero et al. 1990, 1992; Gibbs et al. 1992; Fidel et al. 1994) were very closely associated with spontaneous onset of labor, especially if preterm, and with premature rupture of membranes (Santhanam 1991). At about the same time, the contribution of 'ontogenic' inflammation to normal development was recognized (Yamasu 1989).

Apparently, the recognition that cytokines in amniotic fluid are not only associated with preterm birth, but might also be associated with indicators of brain damage in very preterm infants who survive (Leviton 1993) also prompted renewed attention to fetal inflammation preceding preterm birth. Thus, was born the concept of a 'fetal systemic inflammatory response' (Romero 1998).

Focus No Longer on Endotoxin – Rather on Cytokines, Adhesion Molecules, etc.

Over the decades that followed the initial reports of the adverse effects of LPS on the developing brain, a series of developments influenced how we envisioned the ELGAN study. First, LPS is capable of stimulating the synthesis of inflammation-related proteins (Fontana et al. 1982; Andersson and Matsuda 1989; Dubravec 1990; Munro et al. 1991; Pugin et al. 1999; Jaeschke et al. 1996; Paemen et al. 1997; Jilma et al. 1999; Pagenstecher et al. 2000). Then we found out that these inflammation-related proteins played a role in the central nervous system (Lieberman et al. 1989; Yamasu et al. 1989; Benveniste 1992; Burns e al. 1993), and can contribute to brain damage (Saukkonen et al. 1990; Benveniste 1992; Gruol and Nelson 1997; Zhao and Schwartz 1998; Leib 2000; Rosenberg 1995; Merrill and Benveniste 1996). Documentation that elevated newborn blood concentrations of cytokines and chemokines are associated with indicators of brain damage in humans soon followed (Nelson et al. 1998; Grether et al. 1999; Nelson et al. 2000). These studies, of children born at term or sooner, were able to measure the concentrations of many different proteins in just a drop of blood. We recognized then, that the ability to measure so much with such a small specimen would allow us to use discarded blood (from the end of the needle used to obtain blood for gas measurements), and avoid our having to withdraw blood from fragile newborn strictly for research.

Postnatal Inflammation and the Ability to Characterize It

The realization that perinatal systemic inflammation might be associated with brain damage came with the report of Karin Nelson, Terrie Phillips, and their colleagues that children who were given a diagnosis of cerebral palsy tended to have higher concentrations than their peers of cytokines, chemokines, and coagulation factors in blood specimens in the days immediately following delivery (Nelson et al. 1998). This was among children born at term or sooner, but provided us with assurance that the concentrations of many proteins really could be measured in a drop of blood. This report also gave us confidence that we were more likely now than previously to be able to identify an inflammatory signal if it were present.

Developmental Regulation and Maturation-Dependent Vulnerability

Whether or not the placenta is inflamed, the concentrations of inflammation-related proteins in early blood specimens appear to be developmentally regulated with the most common pattern being a decrease with increasing gestational age (Leviton et al. 2011). We made these findings in our pilot work for the ELGAN study grant application. Others have since found that some aspects of inflammation appear to be more intense the younger the gestational age (Chiesa et al. 2001; Suski et al. 2018). Although we stratified the ELGAN study sample by an indicator of inflammation, our findings and those of others might have had residual confounding associated with inflammation-provoking exposures

(Romero et al. 2015). Unfortunately, the intense inflammation appears not only to compensate for the relative paucity of anti-microbial proteins and peptides (Battersby et al. 2016) and limited neutrophil phagocytic capability, but also appears to be more damaging than protective (Mallard and Wang 2012).

Neurotrophins

Our interest in neurotrophins began in the 1990s with two publications. The first reported that 'massive cell death' is part of the development of the vertebrate nervous system, and that this phenomenon 'is thought to reflect the failure of … neurons to obtain adequate amounts of specific neurotrophic factors that are produced by the target cells and that are required for the neurons to survive. … These survival signals seem to act by suppressing an intrinsic cell suicide program' (Raff et al. 1993: 695). The second, just a year later, proposed that 'some of the developmental problems experienced by preterm newborns reflect a deprivation of placenta-provided hormones and growth factors during crucial stages of neuro-development' (Reuss et al. 1994: 743).

Thus, we were provided with a potential explanation for why ELGANs are at such heightened risk of brain-related dysfunctions and limitations. If ELGANS were not yet able to provide the brain with sufficient neurotrophins to allow normal development, let alone protect against adversity, might exogenous neurotrophins allow normal brain development and protection? We found support within just a few years (Graves 1997; Cheng et al. 1997; Tong and Perez-Polo 1998; Ay et al. 1999). Additional support for BDNF as a protector, followed soon after (Tong and Perez-Polo 1998), as did support for basic fibroblast growth factor (bFGF) as a protector/enhancer of repair (Ay et al. 1999).

These reports prompted us to include in our ELGAN study grant proposal the concept that some biologic response modifiers could function as protectors, minimizing damage by reducing the extent of damage or by enhancing repair (Dammann and Leviton 2000a). We included in our wish list of what we wanted to measure, proteins with oligotrophic and/or neurotrophic properties, such as thyroxine, transforming growth factor-beta 1, vascular endothelial growth factor, nerve growth factor, platelet-derived growth factor, fibroblast growth factor-2, fibroblast growth factor-9, ciliary neurotrophic factor, insulin-like growth factor-I, neurotrophin-3, insulin growth factors, neuregulin, and progesterone. We emphasized proteins with oligotrophic and/or neurotrophic properties because we were beginning to appreciate that white matter damage included damage to axons as well as oligodendrocytes (Dammann et al. 2001).

Cross-Talk between the Immune and Nervous Systems

Our interest in neurotrophins was enhanced by reports that LPS can increase the expression of neurotrophin-3 (NT-3) in microglia (Elkabes et al. 1997), nerve growth factor (NGF) in microglia (Heese et al. 1998), and BDNF in rat microglia (Miwa et al. 1997) and mouse immune cells (Barouch et al. 2000). These findings also further increased our interest in communication between immune and central nervous systems (Lennon 1994; Lotan and Schwartz 1994; Blakemore 1995; Xiao and Link 1998).

Imaging – the Original 'Outcome'/Focus

The earliest studies of the antecedents of cerebral white matter damage in newborns were conducted among children who died and whose brains were examined postmortem (Leviton and Gilles 1973; Leviton et al. 1976; Leviton 1983; Leviton and Gilles 1984). Only with the availability of imaging techniques capable of identifying white matter damage in living human newborns would studies have the capacity to evaluate the occurrence, antecedents, correlates, and consequences of cerebral white matter damage (Paneth et al. 1994). Only with the ability to measure tens of proteins that have inflammation-promoting properties could studies in humans ascertain the role of systemic inflammation in promoting cerebral white matter damage (Nelson et al. 1998; Dammann et al. 2001).

THE NEED FOR THE ELGAN STUDY

In a series of reviews, we outlined our perspective about how inflammation appears to contribute to brain damage in ELGANs, and how anti-inflammatory and neurotrophic processes might limit the brain damage associated with systemic inflammation (Dammann and Leviton 1998, 1999, 2000a, 2000b). Others were providing strong support for some of these ideas (Yoon et al. 1996, 1997a, 1997b, 2000; Nelson et al. 1998; Grether et al. 1999) while thought leaders were just beginning to acknowledge the possibility that inflammation might contribute to perinatal brain damage in ELGANs (Hagberg and Mallard 2000; Inder and Volpe 2000).

IMPLEMENTING THE PLAN

When the advancements in measuring multiple proteins in a drop of blood, identifying cerebral white matter damage in the live newborn, and our understanding of inflammatory phenomena, all came together, we (the ELGAN study team) began in earnest to design and implement the ELGAN study. The design had to achieve several goals.

Study of Those at Highest Risk

The newborns we most wanted to enroll were those at highest risk of brain damage identified early, and dysfunctions evident years later. These were the infants born at the lowest gestational ages who survived, and those who experienced fetal growth restriction. Almost half the infants enrolled were born at or before the 25th week of gestation, and 21% had a birthweight more than one standard deviation below the mean (Table 1.1).

Table 1.1 Demographic characteristics of children enrolled in the ELGAN study

	Number of newborns	Column percents
Gestational age (weeks)		
23	124	8
24	285	19
25	305	20
26	356	24
27	436	29

(Continued)

Table 1.1 Demographic characteristics of children enrolled in the ELGAN study (Continued)

	Number of newborns	Column percents
Birth weight (grams)		
≤750	660	44
751–1000	586	39
1001–1250	237	16
≥ 1250	23	2
Birth weight (Z-score)[a]		
<−2	110	7
≥−2, <−1	211	14
≥−1, 1	1029	68
>1, ≤2	133	9
>2	23	2
Mother's self-identification		
White non-Hispanic	782	52
White Hispanic	43	3
White Unknown	2	<1
Black non-Hispanic	407	27
Black Hispanic	4	<1
Asian non-Hispanic	30	2
Native American non-Hispanic	7	<1
Native American Hispanic	6	<1
Other non-Hispanic	6	<1
Other Hispanic	86	6
Mixed non-Hispanic	30	2
Mixed Hispanic	9	<1
Unknown non-Hispanic	0	0
Unknown Hispanic	20	2
Unknown Unknown	75	5
Zygosity		
Singletons	1007	67
Twins	414	27
Triplets	77	5
Quadruplets	2	<1
Sextuplets	6	<1
TOTAL	1506	100%

[a] The Z-score is the number of standard deviations below or above the mean.

Large Sample Size

After we made calculations about the magnitude of differences we wanted to achieve, we realized that we would need to enroll close to 1800 pregnant women who were likely to deliver before the 28th week of gestation or who had just delivered before the 28th week. To do so over a relatively short period required the enthusiastic participation of colleagues at 10–12 institutions.

Sustained Commitment

We understood that the sustained commitment of our colleagues at these institutions would require logistic assistance and frequent communication. We felt this was best done in what management gurus call a distributed environment. Consequently, we borrowed the spoke and wheel design of airline hubs. Each of the three hubs (New England, North Carolina, and Lake Michigan) would be headed by someone who had successfully carried out a multicenter study intended to identify antecedents of brain damage in newborns, and who was enthusiastic about accepting responsibility for between three and nine subject-enrolling and data-collecting institutions.

The sustained commitment was emphasized repeatedly. We were extraordinarily grateful for the enthusiastic participation of our colleagues and very much wanted to convey gratitude in as many ways as possible. One way was to assure our colleagues that we would do right by them. This included working with them to create the manual and data-collection forms, sharing relevant recent publications, analyzing the data they collected, and working together on manuscripts they wanted to write. This also included our repeatedly demonstrating how close our work was to the cutting edge, documenting that we were on top of the latest literature, and showing how relevant the ELGAN study was to all the topics we were trying to cover.

Another way to show our commitment included providing assurance that together we would seize opportunities to study topics that most interested them. This included an acknowledgement that bronchopulmonary dysplasia (chronic lung disease), necrotizing enterocolitis, and retinopathy of prematurity, would be the foci of analyses and reports.

We also created the equivalent of an internal blog specifically for the entire ELGAN study team. Weekly emails either discussed relevant topics (e.g. an inflammation-related protein) or recent publications (sometimes accompanied by an author's perspective of how her/his study added to our understanding). These were prepared with the intent to inform and inspire.

Distributed Environment

The distributed environment theme was continued by having each neonatologist recruit (at her/his institution) a perinatologist to assist with gaining approval of the other perinatologists to allow their patients to have the opportunity to participate in the ELGAN study. Each neonatologist also recruited a pediatric ophthalmologist (whose specialty was the retina), a pathologist (who had a special interest in the placenta), and a sonologist (a reader of ultrasound scans, usually a radiologist, but not always). Each of the identified people became a member of her/his ELGAN study specialty team, which was responsible for creating a manual and data collection forms, as well as establishing criteria for diagnoses, and working out shared and individual responsibilities.

The distributed environment also applied to the goal of obtaining diversity of subjects in the ELGAN study sample. Attaining this goal was most likely to be important when functions were assessed years later. Among the 873 children who had the 10-year assessment, one quarter had a mother who identified as African-American, while the mother of 11% identified as non-white (not African-American), and

Table 1.2 Associations among socio-economic indicators – except for the bottom row, these are row percents

	Maternal education			Public insurance	KBIT	Non-white	Maternal age		Single
	≤ 12	13–15	≥ 16	Yes	≤ −1	Yes	< 21	21–35	Yes
Maternal education, years ≤ 12				63	20	51	28	63	65
13–15				32	9	43	7	73	40
≥ 16				5	3	16	0	68	11
Public insurance Yes	74	21			18	62	30	63	80
No	23	25			7	23	4	69	18
KBIT-2[a] Z-score ≤ −1	72	19		58		63	17	63	59
> −1	37	24		33		33	13	67	37
Non-white Yes	57	27		60	19		20	69	66
No	32	21		21	6		9	66	24
Maternal age, years < 21	88	12		81	15	58			87
21–35	39	25		33	11	38			36
> 35	19	24		14	11	20			22
Single Yes	67	24		71	17	61	28	61	
No	35	23		12	8	21	3	71	
Column N	359	205		307	95	321	113	585	348

[a] KBIT-2 is the abbreviation for the Kaufman Brief Intelligence Test 2nd Edition, which is a brief, individually administered assessment of verbal and nonverbal cognitive ability.

10% identified as Hispanic. Fully 40% of the 10-year-olds were born to a mother who identified her marital status as single at the time of the delivery, and 35% of mothers were eligible for government-provided medical care then. The mothers' education at the time of delivery level also varied considerably with 40% not having any formal education beyond high school and more than one-third completing 4 years of post-high school study (usually graduating from college). The inter-relationships among these maternal socio-economic characteristics are shown in Table 1.2.

Getting Funding

A single study of the size we envisioned would cost the National Institute of Neurological Disorders and Stroke (NINDS) the same amount of money as would the sum of dozens of pre-clinical studies. NINDS leadership needed to make explicit that the type of observational (non-interventional, clinical) study we wanted to carry out was in keeping with NINDS's mandate. We are forever grateful for their decision to do this, because once this was done NINDS could request a special review panel that was much more appropriate than the previously-assigned study section. The rest is history … almost.

The original ELGAN study grant application was to study the antecedents of abnormal cranial ultrasound scans (i.e. the best indicator then of cerebral white matter damage in the living newborn). ELGANs at all the participating intensive care nurseries routinely had multiple cranial ultrasound assessments, which were essential to avoid biased ascertainment. The reviewers on the special panel suggested that we add clinical neurological and developmental assessments at approximately 6–12 months post term, and at 18–24 months post term. We are also forever grateful for this recommendation.

NINDS uses the cooperative agreement mechanism for large, expensive multicenter studies that involved clinical research. This enabled NINDS to be involved in the conduct of the ELGAN study and to add the two follow up assessments to the study protocol. We are most thankful for this partnership.

CONTENTS OF THIS BOOK

This book is divided into four sections of two to four chapters each. The first section focuses on antenatal risk factors, while the second section deals with postnatal risk factors and correlates. The third and fourth sections differ from these two sections as they focus not on risk factors, but on indicators of brain damage/dysfunction. In the third section the indicators are structural (brain imaging abnormalities), while in the fourth section the indicators are functional (cerebral palsy, cognition limitations, social and communication dysfunctions, and psychiatric disorders).

By and large, the authors of these chapters have eschewed nitty-gritty detail in favor of a relatively broad perspective. These chapters provide an overview. In essence, how did ELGAN study findings influence or even advance our thinking about the topic?

We begin the first section, which deals with antenatal antecedents, by viewing placenta histology and bacteriology as biomarkers of intra-uterine exposures and characteristics that might influence the fetus's risk of brain damage/dysfunction. In addition to a chapter devoted to each, we have a chapter that integrates placenta histology and bacteriology with indications for preterm delivery. The final chapter in the antenatal section discusses the correlates and presumed consequences (Wankhade et al. 2016; Poston et al. 2011) of maternal overweight and obesity (as well as gestational weight gain).

The second section begins with a chapter dealing with one illness severity measure, Score for Neonatal Physiology (SNAP), which conveys risk information about entities that are the subjects of the third and fourth sections. We view SNAP as a postnatal measure because it is a composite of characteristics identified in the first 12 postnatal hours. Nevertheless, the authors of this chapter raise the possibility that SNAP conveys information about maturation above and beyond the maturation information contained within the gestational age variable.

The remainder of the second section is devoted to entities more clearly identified as postnatal, even though each does have antenatal origins. Sepsis, retinopathy of prematurity, and bronchopulmonary dysplasia are three disorders that occur much more commonly in ELGANs than in infants born at term (Chee et al. 2017). Each of these disorders has long-term development consequences in the ELGAN study.

The earliest versions of the ELGAN study had cranial ultrasound abnormalities as the focus of interest. So it should not be surprising that the entire third section of this book is devoted to structural brain disorders. The division into chapters was very easy because only ultrasound assessments were made in the intensive care nursery, while magnetic resonance imaging (MRI) with volume measurements were made only at age 10 years.

Both chapters deal with both antecedents and correlated dysfunctions.

The four chapters in the fourth section deal with indicators of brain dysfunctions. Each offers information about antecedents of the dysfunctions, as well as the relationship between the dysfunctions that are the focus of the chapter and all other dysfunctions. Motor dysfunction classified at age 2 years is the subject of the first chapter in this section. The other three chapters address dysfunctions evident at age 10 years. Limitations of cognition, executive function, and learning are the subject of the second chapter in this section, while the full range of social and communications dysfunctions (from autism spectrum disorders to components and correlates of the preterm behavioral phenotype) are the subject of the third chapter. The wide range of psychiatric dysfunctions reported by parents on the Child Symptom Inventory-4 (CSI-4) are the focus of the last chapter in this section.

We wrote the concluding chapter with the intent of putting the ELGAN study contributions in perspective. Did we make a difference? What if the ELGAN study had never occurred?

Feedback is welcomed! If you cannot connect with us directly, please communicate via Mac Keith Press. Thank you.

REFERENCES

Andersson U, Matsuda T (1989) Human interleukin 6 and tumor necrosis factor alpha production studied at a single-cell level. *Eur J Immunol* **19**: 1157–60.

Arnold CC, Kramer MS, Hobbs CA, McLean FH, Usher RH (1991) Very low birth weight: a problematic cohort for epidemiologic studies of very small or immature neonates. *Am J Epidemiol* **134**: 604–13.

Ay H, Ay I, Koroshetz WJ, Finklestein SP (1999) Potential usefulness of basic fibroblast growth factor as a treatment for stroke. *Cerebrovasc Dis* **9**: 131–5.

Banker BQ, Larroche JC (1962) Periventricular leukomalacia of infancy. A form of neonatal anoxic encephalopathy. *Arch Neurol* **7**: 386–410.

Barouch R, Appel E, Kazimirsky G, Braun A, Renz H, Brodie C (2000) Differential regulation of neurotrophin expression by mitogens and neurotransmitters in mouse lymphocytes. *J Neuroimmunol* **103**: 112–21.

Battersby AJ, Khara J, Wright VJ, Levy O, Kampmann B (2016) Antimicrobial proteins and peptides in early life: ontogeny and translational opportunities. *Frontiers in Immunology* **7**: 309.

Bear JJ, Wu YW (2016) Maternal infections during pregnancy and cerebral palsy in the child. *Pediatr Neurol* **57**: 74–9.

Benveniste EN (1992) Inflammatory cytokines within the central nervous system: sources, function, and mechanism of action. *The American Journal of Physiology* **263**: C1–16.

Blakemore WF (1995) Cross talk between the immune system and the nervous system in response to injury: implications for regeneration. *Human & Experimental Toxicology* **14**: 615–6.

Broman SH (1987) Prenatal risk factors for mental retardation in young children. *Public Health Rep* **102**: 55–7.

Burns TM, Clough JA, Klein RM, Wood GW, Berman NE (1993) Developmental regulation of cytokine expression in the mouse brain. *Growth Factors* **9**: 253–8.

Chee YY, Wong MS, Wong RM, Wong KY (2017) Neonatal outcomes of preterm or very-low-birth-weight infants over a decade from Queen Mary Hospital, Hong Kong: comparison with the Vermont Oxford Network. *Hong Kong Medical Journal = Xianggang yi xue za zhi* **23**: 381–6.

Cheng Y, Gidday JM, Yan Q, Shah AR, Holtzman DM (1997) Marked age-dependent neuroprotection by brain-derived neurotrophic factor against neonatal hypoxic-ischemic brain injury. *Ann Neurol* **41**: 521–9.

Chiesa C, Signore F, Assumma M et al. (2001) Serial measurements of C-reactive protein and interleukin-6 in the immediate postnatal period: reference intervals and analysis of maternal and perinatal confounders. *Clin Chem* **47**: 1016–22.

Dammann O, Hagberg H, Leviton A (2001) Is periventricular leukomalacia an axonopathy as well as an oligopathy? *Pediatr Res* **49**: 453–7.

Dammann O, Leviton A (1998) Infection remote from the brain, neonatal white matter damage, and cerebral palsy in the preterm infant. *Semin Pediatr Neurol* **5**: 190–201.

Dammann O, Leviton A (1999) Brain damage in preterm newborns: might enhancement of developmentally-regulated endogenous protection open a door for prevention? *Pediatrics* **104**: 541–50.

Dammann O, Leviton A (2000a) Brain damage in preterm newborns: biologic response modification as a strategy to reduce disabilities. *J Pediatr* **136**: 433–8.

Dammann O, Leviton A (2000b) Role of the fetus in perinatal infection and neonatal brain damage. *Curr Opin Pediatr* **12**: 99–104.

Dammann O, Phillips TM, Allred EN et al. (2001) Mediators of fetal inflammation in extremely low gestational age newborns. *Cytokine* **13**: 234–9.

Davies PA (1971) Bacterial infection in the fetus and newborn. *Arch Dis Child* **46**: 1–27.

Dubravec DB, Spriggs DR, Mannick JA, Rodrick ML (1990) Circulating human peripheral blood granulocytes synthesize and secrete tumor necrosis factor alpha. *Proc Natl Acad Sci USA* **87**: 6758–61.

Elkabes S, Peng L, Black IB (1998) Lipopolysaccharide differentially regulates microglial trk receptor and neurotrophin expression. *J Neurosci Res* **54**: 117–22.

Fichorova RN, Beatty N, Sassi RRS et al. (2015) Systemic inflammation in the extremely low gestational age newborn following maternal genitourinary infections. *American Journal of Reproductive Immunology* **73**: 162–74.

Fidel PL, Jr, Romero R, Wolf N et al. (1994) Systemic and local cytokine profiles in endotoxin-induced preterm parturition in mice. *Am J Obstet Gynecol* **170**: 1467–75.

Fontana A, Kristensen F, Dubs R, Gemsa D, Weber E (1982) Production of prostaglandin E and an interleukin-1 like factor by cultured astrocytes and C6 glioma cells. *J Immunol* **129**: 2413–9.

Gibbs RS, Romero R, Hillier SL, Eschenbach DA, Sweet RL (1992) A review of premature birth and subclinical infection. *Am J Obstet Gynecol* **166**: 1515–28.

Gilles FH, Averill DR, Jr, Kerr CS (1977) Neonatal endotoxin encephalopathy. *Ann Neurol* **2**: 49–56.

Gilles FH, Leviton A, Dooling EC (1983) *The Developing Human Brain. Growth and Epidemiologic Neuropathology*. Boston: John Wright – PSG Inc.

Gilles FH, Leviton A, Kerr CS (1976) Endotoxin leucoencephalopathy in the telencephalon of the newborn kitten. *J Neurol Sci* **27**: 183–91.

Gilles FH, Murphy SF (1969) Perinatal telencephalic leucoencephalopathy. *J Neurol Neurosurg Psychiatry* **32**: 404–13.

Graves DT (1997) The use of biologic response modifiers in human clinical trials. *Annals of Periodontology* **2**: 259–67.

Grether JK, Nelson KB, Dambrosia JM, Phillips TM (1999) Interferons and cerebral palsy. *J Pediatr* **134**: 324–32.

Gruol DL, Nelson TE (1997) Physiological and pathological roles of interleukin-6 in the central nervous system. *Mol Neurobiol* **15**: 307–39.

Hagberg H, Mallard C (2000) Antenatal brain injury: aetiology and possibilities of prevention. *Semin Neonatol* **5**: 41–51.

Heese K, Fiebich BL, Bauer J, Otten U (1998) NF-kappaB modulates lipopolysaccharide-induced microglial nerve growth factor expression. *Glia* **22**: 401–7.

Inder TE, Volpe JJ (2000) Mechanisms of perinatal brain injury. *Semin Neonatol* **5**: 3–16.

Jaeschke H, Farhood A, Fisher MA, Smith CW (1996) Sequestration of neutrophils in the hepatic vasculature during endotoxemia is independent of beta 2 integrins and intercellular adhesion molecule-1. *Shock* **6**: 351–6.

Jilma B, Blann A, Pernerstorfer T et al. (1999) Regulation of adhesion molecules during human endotoxemia. No acute effects of aspirin. *Am J Respir Crit Care Med* **159**: 857–63.

Lee I, Neil JJ, Huettner PC et al. (2014) The impact of prenatal and neonatal infection on neurodevelopmental outcomes in very preterm infants. *J Perinatol* **34**: 741–7.

Leib SL, Leppert D, Clements J, Tauber MG (2000) Matrix metalloproteinases contribute to brain damage in experimental pneumococcal meningitis. *Infect Immun* **68**: 615–20.

Lennon VA (1994) Cross-talk between nervous and immune systems in response to injury. *Prog Brain Res* **103**: 289–92.

Leviton A (1983) Autopsy data in epidemiologic studies. In: Gilles FH, Leviton A, Dooling EC (eds). *The Developing Human Brain Growth and Epidemiologic Neuropathology*. Boston: John Wright – PSG.

Leviton A (1993) Preterm birth and cerebral palsy: is tumor necrosis factor the missing link? *Dev Med Child Neurol* **35**: 553–8.

Leviton A, Fichorova R, Yamamoto Y et al. (2011) Inflammation-related proteins in the blood of extremely low gestational age newborns. The contribution of inflammation to the appearance of developmental regulation. *Cytokine* **53**: 66–73.

Leviton A, Gilles FH (1971) Custering of the morphological components of perinatal telencephalic leucoencephalopathy. *J Neurol Neurosurg Psychiatry* **34**: 642–5.

Leviton A, Gilles FH (1973) An epidemiologic study of perinatal telencephalic leucoencephalopathy in an autopsy population. *J Neurol Sci* **18**: 53–66.

Leviton A, Gilles FH (1984) Acquired perinatal leukoencephalopathy. *Ann Neurol* **16**: 1–8.

Leviton A, Gilles F, Neff R, Yaney P (1976) Multivariate analysis of risk of perinatal telencephalic leucoencephalopathy. *Am J Epidemiol* **104**: 621–6.

Lotan M, Schwartz M (1994) Cross talk between the immune system and the nervous system in response to injury: implications for regeneration. *FASEB J* **8**: 1026–33.

Lieberman AP, Pitha PM, Shin HS, Shin ML (1989) Production of tumor necrosis factor and other cytokines by astrocytes stimulated with lipopolysaccharide or a neurotropic virus. *Proc Natl Acad Sci USA* **86**: 6348–52.

Mann JR, McDermott S, Bao H, Bersabe A (2009) Maternal genitourinary infection and risk of cerebral palsy. *Dev Med Child Neurol* **51**: 282–8.

Mallard C, Wang X (2012) Infection-induced vulnerability of perinatal brain injury. *Neurol Res Int* **2012**: 102153.

Merrill JE, Benveniste EN (1996) Cytokines in inflammatory brain lesions: helpful and harmful. *Trends Neurosci* **19**: 331–8.

Miller JE, Pedersen LH, Streja E et al. (2013) Maternal infections during pregnancy and cerebral palsy: a population-based cohort study. *Paediatr Perinat Epidemiol* **27**: 542–52.

Miwa T, Furukawa S, Nakajima K, Furukawa Y, Kohsaka S (1997) Lipopolysaccharide enhances synthesis of brain-derived neurotrophic factor in cultured rat microglia. *J Neurosci Res* **50**: 1023–9.

Munro JM, Pober JS, Cotran RS (1991) Recruitment of neutrophils in the local endotoxin response: association with de novo endothelial expression of endothelial leukocyte adhesion molecule-1. *Lab Invest* **64**: 295–9.

Nelson KB, Dambrosia JM, Grether JK, Phillips TM (1998) Neonatal cytokines and coagulation factors in children with cerebral palsy. *Ann Neurol* **44**: 665–75.

Nelson KB, Grether JK, Dambrosia JM, Dickens B, Phillips TM (2000) Cytokine concentrations in neonatal blood of preterm children with cerebral palsy (CP). *Am J Obstet Gynecol* **182**: S95.

Neufeld MD, Frigon C, Graham AS, Mueller BA (2005) Maternal infection and risk of cerebral palsy in term and preterm infants. *J Perinatol* **25**:108–13.

Ornoy A, Altshuler G (1976) Maternal endotoxemia, fetal anomalies, and central nervous system damage: a rat model of a human problem. *Am J Obstet Gynecol* **124**: 196–204.

Pagenstecher A, Stalder AK, Kincaid CL, Volk B, Campbell IL (2000) Regulation of matrix metalloproteinases and their inhibitor genes in lipopolysaccharide-induced endotoxemia in mice. *Am J Pathol* **157**: 197–210.

Paemen L, Jansen PM, Proost P et al. (1997) Induction of gelatinase B and MCP-2 in baboons during sublethal and lethal bacteraemia. *Cytokine* **9**: 412–5.

Paneth N, Rudelli R, Kazam E, Monte W (1994) *Brain Damage in the Preterm Infant*. London: Mac Keith Press.

Philip AG (2005) The evolution of neonatology. *Pediatr Res* **58**: 799–815.

Poston L, Harthoorn LF, Van Der Beek EM (2011) Obesity in pregnancy: implications for the mother and lifelong health of the child. A consensus statement. *Pediatr Res* **69**: 175–80.

Prajitha N, Athira SS, Mohanan PV (2018) Pyrogens, a polypeptide produces fever by metabolic changes in hypothalamus: mechanisms and detections. *Immunology Letters* **204**: 38–46.

Pugin J, Widmer MC, Kossodo S, Liang CM, Preas HLN, Suffredini AF (1999) Human neutrophils secrete gelatinase B in vitro and in vivo in response to endotoxin and proinflammatory mediators. *American Journal of Respiratory Cell and Molecular Biology* **20**: 458–64.

Raff MC, Barres BA, Burne JF, Coles HS, Ishizaki Y, Jacobson MD (1993) Programmed cell death and the control of cell survival: lessons from the nervous system. *Science* **262**: 695–700.

Reuss ML, Paneth N, Susser M (1994) Does the loss of placental hormones contribute to neurodevelopmental disabilities in preterm infants? *Dev Med Child Neurol* **36**: 743–7.

Romero R, Avila C, Brekus CA, Morotti R (1991) The role of systemic and intrauterine infection in preterm parturition. *Ann N Y Acad Sci* **622**: 355–75.

Romero R, Gomez R, Ghezzi F et al. (1998) A fetal systemic inflammatory response is followed by the spontaneous onset of preterm parturition. *Am J Obstet Gynecol* **179**: 186–93.

Romero R, Mazor M, Sepulveda W, Avila C, Copeland D, Williams J (1992) Tumor necrosis factor in preterm and term labor. *Am J Obstet Gynecol* **166**: 1576–87.

Romero R, Miranda J, Chaemsaithong P et al. (2015) Sterile and microbial-associated intra-amniotic inflammation in preterm prelabor rupture of membranes. *J Matern Fetal Neonatal Med* **28**: 1394–409.

Romero R, Parvizi ST, Oyarzun E et al. (1990) Amniotic fluid interleukin-1 in spontaneous labor at term. *J Reprod Med* **35**: 235–8.

Rosenberg GA (1995) Matrix metalloproteinases in brain injury. *J Neurotrauma* **12**: 833–42.

Santhanam U, Avila C, Romero R et al. (1991) Cytokines in normal and abnormal parturition: elevated amniotic fluid interleukin-6 levels in women with premature rupture of membranes associated with intrauterine infection. *Cytokine* **3**: 155–63.

Saukkonen K, Sande S, Cioffe C et al. (1990) The role of cytokines in the generation of inflammation and tissue damage in experimental gram-positive meningitis. *The Journal of Experimental Medicine* **171**: 439–48.

Suski M, Bokiniec R, Szwarc-Duma M et al. (2018) Plasma proteome changes in cord blood samples from preterm infants. *J Perinatol* **38**: 1182–9.

Tong L, Perez-Polo R (1998) Brain-derived neurotrophic factor (BDNF) protects cultured rat cerebellar granule neurons against glucose deprivation-induced apoptosis. *J Neural Transm* **105**: 905–14.

Wankhade UD, Thakali KM, Shankar K (2016) Persistent influence of maternal obesity on offspring health: Mechanisms from animal models and clinical studies. *Mol Cell Endocrinol* **435**: 7–19.

WHO (2019) Preterm birth key facts. Available at https://www.who.int/news-room/fact-sheets/detail/preterm-birth [Accessed February 19, 2019].

Yamasu K, Onoe H, Soma G, Oshima H, Mizuno D (1989) Secretion of tumor necrosis factor during fetal and neonatal development of the mouse: ontogenic inflammation. *Journal of Biological Response Modifiers* **8**: 644–55.

Yoon BH, Jun JK, Romero R et al. (1997b) Amniotic fluid inflammatory cytokines (interleukin-6, interleukin-1beta, and tumor necrosis factor-alpha), neonatal brain white matter lesions, and cerebral palsy. *Am J Obstet Gynecol* **177**: 19–26.

Yoon BH, Kim CJ, Romero R et al. (1997a) Experimentally induced intrauterine infection causes fetal brain white matter lesions in rabbits. *Am J Obstet Gynecol* **177**: 797–802.

Yoon BH, Romero R, Park JS et al. (2000) Fetal exposure to an intra-amniotic inflammation and the development of cerebral palsy at the age of three years. *Am J Obstet Gynecol* **182**: 675–81.

Yoon BH, Romero R, Yang SH et al. (1996) Interleukin-6 concentrations in umbilical cord plasma are elevated in neonates with white matter lesions associated with periventricular leukomalacia. *American Journal of Obstetrics & Gynecology* **174**: 1433–40.

Zhao B, Schwartz JP (1998) Involvement of cytokines in normal CNS development and neurological diseases: recent progress and perspectives. *J Neurosci Res* **52**: 7–16.

Xiao BG, Link H (1998) Immune regulation within the central nervous system. *J Neurol Sci* **157**: 1–12.

PART I

Placenta and Perinatal Risk Factors

Chapter 2   Placental Microorganisms in ELGAN with
Correlation to Pregnancy Outcomes,
Intrauterine Inflammation, and Postnatal
and Later-life Outcomes   17

Chapter 3   Correlations of Placental Histology in
ELGANS with Delivery Indications, Placental
Microbiology, and Childhood Morbidity   27

Chapter 4   Signal Initiators of Early Preterm Birth   35

Chapter 5   Maternal Adiposity   43

PART I

Placenta and Perinatal
Risk Factors

Chapter 2   Placental ...

Chapter 4   ...
             Babies with Delivery Indications, Perinatal
             Microbiology, and Childhood Mortality

Chapter 5   Signal Influence of Early Fetal Death

Chapter 6   Maternal Adiposity

Placental Microorganisms in ELGAN with Correlation to Pregnancy Outcomes, Intrauterine Inflammation, and Postnatal and Later-life Outcomes

Martha Scott Tomlinson and Rebecca C Fry

INTRODUCTION

Inflamed placentas do not always harbor bacteria, just as placentas with organisms in the parenchyma do not always display histologic inflammation. This recognition prompted the ELGAN study designers to plan to assess both placenta histology and placenta bacteriology. The goal was to assess to what extent each contributed to brain damage in the extremely preterm newborn (Leviton et al. 2010a). To make sure the organisms recovered were not contaminants, biopsies of the chorion parenchyma were obtained under sterile conditions after the amnion was incised and pulled away. These biopsies were the source of the bacteria recovered. The laboratory chosen to culture these biopsies had a long-standing and deep interest in the microorganisms common to the vaginal flora (Bartlett et al. 1977; Pybus and Onderdonk 1999), which were a focus of the efforts for the ELGAN study.

After summarizing the microbial findings in the ELGAN study placentas, this chapter presents evaluations of the relationships between placental microorganisms and pregnancy complications, placenta inflammation, placenta epigenetic phenomena, brain ultrasound lesions, microcephaly, retinopathy of prematurity, and later limitations in cognition, attention, and motor function in toddlers.

Some of the major concerns of the ELGAN researchers are the developmental impairments that occur more commonly in preterm children than in those born at term (O'Shea et al. 2009). Bacterial presence in the placenta has been associated with adverse neurological outcomes (Altshuler 1995; Cao et al. 2014), including altered brain structure, as well as cerebral palsy and low scores on the Bayley Scales of Infant Development II (Dammann and Leviton 1997; Polam et al. 2005; Shatrov et al. 2010). However, most of the previous studies have used indicators of infection, such as chorioamnionitis and fetal vasculitis, as a proxy for microbial presence instead of testing for specific microorganisms. The ELGAN study cultured placenta parenchyma biopsies (obtained after the amnion was pulled back under sterile conditions) and identified specific bacterial species that were subsequently assessed for their relationships to a variety of outcomes including pregnancy outcomes, inflammatory responses, brain development, early life neurocognitive function in addition to bronchopulmonary dysplasia (chronic lung disease), necrotizing enterocolitis, and retinopathy of prematurity.

The 'sterile womb paradigm' suggests that the uterus, including the placenta, is sterile and that any microbial presence in the intrauterine environment is the result of infection (Goldenberg et al. 2000; Perez-Munoz et al. 2017). However, the identification of microbial communities in the meconium, the amniotic fluid, the umbilical blood cord, and the placenta of term pregnancies (Stout et al. 2013; Aagaard et al. 2014; Koleva et al. 2015; Neu 2016) challenges this paradigm. In addition, the prenatal microbiome has been associated with altered fetal development as well as heightened risk of developing diseases decades later (Saavedra and Dattilo 2012; Koleva et al. 2015; Stinson et al. 2017; D'Argenio 2018). These findings have contributed to the 'in utero colonization hypothesis' (Perez-Munoz et al. 2017). However, those who oppose this hypothesis cite studies that document or have failed to rule out contamination, and those that have not assessed bacterial viability (Kliman 2014; Lauder et al. 2016; Perez-Munoz et al. 2017).

Summary of Microbial Findings in the Placentas of ELGAN Study Placentas

During the ELGAN enrollment period (2002–2004), women delivering before the 28th week of gestation at one of the 14 participating ELGAN institutions were asked to participate in the study. In total, 1250 mothers of 1506 infants consented to evaluation, of which 1365 placental samples were collected following delivery (Onderdonk et al. 2008a).

Prior to the ELGAN study, the presence of certain species of microbial organisms in the intrauterine environment was associated with increased risk of preterm delivery (Lamont et al. 1987; Alger et al. 1988; Martius et al. 1988; Papiernik 1990; Joste et al. 1994; Klebanoff et al. 1995; Kundsin et al. 1996; Abele-Horn et al. 1997; Krohn et al. 1997; Kataoka et al. 2006). However, it was unclear then whether the organisms needed to enter fetal tissues to initiate the labor process or whether inflammatory stimuli produced elsewhere were sufficient. Therefore, within the ELGAN cohort the microorganisms were recovered from the chorionic parenchyma, a placental tissue of fetal origin. Contamination of the sample from vaginal microorganisms was unlikely since the area biopsied was covered by the amnion (Onderdonk et al. 2008a).

Details about how the samples were handled, and how organisms were cultured and identified are available elsewhere. Overall 51% (696/1365) of the placenta specimens were culture-positive. *Staphylococcus* spp. and *Corynebacterium* sp. were the most frequently recovered organisms, accounting for 42% of all the isolates. Microorganisms associated with bacterial vaginosis, such as *Prevotella* spp. (17%), *Peptostreptococcus* spp. (16%), *Ureaplasma urealyticum* (10%), and *Gardnerella vaginalis* (8%), were also commonly isolated (Table 2.1) (Onderdonk et al. 2008a).

In addition to the culture methods described above, polymerase chain reaction (PCR) methods with universal bacterial primers were used to detect organisms that might not be isolated by the bacteriologic methods. Unfortunately, none of the 154 placental samples assessed demonstrated the presence of an 800-basepair PCR product. Additional PCR analyses were unable to detect bacterial DNA on placentas known to contain high counts of bacteria by culture methods. The researchers also showed that this lack of detection was not due to faulty universal primers. Therefore, the PCR

Table 2.1 Frequency of isolation and mean log count

Organism	No	Frequency, %	Mean count (SD)
Actinomyces	89	13	2.91 (0.80)
Anaerobic *Streptococcus*	72	10	3.08 (0.95)
Bacteroides fragilis	20	3	3.72 (1.21)
Fragilis group	34	5	3.19 (0.97)
Bifidobacterium	16	2	2.87 (0.96)
Corynebacterium	119	17	2.79 (0.77)
E. coli	81	12	3.46 (1.14)
G. vaginalis	58	8	3.53 (0.91)
Lactobacillus	87	12	2.89 (0.85)
Mycoplasma hominis	88	13	3.81 (1.14)
Peptostreptococcus			
anaerobius	8	1	3.34 (0.68)
assacharolyticus	26	4	2.95 (0.75)
magnus	63	9	2.84 (0.77)
prevotii	13	2	3.07 (0.78)
Prevotella bivia	73	10	3.12 (0.96)
Pigmented	36	5	3.02 (0.96)
Other	17	2	3.27 (1.40)
Propionibacterium	94	14	2.51 (0.68)
Staphylococcus aureus	12	2	3.20 (1.30)
Coagulase-negative	175	25	2.56 (0.72)
Streptococcus viridans	82	12	2.90 (1.02)
Group B	58	8	3.47 (1.21)
Group D	64	9	2.86 (0.90)
Ureaplasma urealyticum	69	10	4.13 (0.95)
Total	697		

Reprinted from Onderdonk et al. (2008a), with permission from Elsevier.

methods used in this study were deemed not adequate to detect identification of bacterial DNA in the chorion parenchyma (Onderdonk et al. 2008a). One possible explanation for this is that the placenta may harbor substances that interfere with the detection of bacterial DNA by PCR methods. Naturally occurring substances in cervical specimens interfere with the detection of *Chlamydia trachomatis* by PCR (Toye et al. 1998; Wilcox et al. 2000). In addition, other tissue-specific factors and cell constitutes such as hemoglobin, myoglobin, fat, and glycogen, are thought to influence the amplification kinetics of PCR (Wilson 1997; Belec et al. 1998; Tichopad et al. 2004). Thus, the failure of PCR to document bacterial components might be merely a reflection of placenta biology and not evidence of the absence of bacteria in the placenta.

Relationship between Placental Microorganisms and Pregnancy Complications

Numerous pregnancy complications can lead to preterm birth. The ELGAN study cohort divided the clinical circumstances for preterm delivery into six categories: preterm labor, pre-labor premature rupture of membranes (pPROM), preeclampsia, placental abruption, cervical insufficiency, and intra-uterine growth restriction (IUGR). Three different ELGAN study reports compared microbial presence in the placenta to the clinical subgroups of pregnancy disorder that lead to preterm delivery. The first compared microbial presence in the chorion parenchyma to all six pregnancy complications. Microbial presence was much more common in the placentas from pregnancies complicated by preterm labor (58%), pPROM (69%), placental abruption (55%), and cervical insufficiency (59%) than the placentas from pregnancies complicated by preeclampsia (26%) or fetal indication/IUGR (25%) (McElrath et al. 2008; Onderdonk et al. 2008b). In addition, women whose placentas harbored *U. urealyticum* were at increased risk of pPROM and preterm labor (Olomu et al. 2009).

Within the ELGAN cohort, more than 30% of the placentas from women who had preterm labor, pPROM, placental abruption, or cervical insufficiency harbored multiple microorganisms in contrast to only 4% of preeclamptic placentas and 11% of IUGR placentas (McElrath et al. 2008). These findings support the separation of the six pregnancy complications into two broad groups: intra-uterine inflammation (preterm labor, pPROM, placental abruption, and cervical insufficiency) and abnormal placentation (preeclampsia and IUGR). The placentas that harbored microorganisms in the chorion parenchyma were at higher risk for pregnancy disorders classified by intrauterine inflammation (McElrath et al. 2008).

Relationship between Placental Microorganisms and Inflammation in the Intrauterine Environment

Histologic characteristics, including inflammation of the chorionic plate and vasculitis of the chorionic plate and umbilical cord vessels, were strongly correlated with microorganism recovery in the placenta (Hecht et al. 2008; Onderdonk et al. 2008b). In addition, the more intense the score/grade of the his-tologic chorioamnionitis the more likely it was that a microorganism was recovered from the placenta (Hecht et al. 2008).

Specific microbial species associated with high-grade chorionic plate inflammation included *Actinomyces* spp., *Prevotella bivia, Corynebacterium* spp., *Escherichia coli, Peptostreptococcus magnus, Streptococcus* Group B, *Streptococcus* Group D, alpha-hemolytic *Streptococcus*, and anaerobic *Streptococcus, Mycoplasma* spp., and *Ureaplasma urealyticum* (Hecht et al. 2008; Olomu et al. 2009). These same microorganisms were associated with fetal vasculitis (neutrophilic infiltration of the fetal vessels in the chorionic plate or umbilical cord) (Hecht et al. 2008; Olomu et al. 2009). In contrast, some microorganisms were more prevalent in non-inflamed placentas such as *Lactobacillus* spp., *Propionibacterium* spp., coagulase-negative *Staphylococcus*, and *Gardnerella vaginalis* (Hecht et al. 2008).

In addition to evaluating histologic characteristics, the ELGAN study examined epigenetic mod-ifications within the placenta. Epigenetic modifications, such as DNA methylation, are mechanisms that can alter gene expression. An analysis of 84 ELGAN placentas found 1789 DNA sites were differentially methylated in the presence of placental microorganisms (Tomlinson et al. 2017). The presence of *Streptococcus* Group B was associated with the majority (n = 1229) of the differentially methylated sites. The differentially methylated sites were found to be enriched for inflammatory pathways, specifically the NF-κB pathway (Tomlinson et al. 2017). These epigenetic modifications could potentially trigger the maternal inflammatory response to microorganisms, which then provokes the fetal inflammatory response. If so, then epigenetic phenomena could help explain why ELGANs are at increased risk of so many consequences that are linked to bacteria in the placenta and blood, but not in the brain.

Relationship between Placental Microorganisms and Postnatal Indicators of Inflammation and Brain Development

The presence of bacterial vaginosis (BV)-related microorganisms in the placenta, including *P. bivia*, *G. vaginalis*, anaerobic *Streptococcus*, and *Peptostreptococcus* spp., was associated with a heightened risk of a pro-inflammatory pattern of proteins in the newborn's blood (Fichorova et al. 2011). This pro-inflammatory pattern was also associated with the presence of *E. coli* and alpha-hemolytic *Streptococcus*, facultative anaerobes, as well as the genital mycoplasma species *U. urealyticum* and *Mycoplasma* spp. In contrast, placental recovery of *Lactobacillus* spp. was associated with reduced likelihood of a systemic inflammation. When *Lactobacillus* spp. was the only bacterium recovered from the placenta, most inflammatory proteins were completely undetectable in the newborn blood samples (Fichorova et al. 2011). These findings provide evidence that colonization of the placenta by certain microbial species provokes a systemic inflammatory response in the newborn, while the presence of *Lactobacillus* spp. may suppress this response (Fichorova et al. 2011).

Systemic inflammation in the newborn has been associated with damage in the fetal/newborn brain (Yoon et al. 1996; Dammann and Leviton 1997; Silverstein et al. 1997; Dammann and O'Shea 2008; Malaeb and Dammann 2009). Early brain ultrasound scans can identify echolucent (also known as echopoor or hypoechoic) lesions and ventriculomegaly, both of which are forms of cerebral white matter damage (O'Shea et al. 2005). Within the ELGAN cohort recovery of a single microorganism from the placenta was associated with an increased risk of echolucent lesions, while the presence of multiple microorganisms or skin-associated microorganisms, including *Corynebacterium* spp., *Proionebacterium* spp., and *Staphylococcus* sp., was associated with an increased risk of both echolucent lesions and ventriculomegaly (Leviton et al. 2010a). The presence of *U. urealyticum* in the placenta was also associated with increased risk of both intraventricular hemorrhage and echolucent lesions (Olomu et al. 2009). These findings support the hypothesis that an inflammation-promoting stimulus in the uterus can promote processes that lead to brain damage (Yoon et al. 1997; Bell and Hallenbeck 2002; Debillon et al. 2003; Yuan et al. 2005).

Relationship between Placental Microorganisms and Retinopathy of Prematurity, as well as Small Head Circumference

Neither the presence of bacteria in the placenta alone nor the presence of placenta histologic inflammation alone was associated with retinopathy of prematurity (ROP), a disorder of retinal vasoproliferation in the newborn that can impair vision (Chen et al. 2011b). However, when both were present the risk of ROP was elevated. These findings suggest that ROP pathogenesis is a multi-hit phenomenon (Dammann et al. 2009; Chen et al. 2011a).

Microcephaly at birth (McElrath et al. 2010) and 2 years later (Leviton et al. 2010b), defined as a disproportionately small head circumference (i.e. more than 2 standard deviations below the mean), were not associated with bacterial presence in the placenta among infants delivered vaginally. However, recovery of any *Mycoplasma* spp. or multiple microorganisms in the placenta were associated with increased risk of 'minicephaly' (less severe microcephaly; defined as between 1 and 2 standard deviations below the mean) at birth (McElrath et al. 2010). Infants who were delivered by Cesarean section (C-section) had a reduced risk of microcephaly when multiple microorganisms or vaginal microorganisms (including *Prevotella bivia, Lactobacillus* spp, *Peptostreptococcus magnus*, and *Gardnerella vaginalis*), were found in the placenta (McElrath et al. 2010). In contrast, the presence of *Propionibacterium* spp. and other skin associated organisms, such as *Staphylococcus* spp., in the placenta was associated with increased risk of microcephaly at birth (McElrath et al. 2010) but not at 2 years (Leviton et al. 2010b). At age 2 years, children who were born by C-section were at increased risk of microcephaly if their placenta harbored alpha-hemolytic *Streptococcus*, and were at increased risk of minicephaly if their placenta harbored *Propionibacterium* spp. and skin flora (Leviton et al. 2010b).

Relationship between Placental Microorganisms and Low Bayley Scales Scores and Cerebral Palsy

Organisms recovered from the placenta were not associated with cognitive limitations at age 2 based on the Mental Development Index (MDI) of the Bayley Scales of Infant Development II (BSID-II) (Helderman et al. 2012). However, recovery of a single organism from the placenta was associated with increased risk of attention problems as assessed by the Child Behavior Checklist (CBCL), while the presence of *Mycoplasma* spp. was associated with increased risk of characteristics that are compatible with *Diagnostic and Statistical Manual of Mental Disorders, Fourth Edition* criteria for identifying attention deficit hyperactivity disorder (ADHD[DSM]) in older children (Downey et al. 2015).

Cerebral palsy (CP), a disorder affecting movement, muscle tone, or posture that is caused by damage to the developing brain, preferentially affecting both lower extremities (diparesis or leg-dominated) and all four extremities (quadriparesis). The risk of diparesis was increased among children whose placenta harbored a single and perhaps indicative or a dose-response or equivalent relationship, the presence of multiple microorganisms in the placenta was associated with an increased risk of both diparesis and quadriparesis (Leviton et al. 2010a).

CONCLUSION

In the ELGAN study microbial presence in the placenta has been associated with increased risk of vasculitis in umbilical cord and chorionic plate vessels (Hecht et al. 2008; Onderdonk et al. 2008b), inflammation-related pregnancy disorders that lead to preterm birth (preterm labor, pPROM, placental abruption and cervical insufficiency) (McElrath et al. 2008), differential methylation of inflammatory genes in the placenta (Tomlinson et al. 2017), high concentrations of inflammation-related proteins in the newborn's postnatal blood (Fichorova et al. 2011), retinopathy of prematurity (Chen et al. 2011b), neonatal cerebral white matter damage (Olomu et al. 2009; Leviton et al. 2010a; Downey et al. 2015), and attention problems (Downey et al. 2015).

The majority of the microbial species identified in the ELGAN study are considered pathogenic and pro-inflammatory, except for *Lactobacillus* sp., which has anti-inflammatory properties (Joo et al. 2011; Yeganegi et al. 2010). In the ELGAN study, *Lactobacillus* sp. was prevalent in non-inflamed placentas (Hecht et al. 2008) and was associated with decreased concentrations of inflammation-related proteins in the neonates' blood (Fichorova et al. 2011) as well as a decreased risk of microcephaly (McElrath et al. 2010). These findings highlight the important finding that certain bacteria can be present in the placenta and exert beneficial effects.

REFERENCES

Aagaard K, Ma J, Antony KM, Ganu R, Petrosino J, Versalovic J (2014) The placenta harbors a unique microbiome. *Sci Transl Med* **6**: 237ra65.

Abele-Horn M, Peters J, Genzel-Boroviczeny O, Wolff C, Zimmermann A, Gottschling W (1997) Vaginal ureaplasma urealyticum colonization: influence on pregnancy outcome and neonatal morbidity. *Infection* **25**: 286–91.

Alger LS, Lovchik JC, Hebel JR, Blackmon LR, Crenshaw MC (1988) The association of Chlamydia trachomatis, Neisseria gonorrhoeae, and group B streptococci with preterm rupture of the membranes and pregnancy outcome. *Am J Obstet Gynecol* **159**: 397–404.

Altshuler G (1995) Placental insights into neurodevelopmental and other childhood diseases. *Semin Pediatr Neurol* **2**: 90–9.

Bartlett JG, Onderdonk AB, Drude E et al. (1977) Quantitative bacteriology of the vaginal flora. *J Infect Dis* **136**: 271–7.

Belec L, Authier J, Eliezer-Vanerot MC, Piedouillet C, Mohamed AS, Gherardi RK (1998) Myoglobin as a polymerase chain reaction (PCR) inhibitor: a limitation for PCR from skeletal muscle tissue avoided by the use of Thermus thermophilus polymerase. *Muscle Nerve* **21**: 1064–7.

Bell MJ, Hallenbeck JM (2002) Effects of intrauterine inflammation on developing rat brain. *J Neurosci Res* **70**: 570–9.

Cao B, Stout MJ, Lee I, Mysorekar IU (2014) Placental microbiome and its role in preterm birth. *Neoreviews* **15**: e537–e545.

Chen M, Citil A, McCabe F et al. (2011a) Infection, oxygen, and immaturity: interacting risk factors for retinopathy of prematurity. *Neonatology* **99**: 125–32.

Chen ML, Allred EN, Hecht JL et al. (2011b) Placenta microbiology and histology and the risk for severe retinopathy of prematurity. *Invest Ophthalmol Vis Sci* **52**: 7052–8.

D'Argenio V (2018) The prenatal microbiome: a new player for human health. *High Throughput* **7**: 38.

Dammann O, Brinkhaus MJ, Bartels DB et al. (2009) Immaturity, perinatal inflammation, and retinopathy of prematurity: a multi-hit hypothesis. *Early Hum Dev* **85**: 325–9.

Dammann O, Leviton A (1997) Maternal intrauterine infection, cytokines, and brain damage in the preterm newborn. *Pediatr Res* **42**: 1–8.

Dammann O, O'Shea TM (2008) Cytokines and perinatal brain damage. *Clin Perinatol* **35**: 643–63.

Debillon T, Gras-Leguen C, Leroy S, Caillon J, Roze JC, Gressens P (2003) Patterns of cerebral inflammatory response in a rabbit model of intrauterine infection-mediated brain lesion. *Brain Res Dev Brain Res* **145**: 39–48.

Downey LC, O'Shea TM, Allred EN et al. (2015) Antenatal and early postnatal antecedents of parent-reported attention problems at 2 years of age. *J Pediatr* **166**: 20–5.

Fichorova RN, Onderdonk AB, Yamamoto H et al. (2011) Maternal microbe-specific modulation of inflammatory response in extremely low-gestational-age newborns. *MBio* **2**: e00280–10.

Goldenberg RL, Hauth JC, Andrews WW (2000) Intrauterine infection and preterm delivery. *N Engl J Med* **342**: 1500–7.

Hecht JL, Onderdonk A, Delaney M et al. (2008) Characterization of chorioamnionitis in 2nd-trimester C-section placentas and correlation with microorganism recovery from subamniotic tissues. *Pediatr Dev Pathol* **11**: 15–22.

Helderman JB, O'Shea TM, Kuban KC et al. (2012) Antenatal antecedents of cognitive impairment at 24 months in extremely low gestational age newborns. *Pediatrics* **129**: 494–502.

Joo HM, Hyun YJ, Myoung KS et al. (2011) Lactobacillus johnsonii HY7042 ameliorates Gardnerella vaginalis-induced vaginosis by killing Gardnerella vaginalis and inhibiting NF-kappaB activation. *Int Immunopharmacol* **11**: 1758–65.

Joste NE, Kundsin RB, Genest DR (1994) Histology and Ureaplasma urealyticum culture in 63 cases of first trimester abortion. *Am J Clin Pathol* **102**: 729–32.

Kataoka S, Yamada T, Chou K et al. (2006) Association between preterm birth and vaginal colonization by mycoplasmas in early pregnancy. *J Clin Microbiol* **44**: 51–5.

Klebanoff MA, Regan JA, Rao AV et al. (1995) Outcome of the vaginal infections and prematurity study: results of a clinical trial of erythromycin among pregnant women colonized with group B streptococci. *Am J Obstet Gynecol,* **172**: 1540–5.

Kliman HJ (2014) Comment on 'the placenta harbors a unique microbiome'. *Sci Transl Med* **6**: 254le4.

Koleva PT, Kim JS, Scott JA, Kozyrskyj AL (2015) Microbial programming of health and disease starts during fetal life. *Birth Defects Res C Embryo Today* **105**: 265–77.

Krohn MA, Thwin SS, Rabe LK, Brown Z, Hillier SL (1997) Vaginal colonization by Escherichia coli as a risk factor for very low birth weight delivery and other perinatal complications. *J Infect Dis* **175**: 606–10.

Kundsin RB, Leviton A, Allred EN, Poulin SA (1996) Ureaplasma urealyticum infection of the placenta in pregnancies that ended prematurely. *Obstet Gynecol* **87**: 122–7.

Lamont RF, Taylor-Robinson D, Wigglesworth JS, Furr PM, Evans RT, Elder MG (1987) The role of mycoplasmas, ureaplasmas and chlamydiae in the genital tract of women presenting in spontaneous early preterm labour. *J Med Microbiol* **24**: 253–7.

Lauder AP, Roche AM, Sherrill-Mix S et al. (2016) Comparison of placenta samples with contamination controls does not provide evidence for a distinct placenta microbiota. *Microbiome* **4**: 29.

Leviton A, Allred EN, Kuban KC et al. (2010a) Microbiologic and histologic characteristics of the extremely preterm infant's placenta predict white matter damage and later cerebral palsy. The ELGAN study. *Pediatr Res* **67**: 95–101.

Leviton A, Kuban K, Allred EN et al. (2010b) Antenatal antecedents of a small head circumference at age 24-months post-term equivalent in a sample of infants born before the 28th post-menstrual week. *Early Hum Dev* **86**: 515–21.

Malaeb S, Dammann O (2009) Fetal inflammatory response and brain injury in the preterm newborn. *J Child Neurol* **24**: 1119–26.

Martius J, Krohn MA, Hillier SL, Stamm WE, Holmes KK, Eschenbach DA (1988) Relationships of vaginal Lactobacillus species, cervical Chlamydia trachomatis, and bacterial vaginosis to preterm birth. *Obstet Gynecol* **71**: 89–95.

McElrath TF, Allred EN, Kuban K et al. (2010) Factors associated with small head circumference at birth among infants born before the 28th week. *Am J Obstet Gynecol* **203**: 138 e1–8.

McElrath TF, Hecht JL, Dammann O et al. (2008) Pregnancy disorders that lead to delivery before the 28th week of gestation: an epidemiologic approach to classification. *Am J Epidemiol* **168**: 980–9.

Neu J (2016) The microbiome during pregnancy and early postnatal life. *Semin Fetal Neonatal Med* **21**: 373–9.

O'Shea TM, Allred EN, Dammann O et al. (2009) The ELGAN study of the brain and related disorders in extremely low gestational age newborns. *Early Hum Dev* **85**: 719–25.

O'Shea TM, Counsell SJ, Bartels DB, Dammann O (2005) Magnetic resonance and ultrasound brain imaging in preterm infants. *Early Hum Dev* **81**: 263–71.

Olomu IN, Hecht JL, Onderdonk AO, Allred EN, Leviton A; Extremely Low Gestational Age Newborn Study I (2009). Perinatal correlates of Ureaplasma urealyticum in placenta parenchyma of singleton pregnancies that end before 28 weeks of gestation. *Pediatrics* **123**: 1329–36.

Onderdonk AB, Delaney ML, Dubois AM, Allred EN, Leviton A; Extremely Low Gestational Age Newborns Study I (2008a) Detection of bacteria in placental tissues obtained from extremely low gestational age neonates. *Am J Obstet Gynecol* **198**: 110 e1–7.

Onderdonk AB, Hecht JL, McElrath TF et al. (2008b) Colonization of second-trimester placenta parenchyma. *Am J Obstet Gynecol* **199**: 52 e1–52 e10.

Papiernik E (1990) Preterm labor, preterm delivery, intrauterine infection, and preterm rupture of membranes. *Curr Opin Obstet Gynecol* **2**: 8–12.

Perez-Munoz ME, Arrieta MC, Ramer-Tait AE, Walter J (2017) A critical assessment of the 'sterile womb' and 'in utero colonization' hypotheses: implications for research on the pioneer infant microbiome. *Microbiome* **5**: 48.

Polam S, Koons A, Anwar M, Shen-Schwarz S, Hegyi T (2005) Effect of chorioamnionitis on neurodevelopmental outcome in preterm infants. *Arch Pediatr Adolesc Med* **159**: 1032–5.

Pybus V, Onderdonk AB (1999) Microbial interactions in the vaginal ecosystem, with emphasis on the pathogenesis of bacterial vaginosis. *Microbes Infect* **1**: 285–92.

Saavedra JM, Dattilo AM (2012) Early development of intestinal microbiota: implications for future health. *Gastroenterol Clin North Am* **41**: 717–31.

Shatrov JG, Birch SC, Lam LT, Quinlivan JA, McIntyre S, Mendz GL (2010) Chorioamnionitis and cerebral palsy: a meta-analysis. *Obstet Gynecol* **116**: 387–92.

Silverstein FS, Barks JD, Hagan P, Liu XH, Ivacko J, Szaflarski J (1997) Cytokines and perinatal brain injury. *Neurochem Int* **30**: 375–83.

Stinson LF, Payne MS, Keelan JA (2017) Planting the seed: origins, composition, and postnatal health significance of the fetal gastrointestinal microbiota. *Crit Rev Microbiol* **43**: 352–69.

Stout MJ, Conlon B, Landeau M et al. (2013) Identification of intracellular bacteria in the basal plate of the human placenta in term and preterm gestations. *Am J Obstet Gynecol* **208**: 226 e1–7.

Tichopad A, Didier A, Pfaffl MW (2004) Inhibition of real-time RT-PCR quantification due to tissue-specific contaminants. *Mol Cell Probes* **18**: 45–50.

Tomlinson MS, Bommarito PA, Martin EM et al. (2017) Microorganisms in the human placenta are associated with altered CpG methylation of immune and inflammation-related genes. *PLoS One* **12**: e0188664.

Toye B, Woods W, Bobrowska M, Ramotar K (1998) Inhibition of PCR in genital and urine specimens submitted for Chlamydia trachomatis testing. *J Clin Microbiol* **36**: 2356–8.

Wilcox MH, Reynolds MT, Hoy CM, Brayson J (2000) Combined cervical swab and urine specimens for PCR diagnosis of genital Chlamydia trachomatis infection. *Sex Transm Infect* **76**: 177–8.

Wilson IG (1997) Inhibition and facilitation of nucleic acid amplification. *Appl Environ Microbiol* **63**: 3741–51.

Yeganegi M, Leung CG, Martins A et al. (2010) Lactobacillus rhamnosus GR-1-induced IL-10 production in human placental trophoblast cells involves activation of JAK/STAT and MAPK pathways. *Reprod Sci* **17**: 1043–51.

Yoon BH, Kim CJ, Romero R et al. (1997). Experimentally induced intrauterine infection causes fetal brain white matter lesions in rabbits. *Am J Obstet Gynecol* **177**: 797–802.

Yoon BH, Romero R, Yang SH et al. (1996) Interleukin-6 concentrations in umbilical cord plasma are elevated in neonates with white matter lesions associated with periventricular leukomalacia. *Am J Obstet Gynecol* **174**: 1433–40.

Yuan TM, Yu HM, Gu WZ, Li JP (2005) White matter damage and chemokine induction in developing rat brain after intrauterine infection. *J Perinat Med* **33**: 415–22.

Correlations of Placental Histology in ELGANs with Delivery Indications, Placental Microbiology, and Childhood Morbidity

Jonathan L Hecht

INTRODUCTION

Brain development during the 23rd to 27th weeks of gestation is especially vulnerable to disruption (Ream and Lehwald 2018). The risk is increased by diseases affecting the placenta including histologic chorioamnionitis (Pietrasanta et al. 2019), with or without detectable infection, and maternal or fetal vascular malperfusion (Stoll et al. 2004; Harteman et al. 2012). These diseases can be chronic, affecting fetal growth, or acute, leading to premature indicated or spontaneous delivery.

The ELGAN pathologists were tasked with using consensus criteria to create their own data collection forms and manual (O'Shea et al. 2009). The database that resulted from these efforts to minimize inter-observer variability allowed us to describe the frequency of placental lesions in the ELGAN study cohort, as well as enabling our correlating placenta morphology with maternal factors (indication for delivery), microbiology, neonatal serum markers of inflammation and endothelial injury, as well as clinical outcome in the children.

This chapter is divided into six sections. One summarizes the prevalence of each of the histologic lesions, while the other five describe the relationships between placental lesions and indications for preterm delivery, recovery of microorganisms, post-natal serum concentrations of inflammatory markers, and manifestations of brain structure abnormalities or dysfunction.

Summary of Histologic Findings in the Placentas of ELGAN (Hecht et al. 2008b)

During the enrollment period (2002–2004), 1250 mothers of 1506 infants consented to evaluation, and the 947 placentas from singletons were the focus of most of the histologic work (Hecht et al. 2008a,

2008b). Chorioamnionitis was the most frequent finding with inflammation of the chorionic plate in 43%, neutrophilic infiltration into fetal vessels of the plate in 30%, and inflammation of the cord in 19%. Morphological features associated with poor utero-placental perfusion including infarcts, increased syncytial knots, and abruption were each seen in about 20% of placentas. The frequency of maternal inflammation in the chorionic plate decreased with increasing gestational age, but fetal inflammation in the umbilical cord did not vary substantially with gestational age. The prevalence of lesions of poor utero-placental perfusion increased with gestational age. Poor perfusion and chorioamnionitis were inversely related. For example, in placentas with increased syncytial knots (also known as 'distal villous hypoplasia') (Khong et al. 2016), only 18% also had evidence of inflammation in the chorionic plate, while 50% of placentas that did not have increased syncytial knots had chorionic plate inflammation.

The inclusion criteria for the ELGAN cohort were novel at the time. Patients were enrolled based on gestational age at delivery rather than birth weight. Weight based selection biases the sample toward a population with severe growth restriction at each gestational age, and placental lesions associated with poor utero-placental perfusion and the associated clinical presentations such as pre-eclampsia (Arnold et al. 1991; Evans et al. 2007; Lee et al. 2015). Distortions related to birth weight sampling had previously led to erroneous inferences about the prevalence of histological characteristics in placentas delivered much before term, overemphasizing the role of poor maternal perfusion and preeclampsia.

Across placental histology cohorts that include premature births, the rate of chorioamnionitis is high, and in studies that report a trend across gestational age, there is a shift from inflammation to lesions associated with poor maternal perfusion with increasing gestational age at delivery (Been et al. 2012; Nijman et al. 2016). However, the prevalence of inflammation and poor maternal perfusion in preterm varies considerably among cohort studies (see Table 3.1). This likely reflects both the population studied (e.g. range of gestational age range at delivery, proportion of women presenting with preterm premature rupture of membranes or cervical insufficiency, proportion of women delivered by cesarean-section), and the use of different definitions for histologic chorioamnionitis (Kim et al. 2015). For example, in the ELGAN study, maternal inflammation of the chorionic plate was present in 43%, but fetal inflammation of the cord was seen in only 19% of placentas. Among 44 placentas of infants delivered at high altitude for preterm premature rupture of membranes, acute chorioamnionitis was seen in 59% of placentas, funisitis in 30%, and chorionic plate vasculitis in 45% (Armstrong-Wells et al. 2013). Isolated funisitis occurred in only 10%. Likewise, individual morphological features of poor utero-placental perfusion including infarcts, increased syncytial knots, and abruption were each seen in about 20% of placentas in the ELGAN study, but were not always present together. Use of various combinations of these variables could also lead to discrepant reported rates of poor maternal perfusion.

Table 3.1   Selected studies reporting the prevalence of histologic chorioamnionitis

Number of placentas	Gestational age at delivery (weeks)	Histologic chorioamnionitis (%)	Maternal malperfusion (%)	References
216	23–27	27.3%	72%	(Dogan et al. 2015)
44	24–34	59%	NA	(Armstrong-Wells et al. 2013)
183	<32	44%	NA	(Been et al. 2012)
92	23–32	34%	NA	(Chau et al. 2009)
39	24–27	56%	44%	(Nijman et al. 2016)
947	23–27	43%	20%	(Hecht et al. 2008b)

Relationships between Placental Lesions and Clinical Presentation at Delivery

Placental lesions can be grouped in accordance with their associated clinical presentation at delivery. The ELGAN study initially identified six initiators of preterm delivery (preterm labor, preterm membrane rupture, placental abruption, cervical insufficiency, preeclampsia, and intrauterine growth restriction). However, factor analysis divided these into two broad groups, one with inflammatory characteristics that included preterm labor, preterm membrane rupture, placental abruption, and cervical insufficiency; and one with characteristics attributed to abnormal placentation that included preeclampsia and intrauterine growth restriction. Placental findings can sometimes provide a specific indication for delivery, such as ascending bacterial invasion (i.e. chorioamnionitis), maternal malperfusion including uteroplacental vasculopathy (e.g. pre-eclampsia), fetal vascular malperfusion (e.g. fetal thrombotic vasculopathy, cord entrapment), and abruption/hemorrhage.

Using factor analysis that incorporates placenta histology, placenta bacteriology, clinical characteristics, and newborn serum protein profiles, McElrath et al. (McElrath et al. 2008; Faupel-Badger et al. 2011) divided cases into two groups: intrauterine inflammation (preterm labor, preterm membrane rupture, placental abruption, and cervical insufficiency) and abnormal placentation (preeclampsia and intrauterine growth restriction). This pooled dichotomous approach adds power to studies of preterm risk factors and the risks associated with postnatal interventions and complications such as neonatal sepsis (Savitz, 2008). The dichotomous approach has been incorporated into the design of subsequent cohort studies (Gagliardi et al. 2013; Nijman et al. 2016).

Relationships between Placental Lesions and Recovery of Microorganisms

In the ELGAN cohort, chorioamnionitis was associated with infection, which was often polymicrobial (see Chapter 2 even among placentas delivered by cesarean-section where contamination by vaginal flora is expected to be limited (Hecht et al. 2011). Organism recovery from the placental parenchyma was most likely when the placenta showed intense inflammation, regardless of the pattern of inflammatory infiltrate (Table 3.2). This was true, even for cases with polymicrobial cultures, suggesting that the results are not merely due to vaginal contamination.

Chorioamnionitis was a frequent finding in our population. Inflammation in either the chorionic plate or the cord was found in 26% of specimens, and microorganisms were recovered from more than 67% of those cases. These rates of inflammation and microorganism recovery are comparable to, or

Table 3.2 Histologic pattern of placental inflammation in relation to microorganism recovery in the ELGAN study (cesarean-section only)

Histologic pattern of inflammation		Number of isolates		
		Single (row%)	2+ (row%)	p-value
Stage of chorionic plate inflammation	0–1	22	10	≤.001
	2–3	37	29	
Chorionic plate vasculitis	Absent	23	11	≤.001
	Present	38	31	
Umbilical cord vasculitis	Absent	23	11	≤.001
	Present	37	29	

slightly lower than, other reports about pregnancies that ended prematurely (Hillier et al. 1991; Sherman et al. 1997), but are much higher than that of term gestations when only 25% of placentas with histologic chorioamnionitis and only 17% of placentas with funisitis harbored an organism (Lee et al. 2006; Romero et al. 2016).

The histologic characteristics most strongly correlated with microorganism recovery were high-grade inflammation at the chorionic plate, vasculitis of the fetal stem vessels, as well as vasculitis of umbilical cord vessels. Inflammation of umbilical cord vessels is the histologic hallmark of a fetal inflammatory response, and associated with adverse perinatal outcome (Yoon et al. 2000; Pacora et al. 2002). Chorionic plate infiltration represents the maternal response that is linked to fetal morbidity only if it is severe (Dollner et al. 2002; Redline 2006) or accompanied by cord inflammation (Salafia et al. 1997; Pacora et al. 2002). One third of placentas that were not inflamed in ELGAN harbored a microorganism. Similar findings had been previously reported in third-trimester placentas with microorganisms recovered from 23% to 45% of placentas without inflammation (Zlatnik et al. 1990; Hillier et al. 1991).

Relationships between Placental Lesions and Post-natal Serum Concentrations of Inflammatory Markers

Among 871 ELGANS with cord blood measurements, the majority of the concentrations of 25 inflammation-related proteins were elevated in newborns whose placenta had moderate to severe inflammation (Hecht et al. 2011). The strength of the association varied by protein. For example, high-stage funisitis was associated with an odds ratio of 2.7 (99% CI: 1.4–5.3) for a top-quartile concentration of IL-6 and an odds ratio of 4.7 (99% CI: 2.4–9.2) for a top-quartile concentration of TNF-alpha.

Blood proteins showed a dose-response pattern to inflammation that was best seen with increasing stages of neutrophilic infiltration of the chorionic plate. The concentrations of inflammation-related proteins were not significantly elevated in newborns whose placenta showed evidence of under-perfusion. This is consistent with the inverse relationship between histologic features of inflammation and poor perfusion in our population (McElrath et al. 2008). The concentrations of several growth factors (IGFBP-1 and VEGF-R1) decreased with placental inflammation and increased with histologic indicators of vascular insufficiency (distal villous hypoplasia and infarcts). These proteins are often abnormally high in women who have preeclampsia, a syndrome associated with poor placental vascularization and fetal growth restriction (Levine et al. 2006; Mestan et al. 2009).

We failed to detect organisms in more than 30% of inflamed placentas (Hecht et al. 2011). However, even sterile inflammation was associated with fetal cytokine elevation (Hecht et al. 2008a). Sterile intra-amniotic inflammation accompanied by elevated fetal inflammatory proteins has been described in women with preterm labor (Romero et al. 2014; Lu et al. 2016; Gomez-Lopez et al. 2018). In amniotic fluid samples obtained from 59 women with preterm PROM, inflammation was sterile in 29% as documented by both cultivation and PCR amplification techniques (Romero et al. 2015). Sterile intra-amniotic inflammation might represent diffusion of nonviable bacterial components, which might occur following the death of bacteria induced by antibiotics given very recently.

NEUROLOGIC INJURY ASSOCIATED WITH INFLAMMATION

Inflammation in the chorionic plate was associated with ventriculomegaly when the child was in the intensive care nursery (OR=1.5, 95% CI: 1.02–2.3) and diparetic cerebral palsy at age 2 years (CP) (OR=2.3, 95% CI: 1.1–4.8) (Leviton et al. 2010). The risk of ventriculomegaly was even higher if the histologic inflammation was accompanied by a positive placental culture (OR=2.5, 95% CI: 1.1–5.7).

The association of placental inflammation with neurologic impairments has been confirmed in other large prospective cohorts with extreme prematurity (Gagliardi et al. 2013; Salas et al. 2013; Garcia-Munoz Rodrigo et al. 2014; Roescher 2014; Shevell et al. 2014; Tronnes et al. 2014; Lu et al. 2016; Maisonneuve et al. 2017). The strength of this association is likely dependent on the details of the population studied. The contribution of inflammation to brain dysfunctions/damage is often difficult to separate from the effects of prematurity or subsequent infection/interventions. Recognition of this problem apparently prompted the Quebec cerebral palsy registry study to stratify Quebec births on whether or not they were preterm. The association between chorioamnionitis and CP was seen only among children born preterm.

One conceptual issue that is not easily overcome is the difficulty separating placenta inflammation from its correlates when evaluating risks of disorders and dysfunctions that are recognized after birth. In essence, is placenta inflammation in the causal chain, or is placenta inflammation much more an indication of what more clearly contributes to organ damage/dysfunction? Are the processes that lead to placental inflammation also the processes that lead to elevated postnatal concentrations of inflammation-associated proteins (e.g. cytokines and adhesion molecules)? If elevated postnatal concentrations of cytokines and adhesion molecules provide more specific information about organ damage/dysfunction than that provided by placental inflammation, then protein concentrations are likely to compete with and replace placental inflammation in multivariate models of the risk of organ damage/dysfunction. The result is that placental inflammation will not be identified as a risk factor for organ damage/dysfunction. The ELGAN study provided some support for this (Allred et al. 2017; Leviton et al. 2018a; Leviton et al. 2018b; Leviton et al. 2018c).

The ELGAN study provided some support for another competition, this time between the two groups of 'initiators of preterm delivery', the inflammation group and the abnormal placentation group. To a large extent, all ELGANs were delivered for one or the other indication. Thus, the comparison population for the inflammation group consisted largely of children delivered for an abnormal placentation disorder (preeclampsia and intrauterine growth restriction). In the ELGAN study, children born with fetal growth restriction were at increased risk of numerous neurodevelopmental limitations (Korzeniewski et al. 2017).

Fetal stem vessel thrombosis was the placental histologic characteristic most strongly associated with the combined reading and math learning disorder, while an infarct was the placental histologic characteristic most strongly associated with a math-only learning disorder (Appendix Table 3 of Leviton et al. 2018c). As a consequence, placenta inflammation is not identified as a risk factor for many dysfunctions associated with fetal growth restriction.

Summary of What Histologic Examination of the Placenta in the ELGAN Study Added to Our Knowledge of Placenta Biology and Pathology

The ELGAN study has contributed to our understanding of the natural history and sequelae of placenta abnormalities. First, it provided information about the prevalence of inflammatory and vascular lesions in a sample defined by gestational age and not birth weight. Second, placental lesions could be grouped into two categories. The group characterized by histologic chorioamnionitis and placental microbe recovery was associated with preterm labor, prelabor premature rupture of membranes, placental abruption, and cervical insufficiency. The other, characterized by a paucity of organisms and inflammation and by the presence of histologic features of dysfunctional placentation, was associated with preeclampsia and fetal indications for delivery (largely, intrauterine growth restriction). Third, the inflammatory pattern was an (independent) risk factor for ventriculomegaly and diparetic (also known as leg-dominated) CP, providing support for the claim that antenatal inflammation contributes to the brain (structure and function) abnormalities. Fourth, the associations between histologic inflammation and other indicators/correlates of inflammation (e.g. organism recovery from placenta parenchyma, pregnancy disorders that led to preterm birth, elevated blood concentrations of inflammatory proteins shortly after birth) provided documentation of content validity of the data collected in the ELGAN study.

REFERENCES

Allred EN, Dammann O, Fichorova RN et al. (2017) Systemic inflammation during the first postnatal month and the risk of attention deficit hyperactivity disorder characteristics among 10-year-old children born extremely preterm. *J Neuroimmune Pharmacol* **12**: 531–43. doi: 10.1007/s11481-017-9742-9.

Armstrong-Wells J, Post MD, Donnelly M, Manco-Johnson MJ, Fisher BM, Winn VD (2013) Patterns of placental pathology in preterm premature rupture of membranes. *J Dev Orig Health Dis* **4**: 249–55. doi: 10.1017/S2040174413000056.

Arnold CC, Kramer MS, Hobbs CA, McLean FH, Usher RH (1991) Very low birth weight: a problematic cohort for epidemiologic studies of very small or immature neonates. *Am J Epidemiol* **134**: 604–13.

Been JV, Vanterpool SF, De Rooij JD, Rours GI et al. (2012) A clinical prediction rule for histological chorioamnionitis in preterm newborns. *PLoS One* **7**: e46217. doi: 10.1371/journal.pone.0046217.

Chau V, Poskitt KJ, McFadden DE et al. (2009) Effect of chorioamnionitis on brain development and injury in premature newborns. *Ann Neurol* **66**: 155–64. doi: 10.1002/ana.21713.

Dogan K, Salihoglu O, Sever N, Tombul T, Sari E, Yasar L (2015) Do placental histopathologic characteristics differ with gestational ages in preterm and term deliveries? *Fetal Pediatr Pathol* **34**: 365–74. doi: 10.3109/15513815.2015.1087610.

Dollner H, Vatten L, Halgunset J, Rahimipoor S, Austgulen R (2002) Histologic chorioamnionitis and umbilical serum levels of pro-inflammatory cytokines and cytokine inhibitors. *Bjog* **109**: 534–9.

Evans N, Hutchinson J, Simpson JM, Donoghue D, Darlow B, Henderson-Smart D (2007) Prenatal predictors of mortality in very preterm infants cared for in the Australian and New Zealand Neonatal Network. *Arch Dis Child Fetal Neonatal Ed* **92**: F34–40. doi: 10.1136/adc.2006.094169.

Faupel-Badger JM, Fichorova RN et al. (2011) Cluster analysis of placental inflammatory proteins can distinguish preeclampsia from preterm labor and premature membrane rupture in singleton deliveries less than 28 weeks of gestation. *Am J Reprod Immunol* **66**: 488–94. doi: 10.1111/j.1600-0897.2011.01023.x.

Gagliardi L, Rusconi F, Da Fre M et al. (2013) Pregnancy disorders leading to very preterm birth influence neonatal outcomes: results of the population-based ACTION cohort study. *Pediatr Res* **73**: 794–801. doi: 10.1038/pr.2013.52.

Garcia-Munoz Rodrigo, F, Galan Henriquez, GM, Ospina, CG. 2014. Morbidity and mortality among very-low-birth-weight infants born to mothers with clinical chorioamnionitis. *Pediatr Neonatol* **55**: 381–6. doi: 10.1016/j.pedneo.2013.12.007.

Gomez-Lopez N, Romero R, Panaitescu B et al. (2018) Inflammasome activation during spontaneous preterm labor with intra-amniotic infection or sterile intra-amniotic inflammation. *Am J Reprod Immunol* **80**: e13049. doi: 10.1111/aji.13049.

Harteman JC, Nikkels PG, Kwee A, Groenendaal F, De Vries LS (2012) Patterns of placental pathology in preterm infants with a periventricular haemorrhagic infarction: association with time of onset and clinical presentation. *Placenta* **33**: 839–44. doi: 10.1016/j.placenta.2012.06.014.

Hecht J, Onderdonk A, Delaney M et al. (2008a) Characterization of chorioamnionitis in 2nd trimester C-section placentas and correlation with microorganism recovery from subamniotic tissues. *Pediatric and Developmental Pathology* **11**: 15–22.

Hecht JL, Allred EN, Kliman HJ et al. (2008b) Histological characteristics of singleton placentas delivered before the 28th week of gestation. *Pathology* **40**: 372–6. doi: 10.1080/00313020802035865.

Hecht JL, Fichorova RN, Tang VF et al. (2011) Relationship between neonatal blood protein concentrations and placenta histologic characteristics in extremely low GA newborns. *Pediatr Res* **69**: 68–73. doi: 10.1203/PDR.0b013e3181fed334.

Hillier SL, Krohn MA, Kiviat NB, Watts DH, Eschenbach DA (1991) Microbiologic causes and neonatal outcomes associated with chorioamnion infection. *Am J Obstet Gynecol* **165**: 955–61.

Khong TY, Mooney EE, Ariel I et al. (2016) Sampling and definitions of placental lesions: Amsterdam placental workshop group consensus statement. *Arch Pathol Lab Med* **140**: 698–713. doi: 10.5858/arpa.2015-0225-CC.

Kim SY, Choi CW, Jung E et al. (2015) Neonatal morbidities associated with histologic chorioamnionitis defined based on the site and extent of inflammation in very low birth weight infants. *J Korean Med Sci* **30**: 1476–82. doi: 10.3346/jkms.2015.30.10.1476.

Korzeniewski SJ, Allred EN, Joseph RM et al. (2017) Neurodevelopment at age 10 years of children born <28 weeks with fetal growth restriction. *Pediatrics* **140**: e20170697. doi: 10.1542/peds.2017-0697.

Lee JW, VanderVeen, Allred EN, Leviton A, Dammann O (2015) Prethreshold retinopathy in premature infants with intrauterine growth restriction. *Acta Paediatr* **104**: 27–31. doi: 10.1111/apa.12799.

Lee SE, Romero R, Kim CJ, Shim SS, Yoon BH (2006) Funisitis in term pregnancy is associated with microbial invasion of the amniotic cavity and intra-amniotic inflammation. *J Matern Fetal Neonatal Med* **19**: 693–7.

Levine RJ, Lam C, Qian C et al. (2006) Soluble endoglin and other circulating antiangiogenic factors in preeclampsia. *N Engl J Med* **355**: 992–1005. doi: 10.1056/NEJMoa055352.

Leviton A, Allred EN, Kuban KC et al. (2010) Microbiologic and histologic characteristics of the extremely preterm infant's placenta predict white matter damage and later cerebral palsy. The ELGAN study. *Pediatr Res* **67**: 95–101. doi: 10.1203/PDR.0b013e3181bf5fab.

Leviton A, Dammann O, Allred EN et al. (2018a) Neonatal systemic inflammation and the risk of low scores on measures of reading and mathematics achievement at age 10 years among children born extremely preterm. *Int J Dev Neurosci* **66**: 45–53. doi: 10.1016/j.ijdevneu.2018.01.001.

Leviton A, Hooper SR, Hunter SJ et al. (2018b) Antecedents of screening positive for attention deficit hyperactivity disorder in ten-year-old children born extremely preterm. *Pediatr Neurol* **81**: 25–30. doi: 10.1016/j.pediatrneurol.2017.12.010.

Leviton A, Joseph RM, Allred EN, O'Shea TM, Kuban KKC (2018c) Antenatal and neonatal antecedents of learning limitations in 10-year old children born extremely preterm. *Early Hum Dev* **118**: 8–14. doi: 10.1016/j.earlhumdev.2018.01.020.

Lu HY, Zhang Q, Wang QX, Lu JY (2016) Contribution of histologic chorioamnionitis and fetal inflammatory response syndrome to increased risk of brain injury in infants with preterm premature rupture of membranes. *Pediatr Neurol* **61**: 94–98 e1. doi: 10.1016/j.pediatrneurol.2016.05.001.

Maisonneuve E, Ancel PY, Foix-L'Helias L, Marret S, Kayem G (2017) Impact of clinical and/or histological chorioamnionitis on neurodevelopmental outcomes in preterm infants: A literature review. *J Gynecol Obstet Hum Reprod* **46**: 307–16. doi: 10.1016/j.jogoh.2017.02.007.

Mcelrath TF, Hecht JL, Dammann O et al. (2008) Pregnancy disorders that lead to delivery before the 28th week of gestation: an epidemiologic approach to classification. *Am J Epidemiol* **168**: 980–9. doi: 10.1093/aje/kwn202.

Mestan K, Yu Y, Thorsen P et al. (2009) Cord blood biomarkers of the fetal inflammatory response. *J Matern Fetal Neonatal Med* **22**: 379–87. doi: 10.1080/14767050802609759.

Nijman TA, Van Vliet EO, Benders MJ et al. (2016) Placental histology in spontaneous and indicated preterm birth: A case control study. *Placenta* **48**: 56–62. doi: 10.1016/j.placenta.2016.10.006.

O'Shea TM, Allred EN, Dammann O et al. (2009) The ELGAN study of the brain and related disorders in extremely low gestational age newborns. *Early Hum Dev* **85**: 719–25. doi: 10.1016/j.earlhumdev.2009.08.060.

Pacora P, Chaiworapongsa T, Maymon E et al. (2002) Funisitis and chorionic vasculitis: the histological counterpart of the fetal inflammatory response syndrome. *J Matern Fetal Neonatal Med* **11**: 18–25.

Pietrasanta C, Pugni L, Merlo D et al. (2019) Impact of different stages of intrauterine inflammation on outcome of preterm neonates: gestational age-dependent and -independent effect. *PLoS One* **14**: e0211484. doi: 10.1371/journal.pone.0211484.

Ream MA, Lehwald L (2018) Neurologic consequences of preterm birth. *Curr Neurol Neurosci Rep* **18**: 48. doi: 10.1007/s11910-018-0862-2.

Redline RW (2006) Inflammatory responses in the placenta and umbilical cord. *Semin Fetal Neonatal Med* **11**: 296–301.

Roescher A (2014) *Placental Lesions and Outcome in Preterm Born Children: The Relation Between Placental Lesions, Neonatal Morbidity and Neurological Development*, chapter 5. Doctor of Philosophy, University of Groningen.

Romero R, Chaemsaithong P, Docheva N et al. (2016) Clinical chorioamnionitis at term VI: acute chorioamnionitis and funisitis according to the presence or absence of microorganisms and inflammation in the amniotic cavity. *J Perinat Med* **44**: 33–51. doi: 10.1515/jpm-2015-0119.

Romero R, Miranda J, Chaemsaithong P et al. (2015) Sterile and microbial-associated intra-amniotic inflammation in preterm prelabor rupture of membranes. *J Matern Fetal Neonatal Med* **28**: 1394–409. doi: 10.3109/14767058.2014.958463.

Romero R, Miranda J, Chaiworapongsa T et al. (2014) Prevalence and clinical significance of sterile intra-amniotic inflammation in patients with preterm labor and intact membranes. *Am J Reprod Immunol* **72**: 458–74. doi: 10.1111/aji.12296.

Salafia CM, Sherer DM, Spong CY et al. (1997) Fetal but not maternal serum cytokine levels correlate with histo-logic acute placental inflammation. *Am J Perinatol* **14**: 419–22.

Salas AA, Faye-Petersen OM, Sims B et al. (2013) Histological characteristics of the fetal inflammatory response associated with neurodevelopmental impairment and death in extremely preterm infants. *J Pediatr* **163**: 652–7; e1–2. doi: 10.1016/j.jpeds.2013.03.081.

Savitz DA (2008) Invited commentary: disaggregating preterm birth to determine etiology. *Am J Epidemiol* **168**: 990–2; discussion 993–4. doi: 10.1093/aje/kwn193.

Sherman DJ, Tovbin J, Lazarovich T et al. (1997) Chorioamnionitis caused by gram-negative bacteria as an etiologic factor in preterm birth. *Eur J Clin Microbiol Infect Dis* **16**: 417–23.

Shevell A, Wintermark P, Benini R, Shevell M, Oskoui M (2014) Chorioamnionitis and cerebral palsy: lessons from a patient registry. *Eur J Paediatr Neurol* **18**: 301–7. doi: 10.1016/j.ejpn.2013.12.005.

Stoll BJ, Hansen NI, Adams-Chapman I et al. (2004) Neurodevelopmental and growth impairment among extremely low-birth-weight infants with neonatal infection. *Jama* **292**: 2357–65.

Tronnes H, Wilcox AJ, Lie RT, Markestad T, Moster D (2014) Risk of cerebral palsy in relation to pregnancy disorders and preterm birth: a national cohort study. *Dev Med Child Neurol* **56**: 779–85. doi: 10.1111/dmcn.12430.

Yoon BH, Romero R, Park JS et al. (2000) The relationship among inflammatory lesions of the umbilical cord (funisitis), umbilical cord plasma interleukin 6 concentration, amniotic fluid infection, and neonatal sepsis. *Am J Obstet Gynecol* **183**: 1124–9.

Zlatnik FJ, Gellhaus TM, Benda JA, Koontz FP, Burmeister LF (1990) Histologic chorioamnionitis, microbial infection, and prematurity. *Obstet Gynecol* **76**: 355–9.

Signal Initiators of Early Preterm Birth

Asha N Talati and Tracy A Manuck

INTRODUCTION

Preterm birth accounts for more than 75% of perinatal mortality and greater than 50% of newborn morbidity, such as prolonged hospitalization and development of long-term respiratory disease (Goldenberg et al. 2008). The underlying etiologies of births at such early gestational ages are multifold, as there is a spectrum of disorders and dysfunctions leading to preterm birth (Esplin 2016) that are likely distinct from births at later gestational ages (Manuck et al. 2015).

In this chapter, first we identify the potential initiators of preterm birth at extremely low gestational ages and provide an overview of pregnancy disorders that lead to parturition <28 weeks. Second, we will review the roles of inflammation, uteroplacental ischemia, decidual hemorrhage, stress, and infection as potential catalysts for the labor cascade. Third, we will briefly discuss the associations between intrauterine pathology and early newborn outcomes. In doing so, we show how the ELGAN study has added to our understanding. Finally, we identify areas of future research regarding the initiation of preterm birth.

PREGNANCY DISORDERS IMPLICATED IN THE INITIATION OF PRETERM BIRTH

The disorders that lead to preterm birth have traditionally been sorted into two broad categories: *spontaneous* and *indicated* preterm birth. *Spontaneous* preterm births are deliveries occurring following the spontaneous onset of uterine contractions, preterm prelabor rupture of membranes, or cervical insufficiency. In contrast, *indicated* preterm births are a consequence of maternal or fetal disease necessitating early delivery (e.g. pre-eclampsia, intrauterine growth restriction) (Iams et al. 2012).

The ELGAN study took a fresh look at how the disorders leading to extremely preterm birth sorted out. Clinical, placental histologic, and microbiologic characteristics of 1006 maternal and newborn dyads enrolled in the ELGAN study were evaluated to see what clustered (McElrath et al. 2008). Preterm labor, preterm prelabor rupture of membranes, cervical insufficiency, and placental abruption were most frequently associated with histologic chorioamnionitis and placental microbe recovery; or, more broadly, intrauterine inflammation. In contrast, pre-eclampsia and intrauterine growth restriction were rarely associated with infection and signs of inflammation. Instead, both pre-eclampsia and intrauterine growth restriction were associated with infarcts and an abundance of syncytial knots in the placenta (McElrath et al. 2008).

Findings from 947 singleton placentas further support the distinction between 'inflammatory' and 'placental dysfunction' phenotypes of women who deliver <28 weeks gestation. Lesions attributed to poor uteroplacental circulation, such as abruption, infarction, thrombosis, perivillous fibrin deposition, and increased syncytial knots were inversely related to the presence of inflammation in the membranes or the cord (Hecht et al. 2008). Compared to the infant whose placenta had histologic characteristics associated with placental dysfunction, the infant whose placenta was inflamed was born at an earlier gestational age. The clustering of such disorders suggests that very early preterm birth generally falls into two phenotypes: 'inflammatory' and 'placental dysfunction' (McElrath et al. 2008).

PREGNANCY DISORDERS ASSOCIATED WITH INTRAUTERINE INFLAMMATION

Inflammatory disorders leading to early preterm birth, such as preterm labor, preterm prelabor rupture of membranes (pPROM), cervical insufficiency, and placental abruption are associated with placental evidence of infection and inflammation and a notable absence of indicators of impaired placentation (McElrath et al. 2008). Several theories regarding the pathophysiology of inflammation as a central causal pathway to preterm parturition exist. We will briefly review current evidence about how inflammation may impact the effects of progesterone on the uterus, cervical remodeling, and serve as a signal initiator for the complex neuronal, hormonal, and immune pathways that modulate birth.

Though the precise events leading to the initiation of spontaneous preterm birth are incompletely understood, current theories about labor initiation center on what causes uterine quiescence and how that is altered. Specifically, triggers (environmental, genetic, intrauterine, etc.) can lead to a cascade of cervical remodeling, myometrial change, and, eventually, a functional progesterone withdrawal that contributes to the onset of labor (Talati et al. 2017). Conditions associated with spontaneous preterm delivery <28 weeks are often associated with maternal risk factors such as race, socio-economic status, smoking, or intra-uterine events such as over-distention (e.g. polyhydramnios, multiple gestations), decidual hemorrhage, or infection (Muglia and Katz 2010). Histologic evidence of inflammation and culture proven infection is commonly seen in cases of spontaneous preterm birth, and is found in nearly 50% of deliveries <30 weeks (Esplin 2014). Whether or not this inflammation occurs as an inciting event leading to spontaneous preterm delivery or develops after the preterm birth cascade has begun is difficult to determine. Preterm intrauterine colonization likely initiates an inflammatory cascade similar to what a parturient may experience at term: a release of cytokines and chemokines that promotes tissue level inflammation and ultimately triggers the signaling cascade involved in initiating labor (Menon et al. 2016). Data from the ELGAN cohort support a high rate of intrauterine inflammation in cases of spontaneous preterm birth. Fully two-thirds (333/489) of patients with preterm vaginal birth at 23–27 weeks had evidence of placental microbial invasion (Onderdonk et al. 2008). By contrast, histologic evidence of chorioamnionitis is present in only 16% of placentas delivered at or after 34 weeks' gestation (Lahra and Jeffery, 2004).

Although inflammation remains a prominent pathway of extremely preterm labor initiation, it would be overly simplistic to say it is the primary driver of the process; instead, it is likely a complex interplay of neuronal, hormonal, and immune pathways that together initiate preterm and term birth (Vannuccini et al. 2016). Clinical or histologic bleeding events, such as abruption, may also signal an inflammatory event and increase the risk of preterm birth. Intrauterine bleeding may lead to initiation of the coagulation cascade and thrombin activation. Thrombin activation may promote cytokine (e.g. inter-leukin-8) and matrix-metalloproteinase 9 (MMP-9) expression in the decidua (Lockwood et al. 2005; Stephenson et al. 2005). Together, these changes may increase the overall intrauterine inflammatory load, weaken the fetal membranes, and potentiate progesterone withdrawal (Elovitz et al. 2001; Rosen et al. 2001; Vidaeff et al. 2012). The ELGAN cohort exemplifies the complexity of extremely preterm labor initiation, demonstrating that multiple pathways may lead to preterm birth. However, further studies are necessary to better elucidate the exact mechanisms by which bleeding events are associated with the initiation of spontaneous preterm birth.

The complex maternal-fetal signaling cascade that begins parturition at term is suspected to involve multiple processes, including cortisol and prostaglandin up-regulation and a functional progesterone withdrawal (Menon et al. 2016). However, the effects of steroid hormones on cervical remodeling and myometrial alterations related to preterm birth need further study. Several models have suggested that maternal stressors leading to excess cortisol release lead to up-regulation of pro-inflammatory cytokines that may trigger the common pathway of preterm birth (Mesiano and Welsh 2007). In an assessment of this concept among deliveries <28 weeks, the ELGAN group demonstrated that inflammation itself *without* adrenal activation is an antecedent of preterm delivery for spontaneous indications (Trivedia et al. 2012). Placental CRH expression was significantly elevated among deliveries stemming from placental dysfunction phenotypes of preterm birth when compared to spontaneous phenotypes. The authors concluded that among infants delivered at less than 28 weeks' gestation, delivery for medical indications was associated with more placental corticotropin-releasing hormone expression and less frequent placental inflammation and infection than spontaneous delivery. The relationship between CRH expression and indicated preterm birth requires further elucidation, as CRH expression may be up-regulated by the processes associated with pre-eclampsia and severe fetal growth restriction instead of driving the latter pathologies.

To summarize, preterm labor, pPROM, cervical insufficiency, and placental abruption are pregnancy disorders associated with inflammation and infection (McElrath et al. 2008). Findings from the ELGAN cohort highlight the role of inflammation as a signal initiator of the complex maternal-fetal signaling cascade that leads to the downstream consequence of very early preterm birth. Current evidence has focused on the role of inflammation in progesterone withdrawal, and myometrial and cervical remodeling. Yet, significant further study is necessary to assess the exact mechanisms by which inflammation initiates and potentiates preterm birth in the setting of individual inflammatory preterm birth phenotypes.

PREGNANCY DISORDERS ASSOCIATED WITH PLACENTAL INSUFFICIENCY

Placental insufficiency, defined as a deficiency of nutrient delivery to the fetus due to utero-placental under-perfusion, is an infrequent underlying cause of early preterm birth (McElrath et al. 2008; Morgan, 2016). In this section, we review pregnancy manifestations of suspected placental insufficiency, current knowledge of extreme preterm birth due to placental dysfunction, and what the ELGAN study contributes to our current fund of knowledge regarding these disorders.

Placental insufficiency may result in a number of pregnancy manifestations, including IUGR, Doppler abnormalities of placental blood flow, oligohydramnios, and non-reassuring fetal heart patterns (McElrath et al. 2008). The ELGAN cohort found that pre-eclampsia and intrauterine growth restriction (IUGR), have common placental characteristics including infarcts, an increase in the presence of syncytial knots, and the absence of inflammation (McElrath et al. 2008). Recent data, however, more finely differentiate findings associated with fetal growth restriction from those associated with pre-eclampsia. Placental infarction, syncytial knots, and low placental weight are commonly associated with fetal growth restriction while accelerated villous maturation has been associated with pre-eclampsia and idiopathic preterm birth (Morgan 2016).

The impact of placental insufficiency and subsequent poor nutrient transfer on early life is of significant interest for the ELGAN. Prior literature has demonstrated that preterm newborns with IUGR are more likely to have low concentrations of angiogenic proteins, inflammatory proteins, neurotrophic factors, and growth factors compared to their appropriate for gestational age equivalents (Abd Ellah et al. 2015). Growth factors and neurotrophic factors promote neonatal, brain, and overall growth, suggesting that newborns with a paucity of these factors may be at risk for long-term growth anomalies (Reichardt 2006). Animal models and underpowered studies of humans suggest that neurophic factors are present at lower concentrations in premature newborns with placental dysfunction than in newborns delivered because of an inflammatory pregnancy disorder (Indo 2014). Similarly, concentrations of inflammatory proteins are also lower in premature newborns with placental dysfunction than in newborns delivered because of an inflammatory pregnancy disorder (Keelan and Mitchell 2007; Stephanova et al. 2013). However, such studies had multiple, various limitations. Thus, little was known about how these factors vary in concentration during the neonatal period and how antecedent pregnancy conditions may impact their presence. Further, the association between these factors and neonatal growth and development was not previously explored. The ELGAN cohort provided understanding to these unanswered questions and furthered our understanding, allowing us to postulate how intrauterine events with comorbid extreme prematurity impact neonatal health.

The ELGAN study found that newborns with growth restriction, pre-eclampsia, or fetal indicated delivery had lower concentrations of angiogenic proteins, than newborns delivered for other reasons. These lower concentrations were seen not only low at birth, but also one month later (Leviton et al. 2017a). By contrast, newborns delivered because of an inflammatory pregnancy disorder tended to have elevated concentrations of both inflammatory proteins and neurotrophic growth factors, suggesting a common pathway contributing to persistent elevation of both factors (Leviton et al. 2017b). Insulin-like growth factor-1 (IGF-1) and insulin like growth factor binding protein-1 (IGFBP-1) concentrations were also low among ELGANs who had low levels of inflammatory, neurotrophic, and angiogenic factors and were more likely to be delivered in the setting of suspected placental insufficiency (Leviton et al. 2019). Surprisingly, IUGR newborns were significantly more likely than others to have elevated inflammatory proteins on day of life 14, even after adjusting for delivery indication, bacteremia, and duration of ventilation (McElrath et al. 2013). The exact etiology of rise in protein concentration is unclear, but may be related to the increased morbidity faced by IUGR ELGANs (especially bronchopulmonary dysplasia/chronic lung disease) (Bose et al. 2009).

In summary, placental insufficiency phenotypes such as pre-eclampsia and fetal growth restriction are a significant cause of early preterm birth. The distinct changes to placental fetal circulation associated with these pregnancy disorders ultimately lead to a paucity of neurotrophic and growth-factor proteins. Although such findings have been associated with aberrations of fetal and childhood growth, the exact mechanisms by which placental insufficiency leads to particular fetal adaptations and eventually influences postnatal development require further investigation.

DEVELOPMENTAL CORRELATES OF MATERNAL PREGNANCY DISORDERS

The longitudinal design of the ELGAN study provided an opportunity to correlate maternal disease processes with short and long term outcomes of the ELGANs. Fetuses delivered to mothers with pre-eclampsia or delivered secondary to a fetal indication (e.g. IUGR, non-reassuring status) had a higher mortality rate than a fetus delivered in the setting of an inflammatory pregnancy disorder (McElrath et al. 2008).

The ELGAN study elucidates how the neonatal inflammatory response varies in accordance with antecedent pregnancy disorder, suggesting it is a continuation of fetal events. Infants born spontaneously were more likely than others to have top-quartile concentrations of 25 inflammatory cytokines, chemokines, adhesion molecules, and metalloproteinases on the day of delivery (McElrath et al. 2011). Infants whose placenta had funisitis were more likely than others to have elevated levels of such inflammatory proteins as CRP, MPO, IL1B, IL8, TNF-alpha, ICAM3, and matrix metallopeptidase-9 (MMP9) at the end of the first postnatal week (Leviton et al. 2011b). Similarly, newborns whose placentas had acute inflammatory lesions were more likely than their peers to have elevated blood concentrations of inflammatory cytokines, chemokines, adhesion molecules, matrix metalloproteinases, and angiogenic factors within the first week of life. Further, placental histology characteristics associated with poor perfusion or placentation were associated with significantly lower levels of inflammatory proteins in newborn blood (Hecht et al. 2011). This was in keeping with lower concentrations of inflammatory proteins amongst newborns in the ELGAN cohort delivered for maternal or fetal indications (McElrath et al. 2011).

Heritable changes that do not affect the DNA sequence but alter gene expression are called epimutations. Pre-eclampsia appears to contribute to the development of functional epimutations, specifically in the TGF-B pathway (Martin et al. 2015; Peixoto et al. 2018). In the ELGAN study population, 10% of newborns with IUGR, delivered for pre-eclampsia, or whose placenta had an infarction had microcephaly, instead of the 2% expected from prior literature (McElrath et al. 2010). Moreover, this relationship persisted at 24 months post-delivery (Leviton et al. 2010). Two-year-olds whose placenta had thrombosis of fetal vessels, and those who had severe fetal growth restriction, were at increased risk of low Mental Development Index (MDI) scores (Helderman et al. 2011; Streimish et al. 2012).

Exposure to intrauterine and immediate newborn stressors has been linked to epigenetic modifications that may affect the developmental trajectories of preterm infants (Provenzi et al. 2018). Data from the ELGAN cohort support the developmental origins of health and disease theory. Genome-wide DNA methylation analysis of 84 placentas from the ELGAN study cohort found genetic alterations in the NF-kB inflammatory response pathway associated with the presence of placental micro-organisms. Specifically, the presence of *Streptococcus* sp. likely leads to hypomethylation of CpG sites and subsequent up-regulation of genes of the NF-kB pathway (Tomlinson et al. 2017). A similar analysis of CpG methylation in ELGAN study placentas demonstrated hypermethylation of genes encoding for critical neuro-developmental proteins (Meakin et al. 2018; Tilley et al. 2018). The epigenetic changes were predictive of moderate to severe cognitive impairment at 10 years of age. Similar findings have been reported in other studies of extreme prematurity (Provenzi et al. 2018).

Data from the ELGAN cohort suggest that fetal exposure to intra-uterine stressors may play a large role in complications previously only associated with prematurity. Maternal pregnancy disorders have been associated with each of the following disorders and limitations: bronchopulmonary dysplasia (Bose et al. 2011), chronic lung disease (Bose et al. 2009), retinopathy of prematurity (Lee et al. 2015; Holm et al. 2017), strabismus (VanderVeen et al. 2016), low intelligence (O'Shea et al. 2012; Leviton et al. 2013; O'Shea et al. 2013; Kuban et al. 2017), cerebral palsy (Kuban et al. 2014), executive dysfunctions (Leviton et al. 2018b), learning disorders (Leviton et al. 2018a), attention-deficit disorder (O'Shea et al. 2014; Allred et al. 2017), autism spectrum disorders and impaired social awareness and its correlates) (Korzeniewski et al. 2018).

SUMMARY

'Inflammation-associated' pregnancy disorders such as preterm labor, pPROM, cervical insufficiency, and abruption are often associated with documented intra-uterine infection or maternal systemic inflammation, thereby leading to placental and fetal inflammatory changes. In the context of existing literature, this may lead to an inflammatory cascade that signals a functional progesterone withdrawal and parturition. By contrast, 'placental dysfunction' disorders, such as intra-uterine growth restriction or pre-eclampsia, lead to preterm birth using different mechanisms, with documented lower rates of maternal, placental, or newborn inflammatory proteins. However, the exact pathways of preterm birth remain yet to be elucidated and are likely a complex myriad of neuronal, hormonal, and inflammatory mediators that initiate parturition.

CONCLUSIONS

Future study of the initiators of preterm birth <28 weeks should build upon the data gathered from the ELGAN cohort to better understand the mechanisms by which they lead to the final pathway of parturition. In turn, we hope this would allow identification of pregnant women at risk of delivery much before term and create targeted therapies aimed at the antecedent condition itself, or the processes that lead to delivery.

REFERENCES

Abd Ellah N, Taylor L, Troja W et al. (2015) Development of non-viral trophoblast-specific gene delivery for placental therapy. *PLos One* **10**: e0140878.

Allred EN, Dammann O, Fichorova RN et al. (2017) Systemic inflammation during the first postnatal month and the risk of attention deficit hyperactivity disorder characteristics among 10-year-old children born extremely preterm. *Journal of Neuroimmune Pharmacology* **12**: 531–43.

Bose C, Laughon M, Allred EN et al. (2011) Blood protein concentrations in the first two postnatal weeks that predict bronchopulmonary dysplasia among infants born before the 28th week of gestation. *Pediatr Res* **69**: 347–53.

Bose C, Van Marter LJ, Laughon M et al. (2009) Fetal growth restriction and chronic lung disease among infants born before the 28th week of gestation. *Pediatrics* **124**: e450–8.

Elovitz MA, Baron J, Phillippe M (2001) The role of thrombin in preterm parturition. *American J Obstet and Gynecol* **185**: 1059–63.

Esplin M (2016) The importance of clinical phenotype in understanding and preventing spontaneous preterm birth. *American Journal of Perinatology* **33**: 236–44.

Esplin MS (2014) Overview of spontaneous preterm birth: a complex and multifactorial phenotype. *Clin Obstet Gynecol* **57**: 518–30.

Goldenberg RL, Culhane JF, Iams JD, Romero R (2008) Epidemiology and causes of preterm birth. *The Lancet* **371**: 75–84.

Hecht JL, Allred EN, Kliman HJ et al. (2008) Histological characteristics of singleton placentas delivered before the 28th week of gestation. *Pathology* **40**: 372–6.

Hecht JL, Fichorova RN, Tang VF et al. (2011) The relationship between neonatal blood protein profiles and placenta histologic characteristics in extremely low gestation age newborns. *Pediatr Res* **69**: 68–73.

Helderman JB, O'Shea TM, Kuban KC et al. (2012) Antenatal antecedents of cognitive impairment at 24 months in extremely low gestational age newborns. *Pediatrics* **129**: 494–502.

Holm M, Morken TS, Fichorova RN et al. (2017) Systemic inflammation-associated proteins and retinopathy of prematurity in infants born before the 28th week of gestation. *Investigative Ophthalmology and Visual Science* **58**: 6419–28.

Iams J, Dildy G, Macones G, Silverman N (2012) Prediction and prevention of preterm birth. Practice Bulletin No. 130. American College of Obstetricians and Gynecologists. *Obstet Gynecol* **120**: 964–73.

Indo Y (2014) Neurobiology of pain, interoception, and emotional response: lessons from nerve growth factor-dependent neurons. *Eur J Neurosci* **39**: 375–91.

Keelan J (2007) Placental cytokines and preeclampsia. *Front Biosci* **12**: 2706–27.

Korzeniewski SJ, Allred EN, O'Shea TM et al. (2018) Elevated protein concentrations in newborn blood and the risks of autism spectrum disorder, and of social impairment, at age 10 years among infants born before the 28th week of gestation. *Translational psychiatry* **8**: 115.

Kuban KC, Joseph RM, O'Shea TM et al. (2017) Circulating inflammatory-associated proteins in the first month of life and cognitive impairment at age 10 years in children born extremely preterm. *J Pediatr* **180**: 116–23; e1.

Kuban KCK, O'Shea TM, Allred EN (2014) Systemic inflammation and cerebral palsy risk in extremely preterm infants. *J Child Neurol* **29**: 1692–8.

Lahra MM, Jeffery HE (2004) A fetal response to chorioamnionitis is associated with early survival after preterm birth. *Am J Obstet Gynecol* **190**: 147–51.

Lee JW, VanderVeen D, Allred EN et al. (2015) Prethreshold retinopathy in premature infants with intrauterine growth restriction. *Acta Paediatr* **104**: 27–31.

Leviton A, Allred EN, Fichorova RN et al. (2019) Relationships with indicators of placental insufficiency and with systemic inflammation. *Am J Perinatol* [Epub ahead of print].

Leviton A, Allred EN, Kuban KCK et al. (2011) Blood protein concentrations in the first two postnatal weeks associated with early postnatal blood gas derangements among infants born before the 28th week of gestation. The ELGAN study. *Cytokine* **56**: 392–8.

Leviton A, Allred EN, Yamamoto H et al. (2017) Antecedents and correlates of blood concentrations of neurotrophic growth factors in very preterm newborns. *Cytokine* **94**: 21–8.

Leviton A, Dammann O, Allred EN et al. (2018) Neonatal systemic inflammation and the risk of low scores on measures of reading and mathematics achievement at age 10 years among children born extremely preterm. *Int J Dev Neurosci* **66**: 45–53.

Leviton A, Hecht JL, Allred EN et al. (2011) Persistence after birth of systemic inflammation associated with umbilical cord inflammation. *Journal of Reproductive Immunology* **90**: 235–43.

Leviton A, Fichorova RN, O'Shea TM et al. (2013) Two-hit model of brain damage in the very preterm newborn: small for gestational age and postnatal systemic inflammation. *Pediatr Res* **73**: 362–70.

Leviton A, Joseph RM, Fichorova RN et al. (2018) Executive dysfunction early postnatal biomarkers among children born extremely preterm. *Journal of Neuroimmune Pharmacology* [Epublication].

Leviton A, Kuban K, Allred EN et al. (2010) Antenatal antecedents of a small head circumference at age 24-months post-term equivalent in a sample of infants born before the 28th post-menstrual week. *Early Hum Dev* **86**: 515–21.

Leviton A, Ryan S, Allred EN et al. (2017) Antecedents and early correlates of high and low concentrations of angiogenic proteins in extremely preterm newborns. *Clin Chim Acta* **471**: 1–5.

Lockwood CJ, Toti P, Arcuri F et al. (2005) Mechanisms of abruption-induced premature rupture of the fetal membranes: thrombin-enhanced interleukin-8 expression in term decidua. *The American Journal of Pathology* **167**: 1443–9.

Martin E, Ray PD, Smeester L et al. (2015) Epigenetics and preeclampsia: defining functional epimutations in the preeclamptic placenta related to the TGF-B pathway. *PLoS One* **10**: e0141294.

Manuck TA, Esplin M, Biggio J et al. (2015) The phenotype of spontaneous preterm birth: application of a clinical phenotyping tool. *Am J Obstet Gynecol* **212**: 487.e1–487.e11.

McElrath TF, Allred EN, Kuban K et al. (2010) Factors associated with small head circumference at birth among infants borth before the 28th week. *Am J Obstet Gynecol* **203**: 138e1–8.

McElrath TF, Allred EN, Van Marter L et al. (2013) Perinatal systemic inflammatory responses of growth-restricted preterm newborns. *Acta Paediatr* **102**: e439–42.

McElrath TF, Fichorova RN, Allred EN et al. (2011) Blood protein profiles of infants born before 28 weeks differ by pregnancy complication. *Am J Obstet Gynecol* **204**: 418.e1–418.e12.

McElrath TF, Hecht J, Dammann O et al. (2008) Pregnancy disorders that lead to delivery before the 28th week of gestation: An epidemiologic approach to classification. *American Journal of Epidemiology* **168**: 980–9.

Menon R, Bonney E, Condon J et al. (2016) Novel concepts on pregnancy clocks and alarms: redundancy and synergy in human parturition. *Human Reproduction Update* **22**: 535–60.

Meakin CJ, Martin EM, Santos HP Jr, et al. (2018) Placental CpG methylation of HPA-axis genes is associated with cognitive impairment at age 10 among children born extremely preterm. *Horm Behav* **101**: 29–35. doi:10.1016/j.yhbeh.2018.02.007.

Mesiano S, Welsh TN (2007) Steroid hormone control of myometrial contractility and parturition. *Seminars in Cell & Developmental Biology* **18**: 321–31.

Morgan TK (2016) Role of the placenta in preterm birth: a review. *Am J Perinatol* **33**: 258–66.

Muglia LJ, Katz M (2010) The enigma of spontaneous preterm birth. *The New England Journal of Medicine* **362**: 529–35.

Onderdonk AB, Delaney M, DuBoi A et al. (2008) Detection of bacteria in placental tissues obtained from extremely low gestational age neonates. *Am J Obstet Gynecol* **198**: 110.e1–110.e7.

O'Shea TM, Allred EN, Kuban KC et al. (2012) Elevated concentrations of inflammation-related proteins in postnatal blood predict severe developmental delay at 2 years of age in extremely preterm infants. *J Pediatr* **160**: 395–401; e4.

O'Shea TM, Joseph RM, Kuban KC et al. (2014) Elevated blood levels of inflammation-related proteins are associated with an attention problem at age 24 mo in extremely preterm infants. *Pediatr Res* **75**: 781–7.

O'Shea TM, Shah B, Allred EN et al. (2013) Inflammation-initiating illnesses, inflammation-related proteins, and cognitive impairment in extremely preterm infants. *Brain Behav Immun* **29**: 104–12.

Peixoto AB, Rolo LC, Nardozz LM et al. (2018) Epigenetics and preeclampsia: programming of future outcomes. *Methods Mol Biol* **1710**: 73–83.

Provenzi L, Guida E, Montirosso R (2018) Preterm behavioral epigenetics: a systematic review. *Neurosci Biobehav Rev* **84**: 262–71.

Reichardt LF (2006) Neurotrophin-regulated signalling pathways. *Philos Trans R Soc Lond B Biol Sci* **361**: 1545–64.

Rosen T, Kuczynski E, O'Neill LM (2001) Plasma levels of thrombin-antithrombin complexes predict preterm premature rupture of the fetal membranes. *The Journal of Maternal-fetal Medicine* **10**: 297–300.

Streimish IG, Ehrenkranz RA, Allred EN et al. (2012) Birth weight and fetal weight-growth restriction: impact on neurodevelopment. *Early Hum Dev* **88**: 765–71.

Stephanova OI, Safronova NU, Furaeva KN et al. (2013) Effects of placental secretory factors on cytokine production by endothelial cells. *Bull Exp Biol Med* **154**: 375–8.

Stephenson CD, Lockwood C, Ma Y et al. (2005) Thrombin-dependent regulation of matrix metalloproteinase (MMP)-9 levels in human fetal membranes. *J Maternal-fetal & Neonatal Medicine* **18**: 7–22.

Talati AN, Hackney DN, Mesiano S (2017) Pathophysiology of preterm labor with intact membranes *Semin Perinatol* **41**: 420–6.

Tilley SK, Martin EM, Smeester L, Joseph RM, Kuban KCK, Heeren TC, et al. (2018) Placental CpG methylation of infants born extremely preterm predicts cognitive impairment later in life. *PLoS ONE* **13(3)**: e0193271.

Tomlinson MS, Bommarito PA, Martin EM, Smeester L, Fichorova RN, Onderdonk AB, et al. (2017) Microorganisms in the human placenta are associated with altered CpG methylation of immune and inflammation-related genes. *PLoS ONE* **12(12)**: e0188664.

Trivedia S, Joachim M, McElrath T et al. (2012) Fetal-placental inflammation, but not adrenal activation, is associated with extreme preterm delivery. *Am J Obstet Gynecol* **206**: 236e1–236e8.

VanderVeen DK, Allred EN, Wallace DK et al. (2016) Strabismus at age 2 years in children born before 28 weeks' gestation: antecedents and correlates. *J Child Neurol* **31**: 451–60.

Vannuccini S, Bocchi C, Severi FM et al. (2016) Endocrinology of human parturition. Ann Endocrinol **77**: 105–13.

Vidaeff AC, Monga M, Saade G et al. (2012) Prospective investigation of second-trimester thrombin activation and preterm birth. *Am J Obstet Gynecol* **206**: 333.e1–6.

Maternal Adiposity

Jelske W van der Burg and Elizabeth T Jensen

EPIDEMIOLOGY OF MATERNAL ADIPOSITY

Despite being classified as a medical condition by the World Health Organization (WHO) in 1997 (World Health Organization 2000), obesity among men and women in many countries continues to increase in prevalence (Abarca-Gómez et al. 2017). In 2016, worldwide, an estimated 39% of adults aged 18 years and older were overweight, and 13% were obese (World Health Organization 2018). Thus, more than 1.9 billion adults, 18 years and older, were overweight. Of these, over 650 million were obese in 2016. Prevalence rates ≥30% were observed in North Africa, the Middle East, and North America (World Health Organization 2018).

In 1979, the United States Department of Health and Human Services began the 'Healthy People' initiative. It includes a set of comprehensive 10-year goals and objectives to promote health and prevent disease in the United States. For 2020, the Healthy People initiative has the goal that at least 59% of women experiencing pregnancy will have a normal (body mass index [BMI] of 18.5 to 24.9 kg/m^2) pre-pregnancy weight (Healthy People Gov. 2010). Despite efforts to meet this objective, the prevalence of pre-pregnancy normal weight has decreased from 53% in 2007 to 45% in 2015 (Healthy People Gov. 2010; Deputy et al. 2018). Concomitant with this decline in pre-pregnancy normal weight, the entire BMI distribution shifted toward a higher BMI, leading to an increase in the prevalence of pre-pregnancy overweight and obesity (Deputy et al. 2018). Almost 26% of women were overweight and 26% were obese prior to their pregnancy in 2015 (Deputy et al. 2018). The proportion of all women who are overweight or obese has increased primarily due to an increase in the proportion of pregnant women who are obese (BMI ≥ 30.0 kg/m^2) (Kim et al. 2007; Flegal et al. 2016; Deputy et al. 2018), with excess weight gain during pregnancy a contributing factor (Siega-Riz and Gray 2013; Lindberg et al. 2016).

In Europe, many countries do not systematically report overweight and obesity rates in their pregnant population. However, the prevalence of maternal obesity is estimated to vary from 7% to 25% in European countries (Devlieger et al. 2016). Maternal obesity is not limited to developed countries. A meta-analysis reported that the prevalence of maternal obesity in Africa ranges from 6.5% to 50.7% (Onubi et al. 2016). This high prevalence of maternal adiposity in developed as well as developing countries has implications for the health of future generations.

CONSEQUENCES OF MATERNAL ADIPOSITY

The consequences of overweight or obesity in pregnancy for the mother are well documented and are associated with an increased risk of both short-term and long-term complications for mothers including miscarriage, preeclampsia, dysfunctional labor, wound infection, and gestational diabetes

(O'Brien et al. 2003; Heslehurst et al. 2008; Stothard et al. 2009; Huda et al. 2010; Metwally et al. 2008). Compared with a normal BMI, obesity in pregnancy is associated with higher rates of cesarean section (Marchi et al. 2015; Abenhaim and Benjamin 2011). Regardless of parity, obese women are twice as likely to have a cesarean section as women of normal weight (Pettersen-Dahl et al. 2018). Obesity is also associated with labor dysfunction, in particular decreased uterine contractility, slower progress of cervical dilation, and longer duration of labor (Ehrenberg et al. 2004; Carlson et al. 2015; Lawn et al. 2016). With increasing prevalence in women of childbearing age, overweight and obesity have become among the most common risk factors in obstetric practice, and among the most important challenges in obstetric care.

The consequences of maternal adiposity are not limited to adverse outcomes experienced by the mother. Adverse health outcomes are also noted in the offspring of obese women, including increased risk for congenital anomalies, stillbirth, neonatal death (Heslehurst et al. 2008; Stothard et al. 2009) and adverse neurodevelopmental outcomes (Van Lieshout et al. 2011; Mehta et al. 2014; Van Der Burg et al. 2015; Godfrey et al. 2017; Van Der Burg et al. 2017; Jensen et al. 2017; Sanchez et al. 2018).

MATERNAL ADIPOSITY AND DEVELOPMENTAL OUTCOMES IN TERM BORN CHILDREN

The association between maternal overweight or obesity and neurodevelopment in human offspring has recently been reviewed with evidence from longitudinal, prospective, and observational studies (Rivera et al. 2015; Sullivan et al. 2015; Veena et al. 2016; Van Der Burg et al. 2016; Edlow 2017; Sanchez et al. 2018). In general, maternal overweight or obesity is associated with poorer cognitive performance during childhood (Brion et al. 2011; Hinkle et al. 2012; Eriksen et al. 2013; Bliddal et al. 2014; Huang et al. 2014) and adolescence (Basatemur et al. 2013), including poorer motor (Buss et al. 2012), spatial (Basatemur et al. 2013), and verbal skills (Huang et al. 2014). Furthermore, infants born to overweight or obese mothers are also at increased risk of developing depression and anxiety (Mina et al. 2017; Robinson et al. 2013), as well as ADHD (Andersen et al. 2017).

PREMATURITY AND DEVELOPMENTAL OUTCOMES

Children born extremely preterm (<28 weeks gestational age) perform significantly worse on cognitive measures than, for example, children born at 32 weeks' gestational age (Aarnoudse-Moens et al. 2009). Furthermore, IQ steadily declines with decreasing gestational age (Kerr-Wilson et al. 2012). Prematurity is also associated with behavioral (including attention and emotional) problems, as well as autism spectrum disorders (Johnson et al. 2010). The heightened frequency of 'inattention, anxiety, and social difficulties' among children born extremely preterm, is called 'the preterm behavioral phenotype' (Johnson and Wolke 2013; Korzeniewski et al. 2017). The risk of cerebral palsy (CP), one of the most common causes of chronic motor disabilities in children (Ahlin et al. 2013; Christensen et al. 2014), increases with decreasing gestational age (Joseph et al. 2003). These findings highlight that children born at an increasingly early gestational age are at heightened risk of cognitive, behavior, and motor developmental limitations.

MATERNAL ADIPOSITY AND DEVELOPMENT IN PRETERM OFFSPRING

In our large prospective cohort of ELGANs, infants of obese mothers were more likely to have impaired cognitive function at 2 (Helderman et al. 2012; Van Der Burg et al. 2015) and 10 years (Jensen et al. 2017), than infants of women with lower BMIs. Maternal adiposity during pregnancy was also a risk factor for attention problems at 2 and 10 years of age among children born extremely preterm (Van Der Burg et al. 2017; Leviton et al. 2018c). Others have found that maternal obesity is also associated with autism and language skills at age 2 years in children born preterm (≤30 weeks' gestation) (Reynolds et al. 2014).

MATERNAL ADIPOSITY VERSUS EXCESSIVE WEIGHT GAIN IN PREGNANCY

While most studies examining maternal adiposity in relation to neurodevelopment have focused on maternal pre-pregnancy overweight or obesity status, the few studies that have examined the contribution of excessive weight gain have generally focused on term children. The evidence from these studies is mixed, with some studies suggesting U-shaped associations between weight gain and poorer neurodevelopmental outcomes (Gardner et al. 2015), some suggesting positive associations (Bilder et al. 2013; Huang et al. 2014), and others indicating no association (Tanda et al. 2013). In the ELGAN study population, we observed a U-shaped relationship between pregnancy weight gain and a low score on the Oral and Written Language Scales Oral Expression assessment (Jensen et al. 2017; Van Der Burg et al. 2017; Leviton et al. 2018c). Children whose mother did not gain an adequate amount of weight were also at increased risk of a low score on the Wechsler Individual Achievement Test-III Word Reading assessments. Each of the seven ELGAN study publications that reported associations of maternal weight gain during pregnancy of pre-pregnancy overweight and obesity did do for different child dysfunctions (cognition, attention, motor) (Table 5.1).

POTENTIAL MECHANISMS

The pathway leading from maternal adiposity to impaired neurodevelopment among ELGANs remains to be elucidated. A few promising hypotheses, however, have been explored, including evaluation of the contribution of the pro-inflammatory maternal milieu and impaired synthesis of growth factors. While some of these hypotheses are specific to how maternal adiposity may disturb neurodevelopment through alterations in the in utero environment (Dowling and McAuliffe 2013), others focus on possible epigenetic alterations in maternal or paternal germ cells, even before conception occurs (Dowling and McAuliffe 2013; Contu and Hawkes 2017).

Understanding the mechanisms that potentially mediate neurodevelopmental outcomes can improve surveillance measures and guide interventions to mitigate risk. Trials of preconception interventions are ongoing in several countries to improve maternal health and nutrition, and the health of their offspring (Barker et al. 2018). Further definition of the underlying epigenetic, cellular, metabolic, and physiological mechanisms, which account for the association between maternal adiposity and neurodevelopment in the preterm offspring, is critical for characterizing more specific recommendations for preconception

Table 5.1 Developmental limitations among children who were born extremely preterm and enrolled in the ELGAN study whose mother was overweight obese or had an undesirable weight gain during this pregnancy

	Cognitive problems	Attention problems	Motor problems
2 years	Helderman et al. (2012) Van der Burg et al. (2015)		Van der Burg et al. (2015)
10 years	Jensen et al. (2017)	Van der Burg et al. (2017) Leviton et al. (2018c)	Jensen et al. (2017)

health. Here we describe four potential mechanisms, inflammation, epigenetics, impaired synthesis of growth factors, and gut microbiome diversity.

Inflammation

A prevailing hypothesis is that the inflammatory milieu that accompanies an obese state may lead to a cascading series of events that affect the fetus's and newborn's brain development and subsequent neuro-development. This is supported by multiple observations.

First, obese and overweight gravida expose their fetuses to an inflammatory environment. In the ELGAN study, newborns of overweight and obese women were more likely to have systemic inflammation than their peers born to women with lower BMIs (Van Der Burg et al. 2013). Others have reported that the newborns of women with Class II and III maternal obesity (BMI > 35 kg/m²) tended to have higher concentrations of inflammatory markers (e.g. CRP, TNF-α, IL-1α, IL-1ra, IL-6, and IL-8) (Broadney et al. 2017).

Second, systemic inflammation in the ELGAN appears to increase the risk of later brain dysfunctions. In the ELGAN study, markers of systemic inflammation (Table 5.2) in the first month of life were associated with impaired IQ and overall cognitive function at both age 2 (O'Shea et al. 2012, 2013; Leviton et al. 2016) and 10 (Kuban et al. 2017), as well as with abnormal brain ultrasound images (Leviton et al. 2018a), microcephaly (Leviton et al. 2011, 2016), executive dysfunctions (Leviton et al. 2019), learning disorders (Leviton et al. 2018b, 2018d), attention-deficit disorder (Allred et al. 2017), autism spectrum

Table 5.2   Systemic inflammatory proteins assessed in the preterm neonate in relation to cognitive function at age 2 and 10 years in the ELGAN cohort

Protein	Mental scale score (<55)[a]	DAS IQ Z-score (≤–2)[b]	LPA impairment (severe)[b]
CRP	+	+	+
SAA	+	No assoc.	+
MPO	No assoc.	No assoc.	No assoc.
IL-1β	No assoc.	No assoc.	No assoc.
IL-6	+	+	+
IL-6R	No assoc.	No assoc.	No assoc.
TNF-α	+	+	+
TNF-R2	+	No assoc.	No assoc.
IL-8 (CXCL8)	+	+	+
RANTES (CCL5)	No assoc.	No assoc.	No assoc.
ICAM-1 (CD54)	+	+	+
MMP-9	No assoc.	No assoc.	No assoc.
VEGF	No assoc.	No assoc.	No assoc.
VEGF-R2	+	No assoc.	+
TSH	No assoc.	No assoc.	+
EPO	+	+	No assoc.

[a] *Bayley Scales of Infant Development,* 2nd ed. Assessed at age 2 (Leviton et al. 2016).
[b] DAS (Differential Ability Scales-II); LPA impairment (latent profile analysis). Assessed at age 10 (Kuban et al. 2017).

disorders (Korzeniewski et al. 2018; Leviton et al. 2018d), and other social limitations (Korzeniewski et al. 2018).

Third, ELGANs born to obese women and ELGANs born to overweight women are at increased risk of some of these brain-related dysfunctions. For example, compared to ELGANs born to mothers with normal BMIs, those born to obese mothers (but not those born to overweight mothers) were more likely at age 2 years to have Bayley Scales of Infant and Toddler Development (2Ed) Mental and Motor Developmental Indices that were more than 3 standard deviations below the expected mean (Van Der Burg et al. 2015). Also at age 2 years, former ELGANs born to obese mothers, as well as those born to overweight mothers, were more likely have parent-reported behaviors characteristic of the attention-deficit hyperactivity syndrome (Van Der Burg et al. 2017). At age 10 years, former ELGANs born to obese women were more likely than others to have lower scores on assessments of verbal IQ, processing speed, visual fine motor control, and the WIAT-III Spelling component (Jensen et al. 2017). In addition, children whose mother gained an excessive amount of weight during the pregnancy tended to have low scores on the oral expression component of the Oral and Written Language Scales–Second Edition.

Thus we have all three components of the three-part syllogism. Maternal obesity and overweight are associated with systemic inflammation in the newborn (component 1), systemic inflammation in the newborn is associated with brain-related dysfunctions (component 2), and maternal obesity and over-weight are associated with brain-related dysfunctions (component 3).

Mental scale score (<55) of Bayley Scales of Infant Development II; DAS (Differential Ability Scales-II; LPA impairment (latent profile analysis); CRP (C-reactive protein); SAA (serum amyloid A); MPO (myeloperoxidase); IL-1β (Interleukin) (IL)-1β; IL-6 (Interleukin-6); IL-6R (IL-6 receptor); TNF-α (tumor necrosis factor-alpha); TNF-alpha R2 (one TNF-α receptors); IL-8 (Interleukin-8); RANTES (regulated upon activation, and normal T-lymphocyte expressed) and (presumably) secreted, CCL5 (chemokine (C-C motif) ligand 5); ICAM-1 (intercellular adhesion molecule-1); CD54 (Cluster of Differentiation 54); MMP-9 (matrix metalloproteinase-9); VEGF (vascular endothelial growth factor); VEGF-R2 (one of VEGF-R2's receptors); TSH (thyroid-stimulating hormone); EPO (erythropoietin).

Inflammation and Epigenetic Modifications

Epigenetic changes, such as DNA methylation, histone modification, and chromatin remodeling, are seen more commonly in the placentas of obese women than in those of their peers (Nomura et al. 2014; Soubry et al. 2015; Mitsuya et al. 2017; Nogues et al. 2019). These very same epigenetic changes appear capable of intensifying inflammatory responses (Claycombe et al. 2015). Although maternal adiposity appears to influence the methylation of DNA in the newborn's blood (Sharp et al. 2017), we do not yet know to what extent these methylation differences influence the intensity of inflammatory responses.

Maternal obesity could lead to epigenetic methylation that up-regulates or down-regulates transcription and, ultimately, protein synthesis alterations that contribute to developmental changes in her offspring (Grafodatskaya et al. 2010; Roth et al. 2011; Salbaum and Kappen 2012; Buckman et al. 2014; Radford 2018).

Impaired Synthesis of Growth Factors

Proteins that promote the development and survival of neurons are identified as neurotrophins. They also appear to be capable of repairing damaged brain tissue (Cai et al. 2014; Xiao and Le 2016). Some of these neurotrophic proteins are synthesized by the placenta and enhance placenta growth (Sahay et al. 2017). One of these neurotrophins, brain-derived neutrotrophic factor (BDNF), is less available in the placenta of obese women than in the placenta of their non-obese peers (Prince et al. 2017). In a mouse model of diet-induced maternal obesity, the offspring have impaired early hippocampal BDNF production, and diminished later spatial cognitive function, which is viewed as hippocampus-dependent (Tozuka et al. 2010). In a population-based cohort study, the children of obese mothers were more likely than others to have low BDNF concentrations in newborn-screening blood spots. In the subset of children born preterm, children who had low BDNF concentrations were more likely than others to have impaired communication function as reported by a parent on the Ages & Stages Questionnaire (Ghassabian et al. 2017).

In the ELGAN study, higher first postnatal month concentrations of neurotrophic proteins, including BDNF, were associated with lower risk of cognitive impairment at age 10 years (Kuban et al. 2018). Even when high concentrations of neurotrophins are not associated with reduced risks of brain-related dysfunctions, high concentrations of neurotrophic proteins (including BDNF) are capable of modulating the risk of such adversities associated with systemic inflammation as attention deficit disorder (Allred et al. 2017), reading and mathematics learning limitations (Leviton et al. 2018b), social impairment (Korzeniewski et al. 2018), and executive dysfunctions (Leviton et al. 2019). Consequently, future assessments of the putative mechanisms that explain the relationship between obesity and impaired development may consider evaluating whether these neurotrophic proteins modify the association between maternal obesity and developmental outcomes, as mediated through systemic inflammation.

Microbiome

Gut microbiota influence the risk of obesity via multiple mechanisms, including energy balance, glucose metabolism, and low-grade inflammation (Cani et al. 2012). In addition, infants born to obese women have lower gut microbiota diversity than infants born to women who are not obese (Singh et al. 2017; Sugino et al. 2019). Still unclear, however, is the role of the microbiome in neurocognitive development, although this is a rapidly growing area of scientific inquiry (Sugino et al. 2019).

LIMITATIONS OF THE EXISTING LITERATURE AND FUTURE OPPORTUNITIES

Confounding

Women who are obese are considerably more likely than other women to be at socioeconomic disadvantage (Newton et al. 2017) and this has also been observed in the ELGAN study (Van Der Burg et al. 2015). Socioeconomic disadvantage has been associated with impaired neurocognitive function in offspring (Leviton et al. 2018c, 2018e, 2018f; Joseph et al. 2018). However, socioeconomic disadvantage is a complex construct and characterization of socioeconomic status can be challenging. Numerous factors contribute to socioeconomic status and it is not necessarily socioeconomic status per se that is the driver of the adverse outcomes observed, rather how socioeconomic status influences access to care, diet, exercise, and other health-related behaviors, environmental exposures, neighborhood environment, and other social factors.

Isolating the independent contribution of maternal obesity/overweight from the factors that might confound these association is challenging. Much of the literature on maternal obesity and neurodevelopmental outcomes in the offspring has been conducted using observational study designs and model building strategies that account for possible confounding in the relationships observed. Efforts to control for possible confounding are dependent on (1) adequately identifying all possible confounders of the relationship being examined, (2) completeness of the data collected on confounders, and (3) accuracy and detail on the data collected. When one or more of these criteria are not met, which is almost certainly the case for most observational studies, there is a potential that residual confounding contributes to the associations observed (Liang et al. 2014).

One approach to investigating the potential for socioeconomic status in explaining associations observed has been to examine paternal obesity in relation to neurocognitive outcomes in the offspring. For example, in Gardner et al. (2015) investigators observed a similar magnitude of association between maternal pre-pregnancy and paternal BMI and autism spectrum disorders, suggesting an absence of an in utero effect. Conversely, one study found a stronger association with maternal BMI (Casas et al. 2013). However, this study was underpowered for evaluating a statistical difference between maternal and paternal associations. However, this approach is imperfect in its aim of evaluating possible confounding given the potential epigenetic modifications that can result from paternal obesity. In other words, the absence of a difference in association between maternal or paternal obesity and neurocognitive function in the offspring does not preclude the possibility that obesity is a true causal agent in the associations observed. Future studies should consider evaluation of biomarkers, as mediators in the association between maternal obesity, taking into account complex social factors as possible confounders of the associations observed.

Maternal genetic factors could also act as possible confounders. For example, genotype influences cognitive function. Attributing the child's developmental limitations to maternal obesity when they should be attributed to genetic factors would be another example of confounding.

In conclusion, the prevalence of maternal obesity is increasing worldwide, creating the potential for a parallel increase in adverse neurodevelopmental outcomes in their offspring. Evidence supporting this association must be interpreted with caution, given the potential of residual confounding contributing to the associations observed. Our findings on ELGANs provide support for the role of obesity-induced inflammation and adverse neurodevelopmental outcomes, but this is an emerging area of research and additional, mechanistic studies are needed to further evaluate these hypotheses. The epigenome and microbiome are intriguing, albeit underdeveloped areas of research that might help us understand the contribution of maternal adiposity to the neurodevelopment of ELGANs.

REFERENCES

Aarnoudse-Moens CSH, Weisglas-Kuperus N, Van Goudoever JB, Oosterlaan J (2009) Meta-analysis of neurobehavioral outcomes in very preterm and/or very low birth weight children. *Pediatrics* **124**: 717–28. doi: 0.1542/peds.2008-2816.

Abarca-Gómez L, Abdeen ZA, Hamid ZA et al. (2017) Worldwide trends in body-mass index, underweight, overweight, and obesity from 1975 to 2016: a pooled analysis of 2416 population-based measurement studies in 128·9 million children, adolescents, and adults. *The Lancet* **390**: 2627–42. doi: 10.1016/S0140-6736(17)32129-3.

Abenhaim HA, Benjamin A (2011) Higher caesarean section rates in women with higher body mass index: are we managing labour differently? *J Obstet Gynaecol Can* **33**: 443–8. doi: 10.1016/S1701-2163(16)34876-9.

Ahlin K, Himmelmann K, Hagberg G et al. (2013) Non-infectious risk factors for different types of cerebral palsy in term-born babies: a population-based, case–control study. *BJOG* **120**: 724–31. doi: 10.1111/1471-0528.12164.

Allred EN, Dammann O, Fichorova RN et al. (2017) Systemic inflammation during the first postnatal month and the risk of attention deficit hyperactivity disorder characteristics among 10-year-old children born extremely preterm. *J Neuroimmune Pharmacol* **12**: 531–43. doi: 10.1007/s11481-017-9742-9.

Andersen CH, Thomsen PH, Nohr EA, Lemcke S (2017) Maternal body mass index before pregnancy as a risk factor for ADHD and autism in children. *Eur Child Adolesc Psychiatry* **27**: 139–48. doi: 10.1007/s00787-017-1027-6.

Barker M, Dombrowski SU, Colbourn T et al. (2018) Intervention strategies to improve nutrition and health behaviours before conception. *Lancet* **391**: 1853–64. doi: 10.1016/S0140-6736(18)30313-1.

Basatemur E, Gardiner J, Williams C et al. (2013) Maternal prepregnancy BMI and child cognition: a longitudinal cohort study. *Pediatrics* **131**: 56–63. doi: 10.1542/peds.2012-0788.

Bilder DA, Bakian AV, Viskochil J et al. (2013) Maternal prenatal weight gain and autism spectrum disorders. *Pediatrics* **132**: e1276–83. doi: 10.1542/peds.2013-1188.

Bliddal M, Olsen J, Stovring H et al. (2014) Maternal pre-pregnancy BMI and intelligence quotient (IQ) in 5-year-old children: a cohort based study. *PLoS One* **9**: e94498. doi: 10.1371/journal.pone.0094498.

Brion MJ, Zeegers M, Jaddoe V et al. (2011) Intrauterine effects of maternal prepregnancy overweight on child cognition and behavior in 2 cohorts. *Pediatrics* **127**: e202–11. doi: 10.1542/peds.2010-0651.

Broadney MM, Chahal N, Michels KA et al. (2017) Impact of parental obesity on neonatal markers of inflammation and immune response. *Int J Obes (Lond)* **41**: 30–7. doi: 10.1038/ijo.2016.187.

Buckman LB, Hasty AH, Flaherty DK et al. (2014) Obesity induced by a high-fat diet is associated with increased immune cell entry into the central nervous system. *Brain Behav Immun* **35**: 33–42. doi: 10.1016/j.bbi.2013.06.007.

Buss C, Entringer S, Davis EP et al. (2012) Impaired executive function mediates the association between maternal pre-pregnancy body mass index and child ADHD symptoms. *PLoS One* **7**: e37758. doi: 10.1371/journal.pone.0037758PONE-D-12-02786 [pii].

Cai J, Hua F, Yuan L et al. (2014) Potential therapeutic effects of neurotrophins for acute and chronic neurological diseases. *Biomed Res Int* **2014**: 601084. doi: 10.1155/2014/601084.

Cani PD, Osto M, Geurts L, Everard A (2012) Involvement of gut microbiota in the development of low-grade inflammation and type 2 diabetes associated with obesity. *Gut Microbes* **3**: 279–88. doi: 10.4161/gmic.19625.

Carlson NS, Hernandez TL, Hurt KJ (2015) Parturition dysfunction in obesity: time to target the pathobiology. *Reprod Biol Endocrinol* **13**: 135. doi: 10.1186/s12958-015-0129-6.

Casas M, Chatzi L, Carsin AE et al. (2013) Maternal pre-pregnancy overweight and obesity, and child neuropsychological development: two Southern European birth cohort studies. *Int J Epidemiol* **42**: 506–17. doi: 10.1093/ije/dyt002.

Christensen D, Van Naarden Braun K, Doernberg NS et al. (2014) Prevalence of cerebral palsy, co-occurring autism spectrum disorders, and motor functioning–Autism and Developmental Disabilities Monitoring Network, USA, 2008. *Dev Med Child Neurol* **56**: 59–65. doi: 0.1111/dmcn.12268.

Claycombe KJ, Brissette CA, Ghribi O (2015) Epigenetics of inflammation, maternal infection, and nutrition. *J Nutr* **145**: 1109S–15S. doi: 10.3945/jn.114.194639.

Contu L, Hawkes CA (2017) A Review of the impact of maternal obesity on the cognitive function and mental health of the offspring. *Int J Mol Sci* **18**: 1093. doi: 10.3390/ijms18051093.

Deputy NP, Dub B, Sharma AJ (2018) Prevalence and trends in prepregnancy normal weight – 48 states, New York City, and District of Columbia, 2011–2015. *MMWR. Morb Mortal Mkly Rep* **66**: 1402–7. doi: 10.15585/mmwr.mm665152a3.

Devlieger R, Benhalima K, Damm P et al. (2016) Maternal obesity in Europe: where do we stand and how to move forward?: A scientific paper commissioned by the European Board and College of Obstetrics and Gynaecology (EBCOG). *Eur J Obstet Gynecol Reprod Biol* **201**: 203–8. doi: 10.1016/j.ejogrb.2016.04.005.

Dowling D, McAuliffe FM (2013) The molecular mechanisms of offspring effects from obese pregnancy. *Obes Facts* **6**: 134–45. doi: 10.1159/000350706.

Edlow AG (2017) Maternal obesity and neurodevelopmental and psychiatric disorders in offspring. *Prenat Diagn* **37**: 95–110. doi: 10.1002/pd.4932.

Ehrenberg HM, Durnwald CP, Catalano P, Mercer BM (2004) The influence of obesity and diabetes on the risk of cesarean delivery. *Am J Obstet Gynecol* **191**: 969–74. doi: 10.1016/j.ajog.2004.06.057.

Eriksen HL, Kesmodel US, Underbjerg M et al. (2013) Predictors of intelligence at the age of 5: family, pregnancy and birth characteristics, postnatal influences, and postnatal growth. *PLoS One* **8**: e79200. doi: 10.1371/journal.pone.0079200.

Flegal KM, Kruszon-Moran D, Carroll MD, Fryar CD, Ogden CL (2016) Trends in obesity among adults in the United States, 2005 to 2014. *JAMA* **315**: 2284–91. doi: 10.1001/jama.2016.6458.

Gardner RM, Lee BK, Magnusson C et al. (2015) Maternal body mass index during early pregnancy, gestational weight gain, and risk of autism spectrum disorders: results from a Swedish total population and discordant sibling study. *Int J Epidemiol* **44**: 870–83. doi: 10.1093/ije/dyv081.

Ghassabian A, Sundaram R, Chahal N et al. (2017) Determinants of neonatal brain-derived neurotrophic factor and association with child development. *Dev Psychopathol* **29**: 1499–511. doi: 10.1017/S0954579417000414.

Godfrey KM, Reynolds RM, Prescott SL et al. (2017) Influence of maternal obesity on the long-term health of offspring. *Lancet Diabetes Endocrinol* **5**: 53–64. doi: 10.1016/S2213-8587(16)30107-3.

Grafodatskaya D, Chung B, Szatmari P, Weksberg R (2010) Autism spectrum disorders and epigenetics. *J Am Acad Child Adolesc Psychiatry* **49**: 794–809. doi: 10.1016/j.jaac.2010.05.005.

Healthy People Gov. (2010) *Maternal, Infant, and Child Health* [Online]. Available: https://www.healthypeople.gov/2020/topics-objectives/topic/Maternal-Infant-and-Child-Health/objectives [Accessed May 2019].

Helderman JB, O'Shea TM, Kuban KC et al. (2012) Antenatal antecedents of cognitive impairment at 24 months in extremely low gestational age newborns. *Pediatrics* **129**: 494–502. doi: 10.1542/peds.2011-1796.

Heslehurst N, Simpson H, Ells LJ et al. (2008) The impact of maternal BMI status on pregnancy outcomes with immediate short-term obstetric resource implications: a meta-analysis. *Obes Rev* **9**: 635–83. doi: 10.1111/j.1467-789X.2008.00511.x.

Hinkle SN, Schieve LA, Stein AD et al. (2012) Associations between maternal prepregnancy body mass index and child neurodevelopment at 2 years of age. *Int J Obes (Lond)* **36**: 1312–9. doi: 10.1038/ijo.2012.143.

Huang L, Yu X, Keim S et al. (2014) Maternal prepregnancy obesity and child neurodevelopment in the Collaborative Perinatal Project. *Int J Epidemiol* **43**: 783–92. doi: 10.1093/ije/dyu030.

Huda SS, Brodie LE, Sattar N (2010) Obesity in pregnancy: prevalence and metabolic consequences. *Semin Fetal Neonatal Med* **15**: 70–6. doi: 10.1016/j.siny.2009.09.006.

Jensen ET, Van Der Burg JW, O'Shea TM et al. (2017) The relationship of maternal prepregnancy body mass index and pregnancy weight gain to neurocognitive function at age 10 years among children born extremely preterm. *J Pediatr* **187**: 50–57.e3. doi: 10.1016/j.jpeds.2017.02.064.

Johnson S, Hollis C, Kochhar P et al. (2010) Psychiatric disorders in extremely preterm children: longitudinal finding at age 11 years in the EPICure study. *J Am Acad Child Adolesc Psychiatry* **49**: 453–63 e1. doi: 10.1097/00004583-201005000-00006.

Johnson S, Wolke D (2013) Behavioural outcomes and psychopathology during adolescence. *Early Hum Dev* **89**: 199–207. doi: 10.1016/j.earlhumdev.2013.01.014.

Joseph K, Allen AC, Lutfi S et al. (2003) Does the risk of cerebral palsy increase or decrease with increasing gestational age? *BMC Pregnancy Childbirth* **3**: 8. doi: 0.1186/1471-2393-3-8.

Joseph RM, O'Shea TM, Allred EN, Heeren T, Kuban KK (2018) Maternal educational status at birth, maternal educational advancement, and neurocognitive outcomes at age 10 years among children born extremely preterm. *Pediatr Res* **83**: 767–77. doi: 10.1038/pr.2017.267.

Kerr-Wilson C, Mackay D, Smith G, Pell J (2012) Meta-analysis of the association between preterm delivery and intelligence. *J Public Health (Oxf)* **34**: 209–216. doi: 10.1093/pubmed/fdr024.

Kim SY, Dietz PM, England L, Morrow B, Callaghan WM (2007) Trends in pre-pregnancy obesity in nine states, 1993–2003. *Obesity (Silver Spring)* **15**: 986–93. doi: 10.1038/oby.2007.621.

Korzeniewski SJ, Allred EN, O'Shea TM et al. (2018) Elevated protein concentrations in newborn blood and the risks of autism spectrum disorder, and of social impairment, at age 10 years among infants born before the 28th week of gestation. *Transl Psychiatry* **8**: 115. doi: 10.1038/s41398-018-0156-0.

Korzeniewski SJ, Joseph RM, Kim SH et al. (2017) Social responsiveness scale assessment of the preterm behavioral phenotype in 10-year-olds born extremely preterm. *J Dev Behav Pediatr* **38**: 697–705. doi: 10.1097/DBP.0000000000000485.

Kuban KC, Joseph RM, O'Shea TM et al. (2017) Circulating Inflammatory-associated proteins in the first month of life and cognitive impairment at age 10 years in children born extremely preterm. *J Pediatr* **180**: 116–23 e1. doi: 10.1016/j.jpeds.2016.09.054.

Kuban KCK, Heeren T, O'Shea TM et al. (2018) Among children born extremely preterm a higher level of circulating neurotrophins is associated with lower risk of cognitive impairment at school age. *J Pediatr* **201**: 40–8 e4. doi: 10.1016/j.jpeds.2018.05.021.

Lawn JE, Blencowe H, Waiswa P et al. (2016) Stillbirths: rates, risk factors, and acceleration towards 2030. *Lancet* **387**: 587–603. doi: 10.1016/S0140-6736(15)00837-5.

Leviton A, Allred EN, Fichorova RN et al. (2016) Systemic inflammation on postnatal days 21 and 28 and indicators of brain dysfunction 2 years later among children born before the 28th week of gestation. *Early Hum Dev* **93**: 25–32. doi: 10.1016/j.earlhumdev.2015.11.004.

Leviton A, Allred EN, Fichorova RN et al. (2018a) Circulating biomarkers in extremely preterm infants associated with ultrasound indicators of brain damage. *Eur J Paediatr Neurol* **22**: 440–50. doi: 10.1016/j.ejpn.2018.01.018.

Leviton A, Dammann O, Allred EN et al. (2018b) Neonatal systemic inflammation and the risk of low scores on measures of reading and mathematics achievement at age 10 years among children born extremely preterm. *Int J Dev Neurosci* **66**: 45–53. doi: 10.1016/j.ijdevneu.2018.01.001.

Leviton A, Hooper SR, Hunter SJ et al. (2018c) Antecedents of screening positive for attention deficit hyperactivity disorder in ten-year-old children born extremely preterm. *Pediatr Neurol* **81**: 25–30. doi: 10.1016/j.pediatrneurol.2017.12.010.

Leviton A, Joseph RM, Allred EN et al. (2018d) The risk of neurodevelopmental disorders at age 10 years associated with blood concentrations of interleukins 4 and 10 during the first postnatal month of children born extremely preterm. *Cytokine* **110**: 181–88. doi: 10.1016/j.cyto.2018.05.004.

Leviton A, Joseph RM, Allred EN, O'Shea TM, Kuban KKC (2018e) Antenatal and neonatal antecedents of learning limitations in 10-year old children born extremely preterm. *Early Hum Dev* **118**: 8–14. doi: 10.1016/j.earlhumdev.2018.01.020.

Leviton A, Joseph RM, Allred EN et al. (2018f) Antenatal and neonatal antecedents of executive dysfunctions in extremely preterm children. *J Child Neurol* **33**: 198–208. doi: 10.1177/0883073817750499.

Leviton A, Joseph RM, Fichorova RN et al. (2019) Executive dysfunction early postnatal biomarkers among children born extremely preterm. *J Neuroimmune Pharmacol* **14**: 188–99. doi: 10.1007/s11481-018-9804-7.

Leviton A, Kuban KC, Allred EN et al. (2011) Early postnatal blood concentrations of inflammation-related proteins and microcephaly two years later in infants born before the 28th post-menstrual week. *Early Hum Dev* **87**: 325–30. doi: S0378-3782(11)00080-6 [pii] 10.1016/j.earlhumdev.2011.01.043 [doi].

Liang W, Zhao Y, Lee AH (2014) An investigation of the significance of residual confounding effect. *Biomed Res Int* **2014**: 658056. doi: 10.1155/2014/658056.

Lindberg S, Anderson C, Pillai P et al. (2016) Prevalence and predictors of unhealthy weight gain in pregnancy. *WMJ* **115**: 233–7. doi: PMC5313046

Marchi J, Berg M, Dencker A, Olander EK, Begley C (2015) Risks associated with obesity in pregnancy, for the mother and baby: a systematic review of reviews. *Obes Rev* **16**: 621–38. doi: 10.1111/obr.12288.

Mehta SH, Kerver JM, Sokol RJ, Keating DP, Paneth N (2014) The association between maternal obesity and neurodevelopmental outcomes of offspring. *J Pediatr* **165**: 891–6. doi: 10.1016/j.jpeds.2014.07.003.

Metwally M, Ong KJ, Ledger WL, Li TC (2008) Does high body mass index increase the risk of miscarriage after spontaneous and assisted conception? A meta-analysis of the evidence. *Fertil Steril* **90**: 714–26. doi: 10.1016/j.fertnstert.2007.07.1290.

Mina TH, Lahti M, Drake AJ et al. (2017) Prenatal exposure to very severe maternal obesity is associated with adverse neuropsychiatric outcomes in children. *Psychol Med* **47**: 353–62. doi: 10.1017/S0033291716002452.

Mitsuya K, Parker AN, Liu L et al. (2017) Alterations in the placental methylome with maternal obesity and evidence for metabolic regulation. *PLoS One* **12**: e0186115. doi: 10.1371/journal.pone.0186115.

Newton S, Braithwaite D, Akinyemiju TF (2017) Socio-economic status over the life course and obesity: systematic review and meta-analysis. *PLoS One* **12**: e0177151. doi: 10.1371/journal.pone.0177151.

Nogues P, Dos Santos E, Jammes H et al. (2019) Maternal obesity influences expression and DNA methylation of the adiponectin and leptin systems in human third-trimester placenta. *Clin Epigenetics* **11**: 20. doi: 10.1186/s13148-019-0612-6.

Nomura Y, Lambertini L, Rialdi A et al. (2014) Global methylation in the placenta and umbilical cord blood from pregnancies with maternal gestational diabetes, preeclampsia, and obesity. *Reprod Sci* **21**: 131–7. doi: 10.1177/1933719113492206.

O'Brien TE, Ray JG, Chan WS (2003) Maternal body mass index and the risk of preeclampsia: a systematic overview. *Epidemiology* **14**: 368–74. doi: 10.1097/01.EDE.0000059921.71494.D1.

O'Shea TM, Allred EN, Kuban KC et al. (2012) Elevated concentrations of inflammation-related proteins in postnatal blood predict severe developmental delay at 2 years of age in extremely preterm infants. *J Pediatr* **160**: 395–401. doi: S0022-3476(11)00899-7 [pii] 10.1016/j.jpeds.2011.08.069.

O'Shea TM, Shah B, Allred EN et al. (2013) Inflammation-initiating illnesses, inflammation-related proteins, and cognitive impairment in extremely preterm infants. *Brain Behav Immun* **29**: 104–12. doi: 10.1016/j.bbi.2012.12.012.

Onubi OJ, Marais D, Aucott L, Okonofua F, Poobalan AS (2016) Maternal obesity in Africa: a systematic review and meta-analysis. *J Public Health (Oxf)* **38**: e218–31. doi: 10.1093/pubmed/fdv138.

Pettersen-Dahl A, Murzakanova G, Sandvik L, Laine K (2018) Maternal body mass index as a predictor for delivery method. *Acta Obstet Gynecol Scand* **97**: 212–18. doi: 10.1111/aogs.13265.

Prince CS, Maloyan A, Myatt L (2017) Maternal obesity alters brain derived neurotrophic factor (BDNF) signaling in the placenta in a sexually dimorphic manner. *Placenta* **49**: 55–63. doi: 10.1016/j.placenta.2016.11.010.

Radford EJ (2018) Exploring the extent and scope of epigenetic inheritance. *Nat Rev Endocrinol* **14**: 345–55. doi: 10.1038/s41574-018-0005-5.

Reynolds LC, Inder TE, Neil JJ, Pineda RG, Rogers CE (2014) Maternal obesity and increased risk for autism and developmental delay among very preterm infants. *J Perinatol* **34**: 688. doi: 10.1038/jp.2014.80.

Rivera HM, Christiansen KJ, Sullivan EL (2015) The role of maternal obesity in the risk of neuropsychiatric disorders. *Front Neurosci* **9**: 194. doi: 10.3389/fnins.2015.00194.

Robinson M, Zubrick SR, Pennell CE et al. (2013) Pre-pregnancy maternal overweight and obesity increase the risk for affective disorders in offspring. *J Dev Orig Health Dis* **4**: 42–8. doi: 10.1017/S2040174412000578.

Roth C, Magnus P, Schjølberg S et al. (2011) Folic acid supplements in pregnancy and severe language delay in children. *JAMA* **306**: 1566–73. doi: 10.1001/jama.2011.1433.

Sahay AS, Sundrani DP, Joshi SR (2017) Neurotrophins: role in placental growth and development. *Vitam Horm* **104**: 243–61. doi: 10.1016/bs.vh.2016.11.002.

Salbaum JM, Kappen C (2012) Genetic and epigenomic footprints of folate. *Prog Mol Biol Transl Sci* **108**: 129. doi: 10.1016/B978-0-12-398397-8.00006-X.

Sanchez CE, Barry C, Sabhlok A et al. (2018) Maternal pre-pregnancy obesity and child neurodevelopmental outcomes: a meta-analysis. *Obes Rev* **19**: 464–84. doi: 10.1111/obr.12643.

Sharp GC, Salas LA, Monnereau C et al. (2017) Maternal BMI at the start of pregnancy and offspring epigenome-wide DNA methylation: findings from the pregnancy and childhood epigenetics (PACE) consortium. *Hum Mol Genet* **26**: 4067–85. doi: 10.1093/hmg/ddx290.

Siega-Riz AM, Gray GL (2013) Gestational weight gain recommendations in the context of the obesity epidemic. *Nutr Rev* **71**: S26–S30. doi: 10.1111/nure.12074.

Singh S, Karagas MR, Mueller NT (2017) Charting the maternal and infant microbiome: what is the role of diabetes and obesity in pregnancy? *Curr Diab Rep* **17**: 11. doi: 10.1007/s11892-017-0836-9.

Soubry A, Murphy SK, Wang F et al. (2015) Newborns of obese parents have altered DNA methylation patterns at imprinted genes. *Int J Obes (Lond)* **39**: 650–7. doi: 10.1038/ijo.2013.193.

Stothard KJ, Tennant PW, Bell R, Rankin J (2009) Maternal overweight and obesity and the risk of congenital anomalies: a systematic review and meta-analysis. *JAMA* **301**: 636–50. doi: 10.1001/jama.2009.113.

Sugino KY, Paneth N, Comstock SS (2019) Michigan cohorts to determine associations of maternal pre-pregnancy body mass index with pregnancy and infant gastrointestinal microbial communities: late pregnancy and early infancy. *PLoS One* **14**: e0213733. doi: 10.1371/journal.pone.0213733.

Sullivan EL, Riper KM, Lockard R, Valleau JC (2015) Maternal high-fat diet programming of the neuroendocrine system and behavior. *Horm Behav.* **76**: 153–61. doi: 10.1016/j.yhbeh.2015.04.008.

Tanda R, Salsberry PJ, Reagan PB, Fang MZ (2013) The impact of prepregnancy obesity on children's cognitive test scores. *Matern Child Health J* **17**: 222–9. doi: 10.1007/s10995-012-0964-4.

Tozuka Y, Kumon M, Wada E et al. (2010) Maternal obesity impairs hippocampal BDNF production and spatial learning performance in young mouse offspring. *Neurochem Int* **57**: 235–47. doi: 10.1016/j.neuint.2010.05.015.

Van Der Burg JW, Allred EN, Kuban K et al. (2015) Maternal obesity and development of the preterm newborn at 2 years. *Acta Paediatr* **104**: 900–3. doi: 10.1111/apa.13038.

Van Der Burg JW, Allred EN, Mcelrath TF et al. (2013) Is maternal obesity associated with sustained inflammation in extremely low gestational age newborns? *Early Hum Dev* **89**: 949–55. doi: 10.1016/j.earlhumdev.2013.09.014.

Van Der Burg JW, Jensen ET, Van De Bor M et al. (2017) Maternal obesity and attention-related symptoms in the preterm offspring. *Early Hum Dev* **115**: 9–15. doi: 10.1016/j.earlhumdev.2017.08.002.

Van Der Burg JW, Sen S, Chomitz VR et al. (2016) The role of systemic inflammation linking maternal BMI to neurodevelopment in children. *Pediatr Res* **79**: 3–12. doi: 10.1038/pr.2015.179.

Van Lieshout RJ, Taylor VH, Boyle MH (2011) Pre-pregnancy and pregnancy obesity and neurodevelopmental outcomes in offspring: a systematic review. *Obes Rev* **12**: e548–59. doi: 10.1111/j.1467-789X.2010.00850.x.

Veena SR, Gale CR, Krishnaveni GV et al. (2016) Association between maternal nutritional status in pregnancy and offspring cognitive function during childhood and adolescence; a systematic review. *BMC Pregnancy Childbirth* **16**: 220. doi: 10.1186/s12884-016-1011-z.

World Health Organization (2000) *Obesity: Preventing and Managing the Global Epidemic.* Report of a WHO consultation (WHO technical report series 894). Geneva, Switzerland: WHO.

World Health Organization (2018) *Overweight and Obesity – Fact Sheet* [Online]. [Accessed May 2019] https://www.who.int/nutrition/publications/obesity/WHO_TRS_894/en/.

Xiao N, Le QT (2016) Neurotrophic factors and their potential applications in tissue regeneration. *Arch Immunol Ther Exp (Warsz)* **64**: 89–99. doi: 10.1007/s00005-015-0376-4.

PART II

Neonatal Exposures and Outcomes

Chapter 6   Illness-Severity and Outcomes among
Children Born Extremely Preterm   57

Chapter 7   Bacteremia   73

Chapter 8   Retinopathy of Prematurity   81

Chapter 9   Bronchopulmonary Dysplasia   89

Illness-Severity and Outcomes among Children Born Extremely Preterm

J Wells Logan and Olaf Dammann

INTRODUCTION

Illness-severity scores were developed to control for case mix in research studies, to compare outcomes between centers, and to study the utilization of resources in intensive care settings. Although the use of illness-severity for comparisons of the quality of the care between institutions remains controversial (Vassar and Holcroft 1994; Adams et al. 2017) adjusting for 'case mix' has become the norm (Dorling et al. 2005; Morse et al. 2015; Hentschel et al. 2018). Illness-severity has also been used to predict neurodevelopmental outcomes in surviving preterm infants (Littman and Parmelee 1978; Buhrer et al. 2000; Lodha et al. 2009; Greenwood et al. 2012; Synnes et al. 2017). The ELGAN study provided the opportunity to explore the relationship between the revised Score for Neonatal Acute Physiology (SNAP-II), an illness-severity score derived from *early* postnatal physiologic derangements, and developmental outcomes at follow-up. We sought to determine if early postnatal measures of illness-severity are associated with developmental impairments at follow-up in a large, multicenter cohort of children born extremely preterm.

THE SCORE FOR NEONATAL ACUTE PHYSIOLOGY (SNAP) AND ILLNESS-SEVERITY

The APACHE (Acute Physiology And Chronic Health Evaluation) (Knaus et al. 1981) and Physiologic Stability Index (PSI) (Yeh et al. 1984) scores are illness-severity scores based on measures of 'acute physiology' for critically ill children and adults. SNAP was designed to parallel APACHE and PSI but was developed to evaluate illness-severity in newborns. It includes the 'worst' of 26 physiologic parameters recorded in the preceding 24 hours. Using a scoring system developed by others (Pollack et al. 1987), the degree of physiologic derangement is given by a weighted score of 0 to 5 points. Zero points are assigned for 'missing data', 1 point for data elements deemed 'important enough to record', 3 points for elements 'sufficient to warrant intervention', and 5 points for elements deemed 'life-threatening'. SNAP is calculated as the sum of points for the 24 hours following admission.

SNAP was validated prospectively in 1643 admissions to three Neonatal Intensive Care Units in the United States (Richardson et al. 1993a). It was evaluated at three arbitrary scoring levels, <10, 10–19, and ≥20. There were no differences in illness-severity by gender, but white and outborn infants were significantly more ill on admission than non-white and inborn infants. The usual pattern of declining mortality with increasing birthweight was noted. SNAP was highly predictive of mortality in each of the four birthweight strata and correlated with other indicators of illness-severity such as nursing workload, therapeutic intensity, physician-estimates of mortality, and length of stay. SNAP correlated highly with the Neonatal Therapeutic Intervention Scoring System (NTISS), a therapy-based illness-severity score based on invasiveness and cost of care in the first 24 hours of life (Cullen et al. 1974; Perlstein et al. 1997).

BIRTHWEIGHT AND ILLNESS-SEVERITY: INDEPENDENT PREDICTORS OF MORTALITY

Soon after the original publication (Richardson et al. 1993a), the relationship between SNAP and birthweight was explored further. Using the same cohort of 1621 consecutive admissions (92 deaths), the best of six prediction models was used to develop the SNAP Perinatal Extension (SNAP-PE) (Richardson et al. 1993b). The authors found that while birthweight is a major determinant of neonatal mortality, it fails to explain the large variations in neonatal mortality observed between intensive care units (Richardson et al. 1993b). A significant interaction was noted between illness-severity and birthweight, especially for infants born <750g, but both birth weight and illness severity were independent predictors of mortality across a wide range of birth weights. These findings suggested that in preterm infants, mortality differences can be explained, at least in part, by differences in illness-severity.

The same author team subsequently demonstrated that illness-severity can be used to track improvements in mortality (Richardson et al. 1998), length of stay (Zupancic and Richardson 1998), and cost of care (Zupancic and Richardson 1998). While centers differ by obstetric case-mix characteristics, only gestational age, SGA status, white race, and severe congenital anomalies are associated with a higher SNAP (Richardson et al. 1999). Antenatal steroid administration, Appearance, Pulse, Grimace, Activity, and Respiration (APGAR) score, and hypothermia affected newborn illness-severity and outcomes, suggesting that both antenatal and perinatal events contribute to mortality risk in infants born preterm (Richardson et al. 1999). SNAP's correlation with mortality significantly enhanced our understanding of risk assessments in preterm neonates, suggesting that the contributions of physiologic derangements to mortality risk are additive and that the risk is mediated, in part, by exposures and events in the antenatal and perinatal periods.

SNAP-II AND SNAP PERINATAL EXTENSION (SNAPPE)

SNAP was later revised, and is now known as the 'Revised Score for Neonatal Acute Physiology' (SNAP-II) (Richardson et al. 2001). The validation study included data from 30 neonatal intensive care admissions in Canada, California, and New England. Using the 34 elements of the original SNAP, the authors identified the six clinical and physiologic elements, collected within the first 12 hours, most significantly associated with mortality: lowest serum pH, lowest recorded temperature, lowest recorded mean arterial blood pressure (MBP), lowest recorded oxygen fraction based on arterial blood gas parameters, the presence of one or more seizures, and urine output (Richardson et al. 2001). While APACHE (Knaus et al. 1981) and other illness-severity scores (Yeh et al. 1984) derive from an arbitrary weighting of elements according to the *perceived* importance of each element, SNAP-II derives from the β-coefficients that correspond to physiologic parameters in the logistic regression. Thus, SNAP-II correlates directly with the *strength* of the association between physiologic derangements and mortality risk (Richardson et al. 2001).

In 2007, SNAP-II was re-validated in a sample of approximately 10 000 newborns from 58 Vermont Oxford Neonatal Network centers in North America. The scores performed similarly to those observed previously, suggesting that SNAP-II had not de-calibrated in the years since the original publication (Zupancic et al. 2007). In order to enhance the reliability of SNAP-II for risk adjustment, the authors added three additional components to account for non-physiologic characteristics that potentially contribute to mortality risk. The SNAP Perinatal Extension-II (SNAPPE-II) includes scoring elements for birthweight, SGA status, and APGAR score (Zupancic et al. 2007). With fewer elements in the score, the revised scores (SNAP-II and SNAPPE-II) are simple, robust measures of illness-severity that reliably predict mortality risk in infants born preterm.

SNAP IN THE ELGAN STUDY

Mortality

We explored the relationship between SNAP-II, our indicator of physiologic instability, and mortality risk among infants in the ELGAN cohort (Dammann et al. 2009). The 28-day mortality rate was 13% (range: 7–20%), and the overall mortality was 18% (range: 8–31%). SNAP-II, SNAPPE-II, and mortality were inversely related to gestational age, even within gestational age strata. The median SNAP-II increased with decreasing gestational age between 26 weeks and 23 weeks, suggesting that SNAP-II correlates strongly with gestational age. Inter-institutional differences were present, but these differences were attributed to differences in the frequency of births at lower gestational ages. Specifically, institutions with more infants in lower gestational age groups had more infants with an elevated SNAP-II (Fig. 6.1).

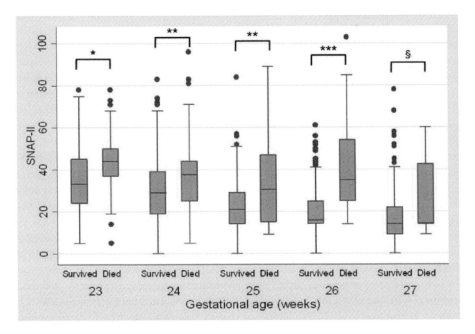

Figure 6.1   Box and whisker plot of SNAP-II at each week of gestational age among those infants who survived and those who died. The median is represented by the line in the middle of the gray box, and the 25th and 75th centiles by the lower and upper limits of the gray box, respectively. Reproduced with permission from Dammann et al. (2009), Copyright © 2009 by the AAP.

A variety of clinical prediction models have been developed to assess mortality risk in critically ill newborns. Some, but not all, have been validated in preterm newborns (Marcin et al. 2000; Pollack et al. 2000; Parry et al. 2003; Gagliardi et al. 2004). Models derived from early postnatal data appear to perform better than those based on birth data alone (Pollack et al. 2000; Lagatta et al. 2011; Meadow et al. 2011; Meadow et al. 2012). Therefore, some have adopted the view that mortality prediction is more reliable when derived from data elements collected in the early postnatal period (i.e. just after delivery, because measures derived from clinical information collected later in the hospital course are more likely to be influenced by medical interventions). Our interpretation of the literature is that the most robust models make use of clinical and laboratory data available in the early postnatal period (Pollack et al. 2000). Therefore, SNAP-II is ideally suited for mortality prediction; it is a simple, robust measure of illness-severity derived from clinical and physiologic data collected within the first 12 hours after birth.

Among very preterm infants, illness-severity is also associated with short-term respiratory outcomes (Escobar et al. 2004), intraventricular hemorrhage (IVH) (Chien et al. 2002), chronic lung disease (CLD) (Chien et al. 2002), necrotizing enterocolitis (NEC) (Carvalho et al. 2011), and retinopathy of prematurity (ROP) (Hagadorn et al. 2007; Fortes Filho et al. 2009). The relationship between illness-severity and these short-term, hospital outcomes suggests that illness-severity could also be associated with developmental outcomes that appear later in life. Our interest in illness-severity, then, is less about mortality prediction than it is about predicting neurodevelopmental outcomes among extremely preterm infants that survived to follow-up.

Structural and Functional Indicators of Brain Damage at Age 2 Years

We evaluated the relationship between SNAP-II components, such as systemic hypotension (Laughon et al. 2007; Logan et al. 2011a, 2011b) and early postnatal blood gas derangements (hypoxemia, hyperoxemia, hypocapnia, hypercapnia, and acidemia), and structural and functional brain disorders in children born extremely preterm (Leviton et al. 2010; Dammann et al. 2010a).

Seventy-eight percent of infants in the ELGAN cohort received some treatment (volume expansion or vasopressor therapy) for *early systemic hypotension* (Laughon et al. 2007). The proportion of infants treated for hypotension varied greatly among the 14 ELGAN centers, even after adjustment for maternal and neonatal risk factors. The rational for treating transitional hypotension is likely the perception that low blood pressure adversely affects oxygen delivery to the tissues, especially the brain (du Plessis 2009). Our findings suggest, however, that if brain injury is related to poor cerebral perfusion, then arterial blood pressure is a poor marker for adequate cerebral perfusion. We found no evidence that early postnatal hypotension was associated with white matter injury (Logan et al. 2011b), developmental delay (Logan et al. 2011a), or cerebral palsy (Logan et al. 2011b) at 2-year follow-up (Fig. 6.2). Thus, while some abnormalities of cerebral blood flow may be associated with abnormal cranial ultrasound lesions (Ment et al. 1984; Meek et al. 1999; Kluckow and Evans 2000; Tsuji et al. 2000; Evans et al. 2002; Osborn et al. 2003; Kissack et al. 2004; Miletin and Dempsey 2008), early postnatal systemic hypotension is not (de Vries et al. 1988; Trounce et al. 1988; Bejar et al. 1992; D'Souza et al. 1995; Perlman et al. 1996; Wiswell et al. 1996; Baud et al. 1998; Cunningham et al. 1999; Dammann et al. 2002; Limperopoulos et al. 2007).

In contrast, *blood gas derangements* (hypoxemia, hyperoxemia, hypocapnia, hypercapnia, and acidemia) noted on at least one of the first three postnatal days are associated with several indicators of brain damage (Fig. 6.3) (Leviton et al. 2010). We found that each of these physiologic derangements corresponds to elements of the SNAP-II score. Infants were classified according to whether they had a blood gas derangement in the highest or lowest quintile for gestational age and postnatal day of blood gas measurement. Infants with blood gas derangements in the extreme quintiles were compared to those in the other four quintiles with regard to whether or not one of several indicators of brain damage was present:

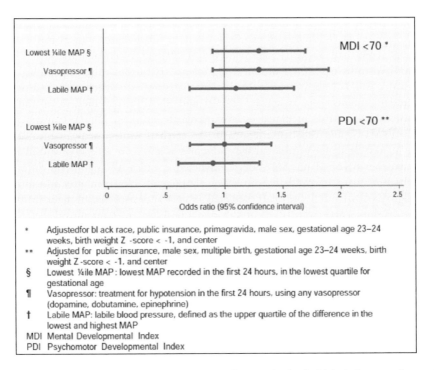

Figure 6.2   ORs (and 95% CIs) of the risk of MDI < 70 and PDI < 70 obtained with logistic regression models that incorporate indicators of hypotension during the first 24 postnatal hours and potential confounders. Reproduced from Logan et al. (2011a) with permission from BMJ Publishing Group Ltd.

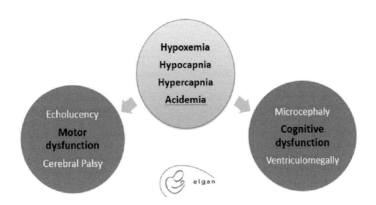

Figure 6.3   Blood gas abnormalities and brain-related outcomes (ELGAN cohort).

(1) ventriculomegaly or echolucency, (2) microcephaly, (3) cerebral palsy, or (4) a low score on a Bayley Scales of Infant Development-II (BSID) test at 24 months corrected gestational age. Every blood gas derangement was associated with multiple indicators of brain damage; for some, associations were seen with only 1 day of exposure, while for others, 2 or more days of exposure were required for an association with adverse outcome (Leviton et al. 2010).

We further examined the relationship between *illness-severity* and the risk of structural and functional brain disorders in children born extremely preterm (Dammann et al. 2010b). Of the 1506 eligible infants, 1435 had SNAP-II data collected, 1399 had a cranial ultrasound examination, and 1149 survived to follow-up. Of the surviving infants, 1014 (88%) had a neurologic exam and 975 (85%) had a BSID-II assessment at 21–24 months corrected gestational age. A total of 1467 extremely preterm infants were assigned SNAP-II and SNAPPE-II scores. After adjustment for gestational age, high SNAP-II predicted intraventricular hemorrhage (IVH), moderate/severe ventriculomegaly (VMEG) and echodense lesions in the cerebral white matter (Table 6.1). SNAP-II scores in the highest decile for gestational age and scores at a Z-score >1 also predicted echolucency (Table 6.1). Neither SNAP-II nor SNAPPE-II predicted a statistically significant difference in the rates of cerebral palsy among children born extremely preterm. However, after adjusting for gestational age, high SNAP-II and SNAPPE-II predicted an mental developmental index (MDI) of <55, a psychomotor developmental index (PDI) of <55, and a positive screen for autism spectrum disorder (Table 6.2) (Dammann et al. 2010a).

Our findings suggest that, in isolation, physiologic derangements in the early postnatal period are less reliable at predicting adversities in extremely preterm infants. However, the cumulative effect of multiple physiologic derangements, as reflected by a composite illness-severity score (SNAP-II), can reliably predict both structural and functional brain disorders in children born extremely preterm.

Neurocognitive Outcomes at Age 10 Years

To our knowledge, the ELGAN study is the only multi-center study to have examined early postnatal illness-severity and school-age outcomes among children born extremely preterm. At age 10 years, 966 of the original cohort were recruited, 889 returned for follow-up, and 874 underwent neurocognitive testing.

Table 6.1   Point estimate (and 95% confidence intervals) of the odds ratio of each ultrasound lesion associated with each of the three different measures of high SNAP-II and SNAPPE-II.

SNAP classification	Cranial ultrasound lesion			
	IVH	VM	ED	EL
SNAP-II				
Score >30	2.0 (1.5, 2.7)	2.0 (1.4, 2.9)	1.5 (1.05, 2.1)	1.2 (0.8, 1.9)
Highest quartile for GA	1.8 (1.4, 2.4)	1.8 (1.2, 2.5)	1.2 (0.9, 1.7)	1.1 (0.7, 1.7)
Highest decile for GA	2.5 (1.7, 3.7)	2.3 (1.5, 3.6)	1.8 (1.1, 2.7)	1.6 (0.9, 2.8)
Z-score >1	2.1 (1.4, 3.1)	2.3 (1.4, 3.5)	1.5 (0.95, 2.3)	1.8 (1.1, 3.1)
SNAPPE-II				
Score >45	1.5 (1.2, 2.1)	1.8 (1.2, 2.6)	1.3 (0.9, 1.8)	1.0 (0.6, 1.6)
Highest quartile for GA	1.6 (1.2, 2.1)	1.6 (1.1, 2.2)	1.4 (0.98, 1.9)	1.1 (0.7, 1.7)
Highest decile for GA	1.5 (0.99, 2.2)	1.5 (0.9, 2.5)	1.4 (0.9, 2.2)	1.4 (0.8, 2.5)
Z-score >1	1.5 (0.98, 2.4)	1.5 (0.8, 2.6)	1.3 (0.8, 2.1)	1.3 (0.7, 2.5)

The referent group for each set of analyses consists of all newborns whose SNAP-II or SNAPPE-II was lower. All models are adjusted for gestational age (23–24, 24–26, and 27 weeks) and include a 'group' term for hospital. GA = gestational age; IVH = intraventricular hemorrhage; VM = ventriculomegaly; ED = echodense lesion; EL = echolucent lesion. Reproduced with permission from Dammann et al. (2010), Copyright © 2010 Karger Publishers, Basel, Switzerland.

Table 6.2 Point estimate (and 95% confidence intervals) of the odds ratio of each category of a low Bayley Scale associated with each of the three different measures of high SNAP-II and the three different measures of high SNAPPE-II.

SNAP classification	MDI		PDI	
	<55	55–69	<55	55–69
SNAP-II				
Score >30	1.4 (0.9, 2.2)	1.4 (0.8, 2.2)	1.7 (1.1, 2.5)	1.6 (1.01, 2.5)
Highest quartile for GA	1.3 (0.9, 2.0)	1.5 (0.96, 2.4)	1.9 (1.3, 2.8)	1.4 (0.9, 2.1)
Highest decile for GA	2.0 (1.1, 3.5)	1.1 (0.5, 2.2)	1.8 (1.1, 3.2)	1.4 (0.8, 2.7)
Z-score >1	1.7 (0.96, 3.1)	1.1 (0.5, 2.2)	1.7 (0.98, 3.0)	1.2 (0.6, 2.2)
SNAPPE-II				
Score >45	2.1 (1.4, 3.3)	1.7 (1.02, 2.7)	2.1 (1.4, 3.1)	2.2 (1.4, 3.4)
Highest quartile for GA	1.8 (1.2, 2.8)	1.4 (0.9, 2.3)	1.8 (1.2, 2.7)	1.6 (1.01, 2.5)
Highest decile for GA	1.6 (0.9, 2.9)	1.2 (0.6, 2.4)	1.9 (1.03, 3.4)	1.8 (0.98, 3.4)
Z-score >1	1.4 (0.7, 3.1)	1.5 (0.7, 3.3)	1.4 (0.7, 3.0)	2.0 (1.00, 4.0)

The referent group for each set of analyses consists of all newborns whose SNAP-II or SNAPPE-II was lower. All models are adjusted for gestational age (GA; 23–24, 25–26, and 27 weeks) and include a 'group' term for hospital. Reproduced with permission from Dammann et al. (2010), Copyright © 2010 Karger Publishers, Basel, Switzerland.

Of the 874 infants in the sample, 53% had a SNAP-II below 20, 25% had a SNAP-II between 20 and 29, and the remaining 23% had a SNAP-II ≥ 30. Examiners who were unaware of the child's medical history assessed a broad range of neurocognitive, behavioral and social outcomes. In the ELGAN sample, an elevated SNAP-II (≥ 30) was associated with an increased risk of cognitive impairment, neurologic adversities, behavioral and social dysfunctions, and education-related adversities at age 10 years as specified in the next paragraph (Logan et al. 2017).

After adjusting for confounders, Z-scores were greater than 1 standard deviation below the normative mean for 11 of 18 cognitive outcomes among children in the highest SNAP-II category, and for six of 18 cognitive outcomes among those in the intermediate (SNAP-II 10-19) SNAP-II category (see Fig. 6.4 for tools used and detailed results). Social dysfunctions were less prominent but were abnormal in two of the eight social dysfunction categories captured by the SRS-2 and ADOS-2 subtests for children in the highest SNAP-II category, and for three of eight in the intermediate SNAP-II category (not shown). Those with a high SNAP-II were also more likely than those with a low SNAP-II to have an individual education plan (IEP), to repeat a grade, to be placed in a remedial class, to be diagnosed or treated for ADHD, ASD, or epilepsy, to need an assistive device to ambulate, and to have diminished parent-reported quality of life.

WHAT IS THE RELATIONSHIP BETWEEN ILLNESS-SEVERITY AND EARLY NEONATAL PHYSIOLOGY?

The characteristic most strongly associated with a high SNAP-II is gestational age. Within each gestational age group, those with a SNAP-II ≥30 are at even greater risk of developmental dysfunctions than those with normal physiologic status (Dammann et al. 2010a; Logan et al. 2017). Infants with

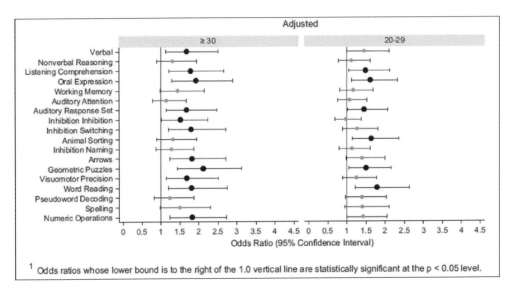

^{1} Odds ratios whose lower bound is to the right of the 1.0 vertical line are statistically significant at the p < 0.05 level.

Figure 6.4   Forest plots of odds ratios (ORs) and 95% confidence intervals of a Z-score ≤ –1 on each DAS-II and NEPSY-II neurocognitive assessment at age 10 associated with a SNAP-II ≥30 or a SNAP-II between 20 and 29. Odds ratios are adjusted for maternal education (≤12 and >12, or <16 years), public insurance, delivery for preeclampsia or fetal indication, gestational age (23–24 and 25–26 weeks) and BW Z-score (<–2 and ≥ –2, <–1). Reproduced with permission from Logan (2017), Copyright © 2017 by the Nature Publishing Group.

higher SNAP-II scores had a greater risk of death or disability, even after adjusting for gestational age (Dammann et al. 2009; Logan et al. 2017). This suggests that illness-severity conveys risk information *over and above* that conveyed by gestational age. We see several possible explanations for this. Because SNAP-II derives from clinical derangements in the early postnatal period, its association with subsequent adversities could be related to factors intrinsic to the pregnancy or delivery, factors that could affect the physiologic status of the newborn after delivery. However, SNAP-II might also convey information about physiologic maturation *not* related to gestational age such as endogenous (genetic or epigenetic) factors not well-described.

Postnatal physiologic depression is common among preterm infants, especially those born extremely preterm (Apgar 1953; Dawson et al. 2010; Saria et al. 2010) Antenatal exposures and events, especially inflammation, can potentially affect the physiologic status of preterm infants (Romero et al. 2007). The adverse effects of inflammation on physiologic status are likely related to the effects of inflammatory cytokines, chemokines, and other inflammatory mediators on end-organ function, including the cardiovascular, pulmonary, renal, endocrine, and hematopoietic systems (Romero et al. 2007). Numerous pregnancy disorders are associated with inflammation, increasing the risk of postnatal physiologic depression (Romero et al. 2007). Even in the absence of infection, inflammation increases the risk of physiologic instability in infants born preterm (Yanowitz et al. 2002; Romero et al. 2007). Therefore, the characteristics of the pregnancy and delivery are potentially important risk factors for physiologic instability in infants born extremely preterm (Villar et al. 2004).

Immature organ function increases the risk of physiologic instability among infants born preterm. Adaptive systems related to respiration, cardiovascular function, thermoregulation, autonomic control, hormone balance, and neuroprotection are often immature or poorly developed in infants born preterm. The physiologic response to resuscitative efforts in preterm infants is frequently delayed when compared to that of infants born at term (Dawson et al. 2010). Evidence suggests, for example, that gestational age significantly affects the time required to reach environment-skin temperature equilibration in very low birthweight infants (Dollberg 2001). Given the high frequency of maturation-dependent events among preterm infants (Saria et al. 2010; Poets et al. 2015), it would not be surprising if clinical prediction models derived from early postnatal clinical data were modified by maturation-dependent physiology (i.e. by factors related to gestational age). Thus, early postnatal physiologic status is related to organ maturation, and by extension, to the gestational age at birth.

However, differences in preterm physiology are potentially related to aspects of maturation that cannot be explained by gestational age alone (Logan et al. 2017). Significant differences in maturation (organ function) are common among infants of the same gestational age. Consider that not all infants born at 25 weeks gestation are alike. Some require intubation and mechanical ventilation, while others do not. Some are born with systemic hypotension, however it might be defined, while others are not (Limperopoulos et al. 2007). Differences in blood pressure, oxygen tension or thermoregulation, then, might reflect differences in end-organ maturation that are unrelated to gestational age. The etiology of these differences could derive from a variety of antenatal or perinatal exposures, as previously discussed. Antenatal steroid administration, for example, is associated with significant improvements in postnatal physiologic stability and outcomes, and the benefits are believed to derive from epigenetic modification of end-organ tissues (Fowden and Forhead 2015). Antenatal steroid administration is an example of an antenatal exposure that has favorable effects on end-organ maturation, but we suspect that pregnancy exposures can have adverse effects on end-organ maturation as well.

Some of our ELGAN colleagues have explored the concept of 'epigenetic age' in infants born less than 30 weeks' gestation (Everson and Marsit 2018). *Epigenetic age* is an estimate of physiologic development conveyed by DNA-based biomarkers (Horvath and Raj 2018). The concept derives from studies suggesting that physical development (end-organ function) is related to epigenetic age in children (Everson and Marsit 2018). Epigenetic age, for example, has been associated with measures of physical development such as stature (Simpkin et al. 2017), pubertal development (Simpkin et al. 2017), and endocrine function (Suarez et al. 2018). This suggests the possibility that epigenetic modifications early in life, perhaps as early as the antenatal period, could be associated with enhancements or decrements in physiologic maturity (Fowden and Forhead 2015). Using this paradigm, then, SNAP-II could be viewed as a marker for physiologic maturation not otherwise conveyed by gestational age.

Why Might Illness-Severity be Related to Developmental Dysfunctions?

One possible explanation for what we found is that physiologic instability is in the causal chain between immaturity (and its correlates) and brain injury in extremely preterm newborns. In this way, SNAP-II could be viewed as a marker for events that lie somewhere along the causal chain. While both hypoxemia and hypotension have been invoked in the pathogenesis of brain damage in very preterm newborns (Costeloe et al. 2000; Wood et al. 2000; Greisen and Vannucci 2001; Back et al. 2007; du Plessis 2009; Kuint et al. 2009; Arduini et al. 2014; Batton et al. 2016), sufficient support for these claims has not been provided (Limperopoulos et al. 2007; Logan et al. 2011a, 2011b; Saugstad and Aune 2014; Manja et al. 2015; Gilles et al. 2018). Despite efforts to improve physiologic stability (Laughon et al. 2007; Laptook and Watkinson 2008; Perlman et al. 2010; Carlo 2012; Smith et al. 2012; Kapadia et al. 2013; Barrington 2014; Saugstad and Aune 2014; Dempsey et al. 2015), the rate of neurodevelopmental limitations among extremely preterm infants remains high in numerous studies (Marlow et al. 2005; Johnson et al. 2009; Logan et al. 2011a, 2011b; Rysavy et al. 2015; Joseph et al. 2016; Plomgaard et al. 2016). Therefore, we are reluctant to adopt this view.

Another explanation is that the associations we observed are explained by unmeasured confounder(s), like bacteremia/sepsis, necrotizing enterocolitis, or chronic lung disease (Gray et al. 1995; Chien et al. 2002), all of which are associated with both inflammation and adverse brain-related outcomes (Shah et al. 2008; Alshaikh et al. 2014; Lee et al. 2014; Barton et al. 2016). In this way, SNAP-II could be viewed as a marker of illness severity that precedes adversities commonly associated with abnormal development. In the same way, SNAP-II could be viewed as a marker for systemic inflammation, which is associated with an increased risk of neurocognitive, behavioral and social dysfunctions (Leviton et al. 2011b; O'Shea et al. 2012; Kuban et al. 2014; O'Shea et al. 2014). Although physiologic derangements, in isolation, were not associated with systemic inflammation in the ELGAN study (Leviton et al. 2011a), preterm infants exposed to inflammatory conditions tend to have higher SNAP-IIs than children with normal or low SNAP-IIs (Gray et al. 1995; Chien et al. 2002) and these conditions are associated with developmental dysfunctions at follow-up (O'Shea et al. 2013).

A third explanation for our findings is that SNAP-II conveys information about immaturity/vulnerability, such as what might be attributed to a paucity of endogenous protectors (Dammann and Leviton 1999). According to this paradigm, SNAP-II provides information about physiologic maturation as a marker for developmentally regulated processes, including the ability to synthesize growth factors and proteins capable of protecting the brain (Dammann and Leviton 1999). For example, SNAP-II has been correlated with corticospinal tract development independent of both gestational age and postnatal risk factors, lending support to the theory that SNAP-II confers information about brain maturation (Zwicker et al. 2013).

CONCLUSION

While it may be difficult to ascertain exactly why illness-severity is associated with an increased risk of developmental dysfunctions in infants born preterm, it clearly provides meaningful information about the risk of subsequent adversities. We favor the view that illness-severity conveys information related to physiologic maturity and/or vulnerability. We suspect that numerous factors interact with the already immature preterm brain to either increase or decrease the risk of subsequent adversities. Those factors that increase organ maturation and physiologic stability, like antenatal steroid administration, will likely result in a more favorable outcome, while factors that interfere with organ maturation and physiologic stability, like bacteremia/sepsis, will likely result in a less favorable outcome.

Taken together, our findings provide support for the view that illness-severity is a developmentally regulated process in extremely preterm newborns. We suspect that numerous mechanisms exist for modification of these developmental processes, especially exposures and events that occur during gestation. For now, we await the results of additional genetic and epigenetic studies into relationships between early exposures and outcomes observed in adolescence and adulthood.

REFERENCES

Adams M, Braun J, Bucher Hu et al. (2017) Comparison of three different methods for risk adjustment in neonatal medicine. *BMC Pediatr* **17**: 106.

Alshaikh B, Yee W, Lodha A, Henderson E, Yusuf K, Sauve R (2014) Coagulase-negative staphylococcus sepsis in preterm infants and long-term neurodevelopmental outcome. *J Perinatol* **34**: 125–9.

Apgar, V (1953) A proposal for a new method of evaluation of the newborn infant. *Curr Res Anesth Analg* **32**: 260–7.

Arduini A, Escobar J, Vento M et al. (2014) Metabolic adaptation and neuroprotection differ in the retina and choroid in a piglet model of acute postnatal hypoxia. *Pediatr Res* **76**: 127–34.

Back SA, Craig A, Kayton RJ et al. (2007) Hypoxia-ischemia preferentially triggers glutamate depletion from oligo-dendroglia and axons in perinatal cerebral white matter. *J Cereb Blood Flow Metab* **27**: 334–47.

Barrington KJ (2014) Management during the first 72 h of age of the periviable infant: an evidence-based review. *Semin Perinatol* **38**: 17–24.

Barton SK, Tolcos M, Miller SL et al. (2016) Ventilation-induced brain injury in preterm neonates: a review of potential therapies. *Neonatology* **110**: 155–62.

Batton B, Li L, Newman NS et al. (2016) Early blood pressure, antihypotensive therapy and outcomes at 18–22 months' corrected age in extremely preterm infants. *Arch Dis Child Fetal Neonatal Ed* **101**: F201–6.

Baud O, Ville Y, Zupan V et al. (1998) Are neonatal brain lesions due to intrauterine infection related to mode of delivery? *Br J Obstet Gynaecol* **105**: 121–4.

Bejar RF, Vaucher YE, Benirschke K, Berry CC (1992) Postnatal white matter necrosis in preterm infants. *J Perinatol* **12**: 3–8.

Bührer C, Grimmer I, Metze B, Obladen M (2000) The CRIB (Clinical Risk Index for Babies) score and neurodevelopmental impairment at one year corrected age in very low birth weight infants. *Intensive Care Med* **26**: 325–9.

Carlo WA (2012) Gentle ventilation: the new evidence from the SUPPORT, COIN, VON, CURPAP, Colombian Network, and Neocosur Network trials. *Early Hum Dev* **88**(Suppl 2): S81–3.

Carvalho PR, Moreira ME, Sa RA, Lopes LM (2011) SNAPPE-II application in newborns with very low birth weight: evaluation of adverse outcomes in severe placental dysfunction. *J Perinat Med* **39**: 343–7.

Chien LY, Whyte R, Thiessen P et al. (2002) SNAP-II predicts severe intraventricular hemorrhage and chronic lung disease in the neonatal intensive care unit. *J Perinatol* **22**: 26–30.

Costeloe K, Hennessy E, Gibson AT, Marlow N, Wilkinson AR (2000) The EPICure study: outcomes to discharge from hospital for infants born at the threshold of viability. *Pediatrics* **106**: 659–71.

Cullen DJ, Civetta JM, Briggs BA, Ferrara LC (1974) Therapeutic intervention scoring system: a method for quantitative comparison of patient care. *Crit Care Med* **2**: 57–60.

Cunningham S, Symon AG, Elton RA, Zhu C, McIntosh N (1999) Intra-arterial blood pressure reference ranges, death and morbidity in very low birthweight infants during the first seven days of life. *Early Hum Dev* **56**: 151–65.

D'Souza SW, Janakova H, Minors D et al. (1995) Blood pressure, heart rate, and skin temperature in preterm infants: associations with periventricular haemorrhage. *Arch Dis Child Fetal Neonatal Ed* **72**: F162–7.

Dammann O, Allred EN, Kuban KC et al. (2002) Systemic hypotension and white-matter damage in preterm infants. *Dev Med Child Neurol* **44**: 82–90.

Dammann O, Leviton A (1999) Brain damage in preterm newborns: might enhancement of developmentally regulated endogenous protection open a door for prevention? *Pediatrics* **104**: 541–50.

Dammann O, Naples M, Bednarek F et al. (2010a) SNAP-II and SNAPPE-II and the risk of structural and functional brain disorders in extremely low gestational age newborns: the ELGAN study. *Neonatology* **97**: 71–82.

Dammann O, Naples M, Bednarek F et al. (2010b) SNAP-II and SNAPPE-II and the risk of structural and functional brain disorders in extremely low gestational age newborns: the ELGAN study. *Neonatology* **97**: 71–82.

Dammann O, Shah B, Naples M et al. (2009) Interinstitutional variation in prediction of death by SNAP-II and SNAPPE-II among extremely preterm infants. *Pediatrics* **124**: e1001–6.

Dawson JA, Kamlin CO, Wong C et al. (2010) Changes in heart rate in the first minutes after birth. *Arch Dis Child Fetal Neonatal Ed* **95**: F177–81.

De Vries LS, Regev R, Dubowitz LM, Whitelaw A, Aber VR (1988) Perinatal risk factors for the development of extensive cystic leukomalacia. *Am J Dis Child* **142**: 732–5.

Dempsey E, Pammi M, Ryan AC, Barrington KJ (2015) Standardised formal resuscitation training programmes for reducing mortality and morbidity in newborn infants. *Cochrane Database Syst Rev* **9**: CD009106.

Dollberg S (2001) Effects of gestation on thermoregulatory transition to extrauterine life. *NeoReviews* 2.

Dorling JS, Field DJ, Manktelow B (2005) Neonatal disease severity scoring systems. *Arch Dis Child Fetal Neonatal Ed* **90**: F11–6.

Du Plessis AJ (2009) The role of systemic hemodynamic disturbances in prematurity-related brain injury. *J Child Neurol* **24**: 1127–40.

Escobar GJ, Shaheen SM, Breed EM et al. (2004) Richardson score predicts short-term adverse respiratory outcomes in newborns >/=34 weeks gestation. *J Pediatr* **145**: 754–60.

Evans N, Kluckow M, Simmons M, Osborn D (2002) Which to measure, systemic or organ blood flow? Middle cerebral artery and superior vena cava flow in very preterm infants. *Arch Dis Child Fetal Neonatal Ed* **87**: F181–4.

Everson TM, Marsit CJ (2018) Integrating -omics approaches into human population-based studies of prenatal and early-life exposures. *Curr Environ Health Rep* **5**: 328–37.

Fortes Filho JB, Dill JC, Ishizaki A, Aguiar WW, Silveira RC, Procianoy RS (2009) Score for neonatal acute physiology and perinatal extension II as a predictor of retinopathy of prematurity: study in 304 very-low-birth-weight preterm infants. *Ophthalmologica* **223**: 177–82.

Fowden AL, Forhead AJ (2015) Glucocorticoids as regulatory signals during intrauterine development. *Exp Physiol* **100**: 1477–87.

Gagliardi L, Cavazza A, Brunelli A et al. (2004) Assessing mortality risk in very low birthweight infants: a comparison of CRIB, CRIB-II, and SNAPPE-II. *Arch Dis Child Fetal Neonatal Ed* **89**: F419–22.

Gilles F, Gressens P, Dammann O, Leviton A (2018) Hypoxia-ischemia is not an antecedent of most preterm brain damage: the illusion of validity. *Dev Med Child Neurol* **60**: 120–5.

Gray JE, Richardson DK, McCormick MC, Goldmann DA (1995) Coagulase-negative staphylococcal bacteremia among very low birth weight infants: relation to admission illness severity, resource use, and outcome. *Pediatrics* **95**: 225–30.

Greenwood S, Abdel-Latif ME, Bajuk B, Lui K (2012) Can the early condition at admission of a high-risk infant aid in the prediction of mortality and poor neurodevelopmental outcome? A population study in Australia. *J Paediatr Child Health* **48**: 588–95.

Greisen G, Vannucci RC (2001) Is periventricular leucomalacia a result of hypoxic-ischaemic injury? Hypocapnia and the preterm brain. *Biol Neonate* **79**: 194–200.

Hagadorn JI, Richardson DK, Schmid CH, Cole CH (2007) Cumulative illness severity and progression from moderate to severe retinopathy of prematurity. *J Perinatol* **27**: 502–9.

Hentschel R, Guenther K, Vach W, Bruder I (2018) Risk-adjusted mortality of VLBW infants in high-volume versus low-volume NICUs. *Arch Dis Child Fetal Neonatal Ed.* **104**: F390–5.

Horvath S, Raj K (2018) DNA methylation-based biomarkers and the epigenetic clock theory of ageing. *Nat Rev Genet* **19**: 371–84.

Johnson S, Hennessy E, Smith R, Trikic R, Wolke D, Marlow N (2009) Academic attainment and special educational needs in extremely preterm children at 11 years of age: the EPICure study. *Arch Dis Child Fetal Neonatal Ed* **94**: F283–9.

Joseph RM, O'Shea TM, Allred EN et al. (2016) Neurocognitive and academic outcomes at age 10 years of extremely preterm newborns. *Pediatrics* **137**: e20154343.

Kapadia VS, Chalak LF, Sparks JE, Allen JR, Savani RC, Wyckoff MH (2013) Resuscitation of preterm neonates with limited versus high oxygen strategy. *Pediatrics* **132**: e1488–96.

Kissack CM, Garr R, Wardle SP, Weindling AM (2004) Postnatal changes in cerebral oxygen extraction in the preterm infant are associated with intraventricular hemorrhage and hemorrhagic parenchymal infarction but not periventricular leukomalacia. *Pediatr Res* **56**: 111–6.

Kluckow M, Evans N (2000) Low superior vena cava flow and intraventricular haemorrhage in preterm infants. *Arch Dis Child Fetal Neonatal Ed* **82**: F188–94.

Knaus WA, Zimmerman JE, Wagner DP, Draper EA, Lawrence DE (1981) APACHE-acute physiology and chronic health evaluation: a physiologically based classification system. *Crit Care Med* **9**: 591–7.

Kuban KC, O'Shea TM, Allred EN et al. (2014) Systemic inflammation and cerebral palsy risk in extremely preterm infants. *J Child Neurol* **29**: 1692–8.

Kuint J, Barak M, Morag I, Maayan-Metzger A (2009) Early treated hypotension and outcome in very low birth weight infants. *Neonatology* **95**: 311–6.

Lagatta J, Andrews B, Caldarelli L, Schreiber M, Plesha-Troyke S, Meadow W (2011) Early neonatal intensive care unit therapy improves predictive power for the outcomes of ventilated extremely low birth weight infants. *J Pediatr* **159**: 384–91 e1.

Laptook AR, Watkinson M (2008) Temperature management in the delivery room. *Semin Fetal Neonatal Med* **13**: 383–91.

Laughon M, Bose C, Allred E et al. (2007) Factors associated with treatment for hypotension in extremely low gestational age newborns during the first postnatal week. *Pediatrics* **119**: 273–80.

Lee I, Neil JJ, Huettner PC (2014) The impact of prenatal and neonatal infection on neurodevelopmental outcomes in very preterm infants. *J Perinatol* **34**: 741–7.

Leviton A, Allred E, Kuban KC et al. (2010) Early blood gas abnormalities and the preterm brain. *Am J Epidemiol* **172**: 907–16.

Leviton A, Allred EN, Kuban KC et al. (2011a) Blood protein concentrations in the first two postnatal weeks associated with early postnatal blood gas derangements among infants born before the 28th week of gestation. The ELGAN study. *Cytokine* **56**: 392–8.

Leviton A, Kuban KC, Allred EN et al. (2011b) Early postnatal blood concentrations of inflammation-related proteins and microcephaly two years later in infants born before the 28th post-menstrual week. *Early Hum Dev* **87**: 325–30.

Limperopoulos C, Bassan H, Kalish LA et al. (2007) Current definitions of hypotension do not predict abnormal cranial ultrasound findings in preterm infants. *Pediatrics* **120**: 966–77.

Littman B, Parmelee AH Jr (1978) Medical correlates of infant development. *Pediatrics* **61**: 470–4.

Lodha A, Sauve R, Chen S, Tang S, Christianson H (2009) Clinical Risk Index for Babies score for the prediction of neurodevelopmental outcomes at 3 years of age in infants of very low birthweight. *Dev Med Child Neurol* **51**: 895–900.

Logan JW, Dammann O, Allred EN et al. (2017) Early postnatal illness severity scores predict neurodevelopmental impairments at 10 years of age in children born extremely preterm. *J Perinatol* **37**: 606–14.

Logan JW, O'Shea TM, Allred EN et al. (2011a) Early postnatal hypotension and developmental delay at 24 months of age among extremely low gestational age newborns. *Arch Dis Child Fetal Neonatal Ed* **96**: F321–8.

Logan JW, O'Shea TM, Allred EN et al. (2011b) Early postnatal hypotension is not associated with indicators of white matter damage or cerebral palsy in extremely low gestational age newborns. *J Perinatol* **31**: 524–34.

Manja V, Lakshminrusimha S, Cook DJ (2015) Oxygen saturation target range for extremely preterm infants: a systematic review and meta-analysis. *JAMA Pediatr* **169**: 332–40.

Marcin JP, Pollack MM, Patel KM, Ruttimann UE (2000) Combining physician's subjective and physiology-based objective mortality risk predictions. *Crit Care Med* **28**: 2984–90.

Marlow N, Wolke D, Bracewell MA, Samara M (2005) Neurologic and developmental disability at six years of age after extremely preterm birth. *N Engl J Med* **352**: 9–19.

Meadow W, Lagatta J, Andrews B, Lantos J (2012) The mathematics of morality for neonatal resuscitation. *Clin Perinatol* **39**: 941–56.

Meadow W, Meadow X, Tanz RR, Lagatta J, Lantos J (2011) The value of a trial of therapy – football as a 'proof-of-concept.' *Acta Paediatr* **100**: 167–9.

Meek JH, Tyszczuk L, Elwell CE, Wyatt JS (1999) Low cerebral blood flow is a risk factor for severe intraventricular haemorrhage. *Arch Dis Child Fetal Neonatal Ed* **81**: F15–8.

Ment LR, Duncan CC, Ehrenkranz RA et al. (1984) Intraventricular hemorrhage in the preterm neonate: timing and cerebral blood flow changes. *J Pediatr* **104**: 419–25.

Miletin J, Dempsey EM (2008) Low superior vena cava flow on day 1 and adverse outcome in the very low birth-weight infant. *Arch Dis Child Fetal Neonatal Ed* **93**: F368–71.

Morse S, Groer M, Shelton MM, Maguire D, Ashmeade T (2015) A systematic review: the utility of the revised version of the score for neonatal acute physiology among critically Ill neonates. *J Perinat Neonatal Nurs* **29**: 315–44; quiz E2.

O'Shea TM, Allred EN, Kuban KC et al. (2012) Elevated concentrations of inflammation-related proteins in postnatal blood predict severe developmental delay at 2 years of age in extremely preterm infants. *J Pediatr* **160**: 395–401, e4.

O'Shea TM, Joseph RM, Kuban KC et al. (2014) Elevated blood levels of inflammation-related proteins are associated with an attention problem at age 24 mo in extremely preterm infants. *Pediatr Res* **75**: 781–7.

O'Shea TM, Shah B, Allred EN et al. (2013) Inflammation-initiating illnesses, inflammation-related proteins, and cognitive impairment in extremely preterm infants. *Brain Behav Immun* **29**: 104–12.

Osborn DA, Evans N, Kluckow M (2003) Hemodynamic and antecedent risk factors of early and late periventricular/intraventricular hemorrhage in premature infants. *Pediatrics* **112**: 33–9.

Parry G, Tucker J, Tarnow-Mordi W (2003) CRIB II: an update of the clinical risk index for babies score. *Lancet* **361**: 1789–91.

Perlman JM, Risser R, Broyles RS (1996) Bilateral cystic periventricular leukomalacia in the premature infant: associated risk factors. *Pediatrics* **97**: 822–7.

Perlman JM, Wyllie J, Kattwinkel J et al. (2010) Neonatal resuscitation: 2010 international consensus on cardiopulmonary resuscitation and emergency cardiovascular care science with treatment recommendations. *Pediatrics* **126**: e1319–44.

Perlstein PH, Atherton HD, Donovan EF, Richardson DK, Kotagal UR (1997) Physician variations and the ancillary costs of neonatal intensive care. *Health Serv Res* **32**: 299–311.

Plomgaard AM, Hagmann C, Alderliesten T et al. (2016) Brain injury in the international multicenter randomized SafeBoosC phase II feasibility trial: cranial ultrasound and magnetic resonance imaging assessments. *Pediatr Res* **79**: 466–72.

Poets CF, Roberts RS, Schmidt B et al. (2015) Association between intermittent hypoxemia or bradycardia and late death or disability in extremely preterm infants. *JAMA* **314**: 595–603.

Pollack MM, Koch MA, Bartel DA et al. (2000) A comparison of neonatal mortality risk prediction models in very low birth weight infants. *Pediatrics* **105**: 1051–7.

Pollack MM, Ruttimann UE, Getson PR (1987) Accurate prediction of the outcome of pediatric intensive care. A new quantitative method. *N Engl J Med* **316**: 134–9.

Richardson DK, Corcoran JD, Escobar GJ, Lee SK (2001) SNAP-II and SNAPPE-II: simplified newborn illness severity and mortality risk scores. *J Pediatr* **138**: 92–100.

Richardson DK, Gray JE, Gortmaker SL, Goldmann DA, Pursley DM, McCormick MC (1998) Declining severity adjusted mortality: evidence of improving neonatal intensive care. *Pediatrics* **102**: 893–9.

Richardson DK, Gray JE, McCormick MC, Workman K, Goldmann DA (1993a) Score for neonatal acute physiology: a physiologic severity index for neonatal intensive care. *Pediatrics* **91**: 617–23.

Richardson DK, Phibbs CS, Gray JE, McCormick MC, Workman-Daniels K, Goldmann DA (1993b) Birth weight and illness severity: independent predictors of neonatal mortality. *Pediatrics* **91**: 969–75.

Richardson DK, Shah BL, Frantz ID, 3rd, Bednarek F, Rubin LP, McCormick MC (1999) Perinatal risk and severity of illness in newborns at 6 neonatal intensive care units. *Am J Public Health* **89**: 511–6.

Romero R, Espinoza J, Goncalves LF, Kusanovic JP, Friel L, Hassan S (2007) The role of inflammation and infection in preterm birth. *Semin Reprod Med* **25**: 21–39.

Rysavy MA, Li L, Bell EF et al. (2015) Between-hospital variation in treatment and outcomes in extremely preterm infants. *N Engl J Med* **372**: 1801–11.

Saria S, Rajani AK, Gould J, Koller D, Penn AA (2010) Integration of early physiological responses predicts later illness severity in preterm infants. *Sci Transl Med* **2**: 48ra65.

Saugstad OD, Aune D (2014) Optimal oxygenation of extremely low birth weight infants: a meta-analysis and systematic review of the oxygen saturation target studies. *Neonatology* **105**: 55–63.

Shah DK, Doyle LW, Anderson PJ et al. (2008) Adverse neurodevelopment in preterm infants with postnatal sepsis or necrotizing enterocolitis is mediated by white matter abnormalities on magnetic resonance imaging at term. *J Pediatr* **153**: 170–5, 175 e1.

Simpkin AJ, Howe LD, Tilling K et al. (2017) The epigenetic clock and physical development during childhood and adolescence: longitudinal analysis from a UK birth cohort. *Int J Epidemiol* **46**: 549–58.

Smith PB, Ambalavanan N, Li L et al. (2012) Approach to infants born at 22 to 24 weeks' gestation: relationship to outcomes of more-mature infants. *Pediatrics* **129**: e1508–16.

Suarez A, Lahti J, Czamara D et al. (2018) The epigenetic clock and pubertal, neuroendocrine, psychiatric, and cognitive outcomes in adolescents. *Clin Epigenetics* **10**: 96.

Synnes A, Luu TM, Moddemann D et al. (2017) Determinants of developmental outcomes in a very preterm Canadian cohort. *Arch Dis Child Fetal Neonatal Ed* **102**: F235–F234.

Trounce JQ, Shaw DE, Levene MI, Rutter N (1988) Clinical risk factors and periventricular leucomalacia. *Arch Dis Child* **63**: 17–22.

Tsuji M, Saul JP, Du Plessis A et al. (2000) Cerebral intravascular oxygenation correlates with mean arterial pressure in critically ill premature infants. *Pediatrics* **106**: 625–32.

Vassar MJ, Holcroft JW (1994) The case against using the APACHE system to predict intensive care unit outcome in trauma patients. *Crit Care Clin* **10**: 117–26; discussion 127–34.

Villar J, Abalos E, Carroli G et al. (2004) Heterogeneity of perinatal outcomes in the preterm delivery syndrome. *Obstet Gynecol* **104**: 78–87.

Wiswell TE, Graziani LJ, Kornhauser MS et al. (1996) Effects of hypocarbia on the development of cystic periventricular leukomalacia in premature infants treated with high-frequency jet ventilation. *Pediatrics* **98**: 918–24.

Wood NS, Marlow N, Costeloe K, Gibson AT, Wilkinson AR (2000). Neurologic and developmental disability after extremely preterm birth. EPICure Study Group. *N Engl J Med* **343**: 378–84.

Yanowitz TD, Jordan JA, Gilmour CH et al. (2002) Hemodynamic disturbances in premature infants born after chorioamnionitis: association with cord blood cytokine concentrations. *Pediatr Res* **51**: 310–6.

Yeh TS, Pollack MM, Ruttimann UE, Holbrook PR, Fields AI (1984) Validation of a physiologic stability index for use in critically ill infants and children. *Pediatr Res* **18**: 445–51.

Zupancic JA, Richardson DK (1998) Characterization of the triage process in neonatal intensive care. *Pediatrics* **102**: 1432–6.

Zupancic JA, Richardson DK, Horbar JD et al. (2007) Revalidation of the Score for neonatal acute physiology in the Vermont Oxford network. *Pediatrics* **119**: e156–63.

Zwicker JG, Grunau RE, Adams E et al. (2013) Score for neonatal acute physiology-II and neonatal pain predict corticospinal tract development in premature newborns. *Pediatr Neurol* **48**: 123–129 e1.

Bacteremia

H Reeve Bright and Kikelomo Babata

INTRODUCTION AND BACKGROUND

Bacteremia is a microbiological finding defined as presence of bacteria in blood (Hagel et al. 2013). Sepsis, on the other hand, is a clinical diagnosis is based on the exhibition of a systemic inflammatory response (manifested by temperature instability, heart rate irregularities, respiratory insufficiency, and leukocyte count abnormalities) (Henneke and Berner 2006) combined with a documented or suspected infection (Girard and Ely 2007). Bacteremia, which disproportionately affects extremely preterm newborns, contributes significantly to their heightened risk of death and multiple lifelong adverse outcomes (Raju et al. 2017; Bright et al. 2017). The risk of death is increased from 7% to 18% in some cohorts (Stoll et al. 2002). The ELGAN study with its gestational age-based cohort and its continued detailed longitudinal assessments provides the opportunity for an in depth understanding of the antecedents, associations and outcomes of bacteremia (Bright et al. 2017).

CLASSIFICATION

Neonatal bacteremia has been classified as early or late, distinguishing infections presumed to have been acquired during labor and delivery from postnatal nosocomial infections (Patel et al. 2011). We defined definite bacteremia as recovery of an organism from the blood. We defined suspected bacteremia as culture negative sepsis requiring antibiotics for more than 72 hours (Patel et al. 2011).

PREVALENCE/INCIDENCE

In the ELGAN study, definite early bacteremia occurred in 6% of newborns, while definite late bacteremia occurred in 24%. Infants with the lowest BW Z-score (< −2) and gestational age (23–24 weeks) were disproportionately affected. Up to 33–34% of them had at least one episode of definite late bacteremia. A trend is evident below with increasing incidence of bacteremia with reducing GA or BW Z-score (Patel et al. 2011; Bright et al. 2017) (Table 7.1).

Interestingly, we also found a higher rate of definite late bacteremia in infants who were born to mothers who had no more than a high school education, who were eligible for government-provided medical care insurance, or identified as black (Bright et al. 2017). This was surprising, but not unreported (Profit et al. 2017).

Widespread Implementation of 2002 CDC Group B Strep guidelines resulted in a significant reduction in early onset Group B strep sepsis in the years 1995–2005 (Phares et al. 2008). The same has not been found for the most frequent early onset sepsis pathogen in the preterm infant, *E. coli* (Stoll et al. 2011).

Table 7.1   Incidence of bacteremia (%) by gestational age (weeks) and birthweight Z-score (Patel et al. 2011; Bright et al. 2017)

	Early bacteremia (%)		Late bacteremia (%)	
	Suspected	**Definite**	**Suspected**	**Definite**
Gestational age (weeks)				
23–24	40	8	19	**33**
25–26	34	8	16	27
27	34	4	11	20
Birthweight Z-score[a]				
< −2	43	9	20	**34**
>/= −2, < −1	39	6	17	32
>/= −1	34	6	14	24

[a] Number of standard deviations.

Between the years of 1993 to 2012, the overall rates of early onset sepsis did not show significant change (Stoll et al. 2015). Late bacteremia, on the other hand, has shown a significant decline (Stoll et al. 2015). This success has been attributed to improvement in hand hygiene, skin care, antibiotic stewardship, early breast milk feeding, and central line bundles (Stoll et al. 2015).

MECHANISM/PATHOPHYSIOLOGY

Inefficient Immature System

Polymorphonuclear (PMNs) cells and macrophages in the extremely preterm infant may be decreased in function (Clapp 2006). Not only is there inadequate recruitment of PMNs to areas with microbial invasion, their phagocytic and microbiocidal functions are limited in times of stress (Clapp 2006). Inhibitory mechanisms to activity of toll-like receptors have been noted. This is thought to prevent inflammation and preterm delivery. Unfortunately, paradoxically, this leaves the extremely preterm exposed and vulnerable to infection (Clapp 2006). This, at least in part, explains why up to one-third of the most immature infants will have an episode of definite bacteremia during their NICU stay (Bright et al. 2017).

Persistent Inflammation

Epidemiologic studies suggest that mediators of inflammation might be the link between infection and brain abnormalities (Dammann and O'Shea 2008). Preterm infants are at risk of impaired resolution of inflammation due to reduced anti-inflammatory proteins. Resistance of activated neutrophils to apoptosis also contributes to this continued cascade. There is also a lack of appropriate developmental regulation leading to a sustained and persistent inflammatory response (Dammann and Leviton 2014).

Immature Vulnerable Brain

Between 23 and 27 weeks of gestational age, the developmental process is particularly vulnerable. Neuronal precursors migrate from the germinal plate to their final destination and oligodendrocyte precursors undergo a maturational process to transform into oligodendrocytes (Leviton and Gressens 2007).

Table 7.2 Number of elevated inflammatory proteins in top quartile for gestational age and the corresponding inflammatory proteins (Leviton et al. 2012a)

	Early bacteremia		Late bacteremia	
	Suspected	**Definite**	**Suspected**	**Definite**
Day 1	–	*CRP, IL-8*	–	–
Day 7	*MMP-9, VEGF*	*CRP, IL-8, SAA, TNF-alpha, TNF-R2, ICAM-1, VEGF-R2*		*CRP, SAA, TNF-R2, IL-8*
Day 14	–	–	–	*CRP, SAA, IL-6, TNF-alpha, TNF-R2, IL-8, MIP-1B, I-TAC, ICAM-1, E-SEL, VEGF-R2*

Furthermore, the immature brain is in a heightened excitatory state, making the brain vulnerable to injury from stress secondary to inflammatory and metabolic disorders (Johnston et al. 2009). The developing brains of ELGANs also lack protection from adversity, as they cannot yet synthesize adequate amounts of neurotrophins to protect neurons and oligodendroglia (Clapp 2006; Dammann et al. 2008).

In the ELGAN study, we have shown the elevation of systemic markers for inflammation is associated with an increased risk for cerebral palsy, ventriculomegaly, and microcephaly at age 2, and cognitive impairment at age 10 (Kuban et al. 2015, 2017). The bacteremia type with the strongest inflammatory foot print was late bacteremia (Table 7.2) (Leviton et al. 2012a), which we have in turn shown to be associated with cognitive and social impairment at 10 years of age (Bright et al. 2017; Babata et al. 2018).

The persistent inflammation due to bacteremia and an immature immune system in the setting of an underdeveloped brain are all a perfect set-up for heightened risk of brain damage. Despite this and the above data, nearly half of all the children in the ELGAN study who had definite late bacteremia had scores within the normal range on their DAS IQ evaluations (Bright et al. 2017). Some predictors of improved outcome in ELGANS include female sex (Dammann et al. 2016), maternal educational achievement, and continued educational advancement (Joseph et al. 2018).

ANTECEDENTS, ASSOCIATIONS, AND OUTCOMES

We studied antenatal and newborn characteristics, along with post-natal exposures (Table 7.3). Not unexpectedly, we found maternal and pregnancy characteristics were associated with early bacteremia. Late bacteremia, on the other hand, was associated with neonatal comorbidities, most important of which were necrotizing enterocolitis (NEC) and isolated intestinal perforation. All forms of bacteremia were associated with the lowest birthweight Z-score and lowest gestational age.

Risk patterns were not significantly different for suspected and definite late bacteremia (Patel et al. 2011). Importantly, we noted that neither the use of antenatal steroids nor the recovery of an organism from the placenta increased the rate of either form of bacteremia. Also, neither preeclampsia nor its histologic correlates were associated with bacteremia.

We studied definite late bacteremia in greater depth as it not only had a higher prevalence than definite early bacteriema (6% vs 24%) (Martin et al. 2010), it also elicited a stronger associated inflammatory response of all four forms of bacteremia (Leviton et al. 2012b). At 2 and 10 years of age, we found that sustained elevation of inflammatory proteins was associated with an increased risk of

Table 7.3   Maternal characteristics, placental histology, infant characteristics, and postnatal exposures associated with presumed and definite early and late bacteremia (Patel et al. 2011)

Early	Presumed	Maternal characteristics	Vaginitis
		Placenta histology	Decidual hemosiderin/fibrin, umbilical cord vasculitis
		Infant characteristics	CNS infection
		Postnatal exposures	Arterial or venous umbilical line
	Definite	Maternal characteristics	Vaginitis, aspirin consumption, prolonged labor, prolonged ROM, cervical insufficiency, and high-risk hospital birth
		Placenta histology	Umbilical cord vasculitis and decidual hemosiderin/fibrin
		Infant characteristics	Fetal indication for delivery, birthweight Z-score <−2, Gestational age 23–24 weeks, CNS infection, and Isolated intestinal perforation
		Postnatal exposures	Central line placement and arterial or venous umbilical line
Late	Presumed	Maternal characteristics	None
		Placenta histology	Placental infarct
		Infant characteristics	Gestational age 23–24 weeks and gestational age 25–26 weeks
		Postnatal exposures	Central line placement, arterial or venous umbilical line, CNS infection, and NEC Stage I-II
	Definite	Maternal characteristics	High-risk hospital birth
		Placenta histology	Umbilical vasculitis
		Infant characteristics	Gestational age 23–24 weeks, gestational age 25–26 weeks, and birthweight Z-score < −1
		Postnatal exposures	Arterial or venous umbilical line, PDA treatment, NEC stage I-II, NEC, Bell stage III, isolated intestinal perforation, pulmonary hemorrhage, and oxygen dependency at 36 weeks GA (chronic lung disease/bronchopulmonary dysplasia)

[a] RR < 1

neurodevelopmental delays/cognitive impairment (Leviton et al. 2013; Kuban et al. 2017). We have also found similar risks of cognitive and social impairment, mostly in ELGANS with definite late bacteremia (Babata et al. 2018). Infants with suspected bacteremia, unsurprisingly, in their outcome profile, were mostly similar to those with no bacteremia (Bright et al. 2017).

ASSESSMENTS AT AGE 2 YEARS

A combination of late bacteremia and surgical NEC was associated with an almost 8-times risk of leg dominated bilateral (diparetic) cerebral palsy, compared to children who had neither late bacteremia nor surgical NEC (Martin et al. 2010). Late bacteremia by itself was associated with an increased risk of an MDI below 70 (Martin et al. 2010). We also studied bacteremia alongside other inflammation initiating illnesses and their accompanying inflammation markers. Interestingly, NEC IIIB, bacteremia, and mechanical ventilation on postnatal day 14 were not individually associated with an MDI <55 on Bayley II. However, bacteremia in combination with mechanical ventilation on day 14 was associated with an elevated risk of an MDI <55 (3 standard deviations below the expected mean) (Leviton et al. 2013), independent of protein elevation (O'Shea et al. 2013).

ASSESSMENTS AT AGE 10 YEARS

Our 10-year follow up studies provided us the opportunity to understand the associations of bacteremia with the finer aspects of cognitive function. Various studies (Luttikhuizen et al. 2013), including ours (O'Shea et al. 2018) have shown that dysfunctions identified at age 2 do not necessarily fully correlate with dysfunctions identified at later ages, with most ELGANs with a low Bayley II MDI at age 2 years having normal cognitive function at 10 years of age.

In comparison to infants with no or suspected bacteremia, those with definite late bacteremia had a higher predominance of lower IQ scores, language, academic achievement and some measures of executive function (Table 7.4). Most of these associations remained after adjustment for sociodemographic

Table 7.4 Age 10 distribution of cognitive abilities (*Differential Ability Scales Second edition DAS-II*), academic achievement (*Wechsler Individual Achievement Test, 3rd edition WIAT-III*), language (*Oral and Written Language Scales OWLS and Child Communication Checklist 2 CCC-2*), social skills (*Social Responsiveness Scale SRS and Autism disorder diagnoses*), and executive function (*DAS-II and NEPSY-II*) by bacteremia category (Bright et al. 2017; Babata et al. 2018)

	Late bacteremia (%)		
	None	**Suspected**	**Definite**
IQ (DAS-II)			
Verbal (Z-score ≤−2)	13	16	28
Nonverbal (Z-score ≤−2)	13	14	20
Academic achievement (WIAT-III)			
Word reading (Z-score ≤−2)	9	13	19
Pseudoword decoding (Z-score ≤−2)	12	14	20
Spelling (Z-score ≤−2)	8	12	18
Numerical operations (Z-score ≤−2)	14	14	24
Language (OWLS and CCC-2)			
OWLS listening comprehension (Z-score ≤−2)	17	20	24
OWLS oral expression (Z-score ≤−2)	17	16	29
Low Q structural language total	19	37	33
Low Q pragmatic language total	21	29	31
Socioemotional outcomes			
SRS total >76	9	17	18
Autism spectrum disorder	5	9	11
Executive function			
DAS-II working memory	15	16	25
NEPSY-II auditory attention	20	26	26
NEPSY-II auditory response set	17	23	25
NEPSY-II inhibition	29	37	41
NEPSY-II inhibition switching	23	30	37
NEPSY-II animal sorting	24	29	39

Data shown are column percentages.

variables (maternal race, maternal education ≤12 years, public insurance, gestational age, and birth weight Z-score), but disappeared after adjusting for IQ. This suggests the possibility that impairments associated with late-bacteremia are a result of low cognitive abilities (Bright et al. 2017).

For socioemotional and social communication impairment, both forms of late bacteremia seemed to have an association, though greater with definite bacteremia (Table 7.2). Interestingly, the socio-emotional impairments we noted with late bacteremia were independent of autism diagnoses. We did not find a statistically significant increased risk of autism with exposure to either form of late bacteremia (Babata et al. 2018).

RECOMMENDATIONS AND IMPLICATIONS OF FUTURE RESEARCH

Aggressive management of preterm labor (Malone 2016), meticulous hand hygiene, skin care, early breast milk nutrition, and improved central line practices all hold great potential for reducing the burden of neonatal bacteremia (Stoll et al. 2015; Bright et al. 2017).

Continued investigation into inflammation modulating therapies offer potential hope in mitigating some of the adverse neurocognitive outcomes we have reported (Martin et al. 2010; Bright et al. 2017).

Judicious antibiotic stewardship will reduce the antibiotic utilization for suspected bacteremia. This would reduce the reported short-term increased risk of NEC, late bacteremia, death, broncho-pulmonary dysplasia (BPD) (Flannery and Puopolo 2018) and the early childhood increased risk of neurobehavioral symptoms (Slykerman et al. 2017).

Lastly, as shown in Table 7.4, roughly 60–90% of children with late bacteremia do not have severe limitations identified on each line It is important to study these infants in comparison to their peers in order to learn more about potential environmental, or other, factors that mitigate the adverse outcomes of late bacteremia.

REFERENCES

Babata K, Bright HR, Allred EN et al. (2018) Socioemotional dysfunctions at age 10 years in extremely preterm newborns with late-onset bacteremia. *Early Human Development* **121**: 1–7.

Bright HR, Babata K, Allred EN et al. (2017) Neurocognitive outcomes at 10 years of age in extremely preterm newborns with late-onset bacteremia. *The Journal of Pediatrics* **187**: 43–9.e1.

Clapp DW (2006) Developmental regulation of the immune system. *Seminars in Perinatology* **30**: 69–72.

Dammann O, Allred EN, Fichorova RN et al. (2016) Duration of systemic inflammation in the first postnatal month among infants born before the 28th week of gestation. *Inflammation* **39**: 672–7.

Dammann O, Bueter W, Leviton A, Gressens P, Dammann CE (2008) Neuregulin-1: a potential endogenous protector in perinatal brain white matter damage. *Neonatology* **93**: 182–7.

Dammann O, Leviton A (2014) Intermittent or sustained systemic inflammation and the preterm brain. *Pediatr Res* **75**: 376–80.

Dammann O, O'Shea TM (2008) Cytokines and perinatal brain damage. *Clinics in Perinatology* **35**: 643–63.

Flannery DD, Puopolo KM (2018) Neonatal antibiotic use: what are we doing and where shall we go? *NeoReviews* **19**: e516–e25.

Girard TD, Ely EW (2007) Bacteremia and sepsis in older adults. *Clinics in Geriatric Medicine* **23**: 633–47, viii.

Hagel S, Pletz MW, Brunkhorst FM, Seifert H, Kern WV (2013) Bacteremia and sepsis. *Der Internist* **54**: 399–407.

Henneke P, Berner R (2006) SIRS and group-B streptococcal sepsis in newborns: pathogenesis and perspectives in adjunctive therapy. *Seminars in Fetal & Neonatal Medicine* **11**: 333–42.

Johnston MV, Ishida A, Ishida WN, Matsushita HB, Nishimura A, Tsuji M (2009) Plasticity and injury in the developing brain. *Brain & Development* **31**: 1–10.

Joseph RM, O'Shea TM, Allred EN, Heeren T, Kuban KK (2018) Maternal educational status at birth, maternal educational advancement, and neurocognitive outcomes at age 10 years among children born extremely preterm. *Pediatr Res* **83**: 767–77.

Kuban KC, Joseph RM, O'Shea TM et al. (2017) Circulating inflammatory-associated proteins in the first month of life and cognitive impairment at age 10 years in children born extremely preterm. *J Pediatr* **180**: 116–23 e1.

Kuban KC, O'Shea TM, Allred EN et al. (2015) The breadth and type of systemic inflammation and the risk of adverse neurological outcomes in extremely low gestation newborns. *Pediatr Neurol* **52**: 42–8.

Leviton A, Fichorova RN, O'Shea TM et al. (2013) Two-hit model of brain damage in the very preterm newborn: small for gestational age and postnatal systemic inflammation. *Pediatr Res* **73**: 362–70.

Leviton A, Gressens P (2007) Neuronal damage accompanies perinatal white-matter damage. *Trends in Neurosciences* **30**: 473–8.

Leviton A, O'Shea TM, Bednarek FJ et al. (2012a) Systemic responses of preterm newborns with presumed or documented bacteraemia. *Acta Paediatrica* **101**: 355–9.

Leviton A, O'Shea TM, Bednarek FJ, Allred EN, Fichorova RN, Dammann O (2012b) Systemic responses of preterm newborns with presumed or documented bacteraemia. *Acta Paediatr* **101**: 355–9.

Luttikhuizen dos Santos ES, de Kieviet JF, Königs M, van Elburg RM, Oosterlaan J (2013) Predictive value of the Bayley scales of infant development on development of very preterm/very low birth weight children: a meta-analysis. *Early Hum Dev*. **89**: 487–96.

Malone FD (2016) What is new in the management of acute preterm labor?: Best articles from the past year. *Obstetrics and Gynecology* **127**: 398–9.

Martin CR, Dammann O, Allred EN et al. (2010) Neurodevelopment of extremely preterm infants who had necrotizing enterocolitis with or without late bacteremia. *The Journal of Pediatrics* **157**: 751–6, e1.

O'Shea TM, Joseph RM, Allred EN et al. (2018) Accuracy of the Bayley-II mental development index at 2 years as a predictor of cognitive impairment at school age among children born extremely preterm. *Journal of Perinatology: Official Journal of the California Perinatal Association* **38**: 908–16.

O'Shea TM, Shah B, Allred EN et al. (2013) Inflammation-initiating illnesses, inflammation-related proteins, and cognitive impairment in extremely preterm infants. *Brain Behav Immun* **29**: 104–12.

Patel S, Dammann O, Martin CR, Allred EN, Leviton A, Investigators ES (2011) Presumed and definite bacteremia in extremely low gestational age newborns. *Acta Paediatrica* **100**: 36–41.

Phares CR, Lynfield R, Farley MM et al. (2008) Epidemiology of invasive group B streptococcal disease in the United States, 1999–2005. *Jama* **299**: 2056–65.

Profit J, Gould JB, Bennett M et al. (2017) Racial/ethnic disparity in NICU quality of care delivery. *Pediatrics* **140**: e20170918.

Raju TNK, Buist AS, Blaisdell CJ, Moxey-Mims M, Saigal S (2017) Adults born preterm: a review of general health and system-specific outcomes. *Acta Paediatrica* **106**: 1409–37.

Slykerman RF, Thompson J, Waldie KE, Murphy R, Wall C, Mitchell EA (2017) Antibiotics in the first year of life and subsequent neurocognitive outcomes. *Acta Paediatrica* **106**: 87–94.

Stoll BJ, Hansen N, Fanaroff AA et al. (2002) Late-onset sepsis in very low birth weight neonates: the experience of the NICHD Neonatal Research Network. *Pediatrics* **110**: 285–91.

Stoll BJ, Hansen NI, Bell EF et al. (2015) Trends in care practices, morbidity, and mortality of extremely preterm neonates, 1993–2012. *Jama* **314**: 1039–51.

Stoll BJ, Hansen NI, Sanchez PJ et al. (2011) Early onset neonatal sepsis: the burden of group B Streptococcal and E. coli disease continues. *Pediatrics* **127**: 817–26.

Retinopathy of Prematurity

Mari Holm, Deborah VanderVeen, and Olaf Dammann

INTRODUCTION

Retinopathy of prematurity (ROP) is a retinal vascular disease in preterm newborns. While the milder forms of ROP usually regress and leave the child with no sight-threatening injury, severe ROP can lead to blindness or other visual disability such as low vision, visual field restriction, significant refractive error (myopia or astigmatism), and strabismus later in childhood (Blencowe et al. 2013; Holmstrom and Larsson 2013). Low gestational age, low birth weight, exposure to oxygen supplements, poor intrauterine and postnatal growth, and exposure to inflammation are established risk factors for ROP (Hellstrom et al. 2013). In multicenter trials that include infants with birthweight ≤1250g in high-income countries, the rates of moderately severe (pre-threshold) ROP have been fairly stable over the last three decades, ranging from 18% in the CRYO-ROP study in 1986, 12% in the ET-ROP study in 2000–2002, and 19% in the e-ROP study in 2011–2013 (Quinn et al. 2016). However, incidence increases in low- and middle-income countries have been attributed in part to the increased survival of infants born preterm (Blencowe et al. 2013).

The development of ROP is biphasic. The first phase, characterized by interrupted retinal vessel growth, is followed by a second phase of pathological neovascularization. The first phase is initiated in response to transfer from the relatively low oxygen tension in utero with a fetal blood saturation of 70%, to relative hyperoxia in the extrauterine environment, where oxygen saturation often reaches 95–100%. At the same time, the newborn loses the maternal supply of nutrients and growth factors. Both factors limit the availability of vascular endothelial growth factor (VEGF), a major promoter of retinal vessel growth. From approximately gestational age (GA) week 30, the metabolic requirement of the maturing retina increases the need for oxygen, while vascular immaturity contributes to retinal hypoxia. Dysregulation of VEGF production and other angiogenetic growth factors, such as insulin-like growth factor (IGF) and erythropoietin (EPO), result in the second (proliferative) phase. In some cases, severe retinal fibrovascular proliferation can lead to traction on the retina and retinal detachment, which is the main cause of ocular blindness from ROP (Hartnett and Penn 2012).

ROP CLASSIFICATION AND TREATMENT

The classification of ROP is defined by the International Committee for Classification of Retinopathy of Prematurity (Committee for the Classification of Retinopathy of Prematurity 1984) (Table 8.1). The guidelines suggest that the first ophthalmologic examination be performed within the 31st to 33rd post-menstrual week, and follow-up exams until normal vascularization begins in zone 3 (American Academy of Pediatrics 2001).

Table 8.1	Classification of retinopathy of prematurity (8)		
Location	Zone I	The inner zone or posterior pole. Consists of the radius from the disk to twice the distance from the disk to the center of the macula.
	Zone II	The circle from the edge of zone I to the tangent of the nasal ora serrata at 3 o'clock right eye and 9 o'clock left eye.
	Zone III	The residual temporal crescent not included in zones I and II.
Extent of disease	Clock hours	The specified clock hours with present disease.
Severity	Stage 1	Presence of a demarcation line separating the vascular to the avascular retina. Abnormal vasculature leading up to the line.
	Stage 2	Presence of a vascular ridge separating the vascular to the avascular retina.
	Stage 3	Presence of a vascular ridge including extraretinal fibrovascular proliferation.
	Stage 4	Partial retinal detachment.
	Stage 5	Full retinal detachment.
Plus disease		Presence of engorgement and tortuosity of venules and arterioles in at least two quadrants of the posterior retina.
Threshold ROP		Presence of plus disease or stage 3 without plus disease in zone I; five contiguous or eight cumulative clock hours of stage 3 in zone II.
Prethreshold ROP		Presence of stages 1 or 2 without plus disease in zone I; less than five contiguous or eight cumulative clock hours of stage 3 or stage 2 with plus disease in zone II.

Historically, treatment for ROP was performed based on eyes meeting 'threshold' criteria (Cryotherapy for Retinopathy of Prematurity Cooperative Group 2001), and eyes with 'prethreshold' ROP were watched carefully because of the risk of progression to threshold disease. Threshold ROP was defined as five contiguous or eight cumulative clock hours of stage 3 ROP in zone I or II in the presence of plus disease, and prethreshold ROP is any ROP in zone I less than threshold criteria, or in zone II, plus disease but with stage 2 or less than five contiguous or eight interrupted clock hours of stage 3, or any stage 3 without plus disease. In 2003, updated guidelines were published, recommending that treatment should be considered if clinical criteria for Type 1 ROP are met: in zone I, any ROP with plus disease or stage 3 with or without plus disease, and in zone II, stage 2 ROP with plus disease (ETROP 2003). Conventional treatment is peripheral retinal ablation with laser photocoagulation. Because enrollment for the ELGAN study spanned the period when guidelines for treatment changed, classifications of ROP used the study criteria as an indicator of severe ROP (typically, prethreshold or worse). It should also be noted, therefore, that subcategories of ROP in zone 1, presence of stage 3, and presence of plus disease are also used as markers of severe ROP. Plus disease is dilatation and tortuosity of posterior retinal vessels in at least two quadrants, meeting or exceeding that of a standard image.

EYE EXAMINATIONS IN THE ELGAN STUDY

Experienced ELGAN study ophthalmologists helped to prepare a manual and data collection form, and also performed ROP screening. Conference calls were held to review representative retinal images with ROP in an effort to minimize observer variability. The ophthalmologists were encouraged to take photographs if in doubt of disease classification. Definitions of terms were those accepted by the International Committee for Classification of Retinopathy of Prematurity (Table 8.1) (Committee for the Classification of Retinopathy of Prematurity 1984). In keeping with guidelines, the first ophthalmologic examination was within the 31st to 33rd post-menstrual week, or by the 4th postnatal week, whichever was later (American Academy of Pediatrics 2001). Follow-up exams were performed weekly for infants at high ROP risk, while others were examined every 2–3 weeks. Retinal exams were conducted until normal vascularization began in zone III. Information about ROP treatment was not included in our study, as guidelines for laser treatment changed during the recruitment period (Early Treatment for Retinopathy of Prematurity Cooperative Group 2003).

RISK FACTORS FOR ROP IN PREGNANCY

Bacteria in the placenta and signs of histological placental inflammation were not associated with severe ROP in univariable analyses. However, the interaction between placenta inflammation with either low gestational age (23/24 weeks) or postnatal hyperoxemia was associated with a 2.4–10-fold risk increase among infants with bacteria recovered from their placentas (Chen et al. 2011).

We explored the relationships between pregnancy disorders that led to preterm birth and ROP (Lee et al. 2013). Disorders were classified as being related to intrauterine inflammation (preterm labor, prelabor premature rupture of membranes, placental abruption, and cervical insufficiency) or to placenta dysfunction (preeclampsia and fetal indication/intrauterine growth restriction) (McElrath et al. 2008). We hypothesized that pregnancy disorders involving inflammation are associated with an increased risk for ROP and/or that they modified the ROP risk associated postnatal risk factors, such as hyperoxemia and bacteremia.

Inflammation-associated and placentation disorders were both associated with a 14–15% crude risk for prethreshold/threshold ROP. In comprehensively adjusted multivariable models, all pregnancy disorders except fetal indication (OR range 0.9–1.8) were associated with a reduced ROP risk (OR range 0.2–0.8) compared to the reference group defined by preterm labor. Individually, postnatal hyperoxemia and bacteremia were not associated with increased ROP risk, but their combination (interaction) was associated with a prominently increased risk for severe ROP (OR range 3–6). This risk increase was more prominent in the stratum defined by placental dysfunction disorders (OR range 11–78) than in the stratum of inflammation-associated disorders (3–5). In separate analyses we found that the risk for prethreshold ROP is highest (60%) in infants with a gestational age of 23/24 weeks who are also severely growth restricted (birthweight Z-score <−2) (Lee et al. 2015).

RISK FACTORS FOR ROP DEVELOPMENT IN THE NEONATAL PERIOD

The newborn with ROP is also at risk for other complications of prematurity (Leviton et al. 2010). In the ELGAN study, severe ROP was associated with ultrasound-defined cerebral ventriculomegaly, respiratory difficulties, as well as early and late bacteremia. Postnatal growth velocity in the lowest quartile was associated increased ROP risk.

Nutrition might also be important in ROP etiology. Development of zone 1 ROP was associated with receipt of a relatively low lipid or total calorie intake, and development of stage 3 ROP was associated with the lowest quartile of total calorie intake (VanderVeen et al. 2013).

Receipt of oxygen is a well-known risk factor for ROP. In the ELGAN cohort, a PaO_2 as well as a PCO_2 in the highest quartile for GA on at least two of the first three postnatal days was associated an increased risk of severe ROP. The same holds true for infants in the lowest pH quartile for gestational age (Hauspurg et al. 2011).

ROP AND INFLAMMATION

Inflammatory phenomena including clinical and histological chorioamnionitis (Chen et al. 2011; Woo et al. 2012), occurrence of bacteria in the placenta (Chen et al. 2011), and postnatal systemic infections and sepsis (Klinger et al. 2010; Silveira et al. 2011; Tolsma et al. 2011; Lundgren et al. 2016) appear to contribute to the onset and/or severity of ROP. Angiogenesis and inflammation are closely related (Ribatti and Crivellato 2009; Szade et al. 2015), and altered retinal vascularization follows exposure to systemic inflammation (Tremblay et al. 2013; Hong et al. 2014). Hyperoxia, which is responsible for the initial arrest of retinal vascularization in ROP development, has also been reported to invoke an upregulation of the inflammatory response in the brain (Davies et al. 2006; Baburamani et al. 2014; Wollen et al. 2014). Finally, inflammation seems to reduce the newborn's IGF-1 production, which may contribute to ROP occurrence (Hansen-Pupp et al. 2007).

Numerous studies have made attempts at clarifying the role for specific inflammatory biomarkers of preterm brain injury and ROP. In the ELGAN study, we explored the relationships between prethreshold ROP and being in the top quartile of 27 different proteins measured in systemic blood on postnatal days 1, 7, 14, 21, and 28 (Holm et al. 2017). Each protein was evaluated individually. The risk for ROP was increased when some of the inflammation-related proteins were elevated in postnatal weeks 3 and 4, while the risk was reduced in infants who had top quartile concentrations of growth factors, angiogenic proteins, and neurotrophins.

Among the cytokines associated with an *increased* prethreshold ROP risk were MPO, IL-6, TNF-α and its receptors, IL-8, and ICAM-1. This is in keeping with previous findings. High concentrations of IL-6 (Sood et al. 2010), IL-8, and TNF-α in systemic circulation were associated with ROP in other studies (Silveira et al. 2011). While some found a relationship between ROP and increased concentrations of IL-7, MCP-1, MIP-1α, and MIP-1β in cord blood (Yu et al. 2014), others failed to confirm that cord blood cytokines are associated with ROP (Takahashi et al. 2010; Woo et al. 2013).

Several proteins were associated with a *decreased* ROP risk. High concentrations of RANTES were associated with lower ROP risk only during the first two postnatal weeks. This finding corresponds to RANTES's proposed protective effect in the preterm retina (Sato et al. 2009; Hellgren et al. 2010; Sood et al. 2010). Of the angioneurins studied, ANG-1 was one of the most consistent predictors of reduced ROP risk on all days, except day 1. On days 21 and 28, high concentrations of the neurotrophins NT-4 and BDNF appeared to be protective of later ROP. Others have also found support for reduced ROP risk associated with NT-4 (Sood et al. 2010) and BDNF (Rao et al. 2009; Sood et al. 2010). Our results support the hypothesis that angioneurins are biomarkers of protection in ROP etiology.

We also explored the relationship of top quartile concentrations of proteins with ROP risk in light of the top quartile concentrations of protein associated with reduced risk was explored. While IGF-1, IGFBP-1, and VEGFR-2 were not associated with a risk decrease when analyzed individually, the risk of ROP was elevated when IGF-1, IGFBP-1, and VEGFR-2 were in the lower three quartiles only in the concurrent presence of high concentrations of IL-6, TNF-α, and ICAM-1.

IGF-1 is important for fetal growth, including healthy retinal angiogenesis (Smith et al. 1997; Hellstrom et al. 2001, 2002, 2003). IGF-1 binding protein (IGFBP-3) has been found to be lower in premature infants, and possibly contributing to retinal vessel depletion (Lofqvist et al. 2007). Elevated IGF-1 or IGFBP-1 were protective of ROP. However, of special interest in light of our results, is that inflammation is a factor that might further reduce the preterm newborn's limited IGF-1 production (28). This corresponds to our finding that the infants in the lower three IGF-1/IGFBP-1 quartiles were vulnerable when the inflammatory mediators IL-6 and TNF-α were elevated.

In summary, top quartile concentrations of proteins with neurotrophic and/or angiogenic potential were found to modulate the increased ROP risk associated with top quartile concentrations of the inflammation-associated cytokines, chemokines, and adhesion molecules.

ROP AND LONG-TERM OUTCOMES

Abnormalities in the developing brain appear to accompany retinal damage (Msall 2006). In the ELGAN study, children with severe ROP were more likely than their peers to have cognitive impairment at 2 years corrected age. Having a head circumference of 1–2 standard deviations below the mean was associated with zone I ROP (Allred et al. 2014). This is in keeping with other studies where ROP has been identified as a neonatal risk factor for impaired executive functions, especially visual tasks (Bohm et al. 2004), and for difficulties with learning, attention, and behavior (Termote et al. 2003; Msall et al. 2004; Farooqi et al. 2011).

Neonatal ROP is associated with abnormal visual function at age 2. Prethreshold ROP was one of the strongest predictors, in addition to cerebral ventriculomegaly, of having a visual field deficit at 2 years of age (Holm et al. 2015). Previous studies have also identified ROP as a risk factor of visual field deficit. This is probably mediated both via the pathological process of ROP itself, and the iatrogenic effect of peripheral retinal ablation by either cryotherapy or laser treatment (Cryotherapy for Retinopathy of Prematurity Cooperative Group 2001; Larsson et al. 2004; Quinn et al. 2011). Visual field deficits following ROP treatment are typically that of overall constriction, and not that of a loss of a whole visual field quadrant (Larsson et al. 2004; McLoone et al. 2007); quadrantic of inferior visual field deficits are often attributed to cerebral injury in the setting of periventricular leukomalacia. Improved knowledge about the impact of ROP on the developing neuroretina might also play a role in cases of subnormal visual acuity or less severe visual field deficits (Rivera et al. 2016).

We found that children with a history of type I ROP are at heightened risk of strabismus at age 2 (esotropic or exotropic). Other important risk factors for strabismus were the presence of impairment in other visual functions such as fixation or visual field deficit (VanderVeen et al. 2015). A similar pattern was present in children with impaired visual fixation at age 2 years, where prethreshold ROP was an important risk factor (Phadke et al. 2014).

IMPLICATIONS FOR FUTURE RESEARCH

Many of the pathophysiological processes associated with preterm birth are complex, and this includes the complex pathways leading to ROP and impaired visual function. Some of the biomarkers measured in the ELGAN study are probably markers of parts of this complex pathogenesis of ROP. Regulation of other factors such as VEGF, EPO, and IGF-1 might prove to be directly protective, and have begun to be used in ROP treatment or have at least been studied in clinical trials (Stahl et al. 2014). However, most of our knowledge about molecular mechanisms of ROP pathogenesis comes from animal models. More and improved epidemiological studies with a molecular dimension will help in closing the translation gap from bench to bedside.

REFERENCES

Allred EN, Capone A Jr, Fraioli A et al. (2014) Retinopathy of prematurity and brain damage in the very preterm newborn. *Journal of AAPOS* **18**: 241–7.

American Academy of Pediatrics (2001) Screening examination of premature infants for retinopathy of prematurity. *Pediatrics* **108**: 809–11.

Baburamani AA, Supramaniam VG, Hagberg H, Mallard C (2014) Microglia toxicity in preterm brain injury. *Reprod Toxicol* **48**: 106–12.

Blencowe H, Lawn JE, Vazquez T, Fielder A, Gilbert C (2013) Preterm-associated visual impairment and estimates of retinopathy of prematurity at regional and global levels for 2010. *Pediatric Research* **74**: 35–49.

Bohm B, Smedler AC, Forssberg H (2004) Impulse control, working memory and other executive functions in preterm children when starting school. *Acta Paediatrica* **93**: 1363–71.

Chen ML, Allred EN, Hecht JL et al. (2011) Placenta microbiology and histology, and the risk for severe retinopathy of prematurity. *Invest Ophthalmol Vis Sci* **52**: 7052–8.

Committee for the Classification of Retinopathy of Prematurity (1984) An international classification of retinopathy of prematurity. The Committee for the Classification of Retinopathy of Prematurity. *Arch Ophthalmol* **102**: 1130–4.

Cryotherapy for Retinopathy of Prematurity Cooperative Group (2001) Effect of retinal ablative therapy for threshold retinopathy of prematurity: results of Goldmann perimetry at the age of 10 years. *Arch Ophthalmol* **119**: 1120–5.

Davies MH, Eubanks JP, Powers MR (2006) Microglia and macrophages are increased in response to ischemia-induced retinopathy in the mouse retina. Molecular vision **12**: 467–77.

Early Treatment for Retinopathy of Prematurity Cooperative Group (2003) Revised indications for the treatment of retinopathy of prematurity: results of the early treatment for retinopathy of prematurity randomized trial. *Arch Ophthalmol* **121**: 1684–94.

ETROP: Early Treatment for Retinopathy of Prematurity Cooperative Group (2003) Revised indications for the treatment of retinopathy of prematurity: results of the early treatment for retinopathy of prematurity randomized trial. *Arch Ophthalmol* **121**: 1684–94.

Farooqi A, Hagglof B, Sedin G, Serenius F (2011) Impact at age 11 years of major neonatal morbidities in children born extremely preterm. *Pediatrics* **127**: e1247–57.

Hansen-Pupp I, Hellstrom-Westas L, Cilio CM, Andersson S, Fellman V, Ley D. (2007) Inflammation at birth and the insulin-like growth factor system in very preterm infants. *Acta Paediatrica* **96**: 830–6.

Hartnett ME, Penn JS (2012) Mechanisms and management of retinopathy of prematurity. *The New England Journal of Medicine* **367**: 2515–26.

Hauspurg AK, Allred EN, VanderVeen DK et al. (2011) Blood gases and retinopathy of prematurity: the ELGAN study. *Neonatology* **99**: 104–11.

Hellgren G, Willett K, Engstrom E et al. (2010) Proliferative retinopathy is associated with impaired increase in BDNF and RANTES expression levels after preterm birth. *Neonatology* **98**: 409–18.

Hellstrom A, Carlsson B, Niklasson A et al. (2002) IGF-I is critical for normal vascularization of the human retina. *J Clin Endocrinol Metab* **87**: 3413–6.

Hellstrom A, Engstrom E, Hard AL et al. (2003) Postnatal serum insulin-like growth factor I deficiency is associated with retinopathy of prematurity and other complications of premature birth. *Pediatrics* **112**: 1016–20.

Hellstrom A, Perruzzi C, Ju M et al. (2001) Low IGF-I suppresses VEGF-survival signaling in retinal endothelial cells: direct correlation with clinical retinopathy of prematurity. *Proc Natl Acad Sci USA* **98**: 5804–8.

Hellstrom A, Smith LE, Dammann O (2013) Retinopathy of prematurity. *Lancet* **382**: 1445–57.

Holm M, Morken TS, Fichorova RN et al. (2017) Systemic inflammation-associated proteins and retinopathy of prematurity in infants born before the 28th week of gestation. *Invest Ophthalmol Vis Sci* **58**: 6419–28.

Holm M, Msall ME, Skranes J, Dammann O, Allred E, Leviton A (2015) Antecedents and correlates of visual field deficits in children born extremely preterm. *European Journal of Paediatric Neurology* **19**: 56–63.

Holmstrom G, Larsson E (2013) Outcome of retinopathy of prematurity. *Clinics in Perinatology* **40**: 311–21.

Hong HK, Lee HJ, Ko JH et al. (2014) Neonatal systemic inflammation in rats alters retinal vessel development and simulates pathologic features of retinopathy of prematurity. *Journal of Neuroinflammation* **11**: 87.

Klinger G, Levy I, Sirota L, Boyko V, Lerner-Geva L, Reichman B (2010) Outcome of early-onset sepsis in a national cohort of very low birth weight infants. *Pediatrics* **10;125**: e736–40.

Larsson E, Martin L, Holmstrom G (2004) Peripheral and central visual fields in 11-year-old children who had been born prematurely and at term. *Journal of Pediatric Ophthalmology and Strabismus* **41**: 39–45.

Lee JW, McElrath T, Chen M et al. (2013) Pregnancy disorders appear to modify the risk for retinopathy of prematurity associated with neonatal hyperoxemia and bacteremia. *The Journal of Maternal-fetal & Neonatal Medicine* **26**: 811–8.

Lee JW, VanderVeen D, Allred EN, Leviton A, Dammann O (2015) Prethreshold retinopathy in premature infants with intrauterine growth restriction. *Acta Paediatrica* **104**: 27–31.

Leviton A, Dammann O, Engelke S et al. (2010) The clustering of disorders in infants born before the 28th week of gestation. *Acta Paediatrica* **99**: 1795–800.

Lofqvist C, Chen J, Connor KM et al. (2007) IGFBP3 suppresses retinopathy through suppression of oxygen-induced vessel loss and promotion of vascular regrowth. *Proc Natl Acad Sci USA* **104**: 10589–94.

Lundgren P, Lundberg L, Hellgren G et al. (2016) Aggressive posterior retinopathy of prematurity is associated with multiple infectious episodes and thrombocytopenia. *Neonatology* **111**: 79–85.

McElrath TF, Hecht JL, Dammann O et al. (2008) Pregnancy disorders that lead to delivery before the 28th week of gestation: an epidemiologic approach to classification. *Am J Epidemiol* **168**: 980–9.

McLoone E, O'Keefe M, McLoone S, Lanigan B (2007) Effect of diode laser retinal ablative therapy for threshold retinopathy of prematurity on the visual field: results of Goldmann perimetry at a mean age of 11 years. *Journal of Pediatric Ophthalmology and Strabismus* **44**: 170–3.

Msall ME (2006) The retina as a window to the brain in vulnerable neonates. *Pediatrics* **117**: 2287–9.

Msall ME, Phelps DL, Hardy RJ et al. (2004) Educational and social competencies at 8 years in children with threshold retinopathy of prematurity in the CRYO-ROP multicenter study. *Pediatrics* **113**: 790–9.

Phadke A, Msall ME, Droste P et al. (2014) Impaired visual fixation at the age of 2 years in children born before the twenty-eighth week of gestation. Antecedents and correlates in the multicenter ELGAN study. *Pediatric Neurology* **51**: 36–42.

Quinn GE, Barr C, Bremer D et al. (2016) Changes in course of retinopathy of prematurity from 1986 to 2013: comparison of three studies in the United States. *Ophthalmology* **123**: 1595–600.

Quinn GE, Dobson V, Hardy RJ, Tung B, Palmer EA, Good WV (2011) Visual field extent at 6 years of age in children who had high-risk prethreshold retinopathy of prematurity. *Arch Ophthalmol* **129**: 127–32.

Rao R, Mashburn CB, Mao J, Wadhwa N, Smith GM, Desai NS (2009) Brain-derived neurotrophic factor in infants <32 weeks gestational age: correlation with antenatal factors and postnatal outcomes. *Pediatric Research* **65**: 548–52.

Ribatti D, Crivellato E (2009) Immune cells and angiogenesis. *Journal of Cellular and Molecular Medicine* **13(9A)**: 2822–33.

Rivera JC, Madaan A, Zhou TE, Chemtob S (2016) Review of the mechanisms and therapeutic avenues for retinal and choroidal vascular dysfunctions in retinopathy of prematurity. *Acta Paediatrica* **105**: 1421–33.

Sato T, Kusaka S, Shimojo H, Fujikado T (2009) Simultaneous analyses of vitreous levels of 27 cytokines in eyes with retinopathy of prematurity. *Ophthalmology* **116**: 2165–9.

Silveira RC, Fortes Filho JB, Procianoy RS (2011) Assessment of the contribution of cytokine plasma levels to detect retinopathy of prematurity in very low birth weight infants. *Investigative Ophthalmology & Visual Science* **52**: 1297–12301.

Smith LE, Kopchick JJ, Chen W et al. (1997) Essential role of growth hormone in ischemia-induced retinal neovascularization. *Science* **276**: 1706–9.

Sood BG, Madan A, Saha S et al. (2010) Perinatal systemic inflammatory response syndrome and retinopathy of prematurity. *Pediatric Research* **67**: 394–400.

Stahl A, Hellstrom A, Smith LE (2014) Insulin-like growth factor-1 and anti-vascular endothelial growth factor in retinopathy of prematurity: has the time come? *Neonatology* **106**: 254–60.

Szade A, Grochot-Przeczek A, Florczyk U, Jozkowicz A, Dulak J (2015) Cellular and molecular mechanisms of inflammation-induced angiogenesis. *IUBMB Life* **67**: 145–59.

Takahashi N, Uehara R, Kobayashi M et al. (2010) Cytokine profiles of seventeen cytokines, growth factors and chemokines in cord blood and its relation to perinatal clinical findings. *Cytokine* **49**: 331–7.

Termote J, Schalij-Delfos NE, Donders AR, Cats BP (2003) The incidence of visually impaired children with retinopathy of prematurity and their concomitant disabilities. *Journal of AAPOS* **7**: 131–6.

Tolsma KW, Allred EN, Chen ML et al. (2011) Neonatal bacteremia and retinopathy of prematurity: the ELGAN study. *Arch Ophthalmol* **129**: 1555–63.

Tremblay S, Miloudi K, Chaychi S et al. (2013) Systemic inflammation perturbs developmental retinal angiogenesis and neuroretinal function. *Invest Ophthalmol Vis Sci* **54(13)**: 8125–39.

VanderVeen DK, Allred EN, Wallace DK, Leviton A (2015) Strabismus at age 2 years in children born before 28 weeks' gestation: antecedents and correlates. *Journal of Child Neurology* **31**: 451–60.

VanderVeen DK, Martin CR, Mehendale R et al. (2013) Early nutrition and weight gain in preterm newborns and the risk of retinopathy of prematurity. *PloS One* **8**: e64325.

Wollen EJ, Sejersted Y, Wright MS et al. (2014) Transcriptome profiling of the newborn mouse brain after hypoxia-reoxygenation: hyperoxic reoxygenation induces inflammatory and energy failure responsive genes. *Pediatric Research* **75(4)**: 517–26.

Woo SJ, Park KH, Jung HJ et al. (2012) Effects of maternal and placental inflammation on retinopathy of prematurity. *Graefe's Archive for Clinical and Experimental Ophthalmology = Albrecht von Graefes Archiv fur klinische und experimentelle Ophthalmologie* **250**: 915–23.

Woo SJ, Park KH, Lee SY et al. (2013) The relationship between cord blood cytokine levels and perinatal factors and retinopathy of prematurity: a gestational age-matched case-control study. *Invest Ophthalmol Vis Sci* **54**: 3434–9.

Yu H, Yuan L, Zou Y et al. (2014) Serum concentrations of cytokines in infants with retinopathy of prematurity. *APMIS: Acta Pathologica, Microbiologica, et Immunologica Scandinavica* **122**: 818–23.

Bronchopulmonary Dysplasia

Wesley M Jackson and Matthew M Laughon

CHAPTER SUMMARY

The ELGAN study has contributed to our understanding of the natural history and sequelae of bronchopulmonary dysplasia (BPD). First, it identified risk factors for BPD, primarily fetal growth restriction: patterns of early lung disease based on receipt of supplemental oxygen in the first 14 postnatal days: elevations in blood concentrations of pro-inflammatory proteins in the first two postnatal weeks and abnormal blood gas measurements in the first three postnatal days. Second, it documented that BPD is an independent risk factor for poor neurodevelopmental outcomes. Third, it showed that BPD is a risk factor for preschool wheezing, but not childhood asthma. This chapter also provides context for these findings in the current field of BPD research.

BRONCHOPULMONARY DYSPLASIA – IMPORTANCE AND DEFINITIONS

Bronchopulmonary dysplasia (BPD; also called chronic lung disease, or CLD) is the most common pulmonary morbidity among preterm infants and its incidence is stable, despite: and in part due to: improved survival at earlier gestational ages (Zysman-Colman et al. 2013; Stoll et al. 2015). Since BPD was first described by Northway in 1967 as a chronic disease related to pulmonary injury following respiratory distress syndrome in neonates, the definition has evolved in an effort to improve its reliability, accuracy, and prognostic capacity (Northway et al. 1967; Higgins et al. 2018). Although the National Institutes of Health offered a severity-based, clinical definition of BPD (Jobe and Bancalari 2001; Higgins et al. 2018), the most common definition of BPD that continues to be used in research studies is based on the Shennan (Shennan et al. 1988) definition of supplemental oxygen at 36 weeks postmenstrual age (PMA) (Beam et al. 2014). The ELGAN study defined BPD as the need for oxygen therapy at 36 weeks PMA as determined by the clinician caring for the infant: and not based on standardized oxygen saturation goals. Infants with BPD were further classified as mild/moderate if not receiving mechanical ventilation at 36 weeks PMA, and as severe BPD if receiving mechanical ventilation at that time point.

FETAL GROWTH RESTRICTION IS A RISK FACTOR FOR BPD

When BPD was first described, the disease was primarily diagnosed in preterm infants >30 weeks' gestation who had surfactant deficiency and subsequently developed lung injury, inflammation, and parenchymal fibrosis attributed to prolonged exposure to mechanical ventilation and high fractions of inspired supplemental oxygen (Ambalavanan and Carlo 2004). In the following decades, improvements in the survival of ELGANs and the use of less injurious ventilation modalities, including nasal continuous positive airway pressure and aggressive weaning from mechanical ventilation, has diminished the inflammatory component of the disease. The 'new' BPD observed in these more preterm infants is characterized by arrested alveolar and pulmonary vascular development (Jobe 2011). As a result, researchers explored which perinatal factors, aside from gestational age, influence lung maturity and therefore confer the highest risk of the 'new' BPD in ELGANs.

In an effort to identify exposures and events before delivery that predict BPD in extremely preterm, ELGAN investigators used logistic regression models to examine which antenatal and neonatal variables were associated with BPD risk (Bose et al. 2009). Among the 1241 infants in the ELGAN study who survived to 36 weeks PMA and for whom the BPD status was known: fetal growth restriction (FGR) (defined as birthweight Z-score <−1) conveyed the most information for BPD risk, followed by gestational age, birth weight, and sex. When the analysis was stratified by gestational age, FGR was not associated with BPD in the least mature group (23–24 weeks): and most prominently among the most mature group (27 weeks). After controlling for potential confounders, including delivery indication and gestational age, the overall BPD odds ratios (95% confidence interval) for infants with FGR (birthweight Z-score ≥−2, <−1) was 3.2 (2.1–5.0), and for infants with severe FGR (birthweight Z-score <−2) was 4.4 (2.3–8.2).

The finding of FGR as a risk factor for BPD in preterm infants is consistent with previous studies (Lal et al. 2003; Reiss et al. 2003; Garite et al. 2004), and has been validated in subsequent cohort studies (Eriksson et al. 2015; Sasi et al. 2015; Klevebro et al. 2016; Torchin et al. 2016). Several mechanisms have been proposed which might explain this association in the era of 'new' BPD. First, the processes that reduce fetal somatic growth might also reduce/delay alveolar and vascular lung development (Jobe and Ikegami 1998). Placenta-mediated maternal disorders, such as gestational hypertension and preeclampsia, are associated with an imbalance in the placental release of pro-angiogenic and anti-angiogenic factors, which influence fetal lung vasculature development (Kovo et al. 2013). Furthermore, intrauterine growth restriction occurs when the placenta fails to meet the oxygen and nutrient needs of the fetus. The resulting deleterious effects on the developing lung have been attributed to inhibition of transforming growth factor beta (TGF-β) signaling leading to dysregulated alveolar growth (Ambalavanan et al. 2008; Alejandre Alcazar et al. 2011). Finally, FGR may lead to abnormal fetal programming resulting in poor growth and development of the lung in utero and throughout infancy and childhood. Children born at term with FGR have reduced lung function on spirometry and have higher risk of asthma compared to peers who were not born with growth restriction (Metsala et al. 2008; Kotecha et al. 2010).

PATTERNS OF EARLY LUNG DISEASE PREDICT RISK FOR BPD

While nearly all ELGANs require some form of respiratory support shortly after birth, often in the form of mechanical ventilation and supplemental oxygen, the amount and duration of support varies. Based on supplemental oxygen requirements, the ELGAN investigators described three patterns of lung disease in the first two postnatal weeks (Laughon et al. 2009a). These patterns were used to classify ELGANs into three mutually exclusive groups. Infants in the first group had consistently low fractions of inspired oxygen (FiO2 consistently <0.23 on postnatal days 3–7, and FiO2 ≤ 0.25 on day 14). These infants had relatively normal pulmonary function throughout the first two postnatal weeks. In the second group were infants with pulmonary deterioration (PD), characterized by an FiO2 consistently <0.23 on *any* day between days 3–7 and FiO2 > 0.25 on day 14. After briefly recovering pulmonary function in the first week, they decompensated and required increased supplemental oxygen and/or mechanical ventilation in the second week. Those in the third group had early and persistent pulmonary dysfunction (EPPD) (i.e. an FiO2 consistently ≥0.23 on postnatal days 3–7 and FiO2 > 0.25 on day 14). These infants required mechanical ventilation and high concentrations of oxygen throughout the first two postnatal weeks. The FiO2 value for each infant was assigned based on the modal FiO2 for that day.

In the cohort of 1340 infants, 20% had consistently low FiO2, 38% had PD, and 43% had EPPD (Figure 9.1). Compared to infants with consistently low FiO2, infants with PD had lower gestational ages and birth weights, and higher Scores for Neonatal Acute Physiology II (SNAP-II), an indicator of illness severity in the first 12 hours of life (Richardson et al. 2001). Infants with EPPD had still lower gestational ages and birth weights, and higher SNAP-IIs. Multivariable analyses identified mechanical ventilation on day 7 as a modifiable risk factor for PD.

While PD in ELGANs had been previously described as 'atypical BPD' (i.e. BPD not preceded by respiratory distress syndrome), in retrospective cohort studies (Panickar et al. 2004; Streubel et al. 2008) the ELGAN study was the first to use prospectively collected data to describe early patterns of lung disease, defined by FiO2 that might predict different levels of BPD risk. And indeed it did. The incidence of BPD increased progressively from 17% in the low FiO2 to 51% among infants with PD, to 67% among infants who had EPPD.

Nearly one-fifth of ELGANs in the low FiO2 group developed BPD, despite minimal, if any, exposure to mechanical ventilation and supplemental oxygen in the first two postnatal weeks. This observation led investigators to compare antecedents of BPD in each group, in light of the hypothesis that pathophysiological mechanisms other than lung injury from respiratory support may explain differences in BPD incidence among groups (Laughon et al. 2011b). In time-oriented risk models, FGR is a risk factor

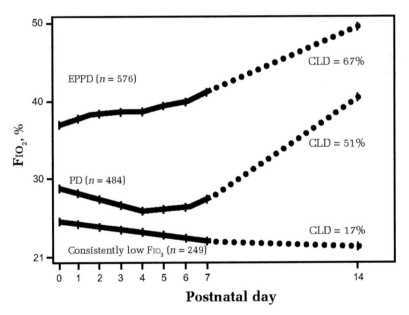

Figure 9.1 Early patterns of lung disease in ELGANs Median of the mode fraction of inspired oxygen (FiO2) on postnatal days 0–7 and on postnatal day 14 and frequency of CLD (chronic lung disease; or BPD) among 1340 ELGANs with three patterns of respiratory disease (low FiO2, PD, and EPPD) during the first two postnatal weeks. Printed with permission from Laughon M, Allred EN, Bose C, O'Shea TM, Van Marter LJ, Ehrenkranz RA, Leviton A (2009) Patterns of respiratory disease during the first 2 postnatal weeks in extremely premature infants. Reproduced with permission from Laughon (2009a), Copyright © 2009 by the AAP.

for BPD in all three groups, consistent with previous findings from the ELGAN study. Furthermore, the association of FGR and BPD risk is most pronounced in the low FiO2 group, indicating that this mechanism might occur even in the absence of early lung injury. In addition to FGR, two of the three other predominant antecedents of BPD in the PD group are antenatal (gestational age and male sex), and only one is postnatal (mechanical ventilation). In the EPPD group, mechanical ventilation at 7 days, pulmonary interstitial emphysema, and, to a lesser extent, gestational age and FGR, are the primary risk factors for BPD. In the ELGAN study, BPD was not associated with histologic markers of placental inflammation or microbiologic evidence of placental infection in any of the three groups. To what extent placental inflammation is causally associated with increased or decreased risk of BPD remains controversial (Lacaze-Masmonteil 2014; Thomas and Speer 2014; Choi 2017).

SYSTEMIC INFLAMMATION IS A RISK FACTOR FOR BPD

Exposures that result in systemic inflammation, both in the antenatal and postnatal environment, contribute to neonatal lung injury (Kallapur and Jobe 2006; Viscardi 2012; Balany and Bhandari 2015). Antenatal inflammation can occur in the setting of chorioamnionitis (or other infection) and is often associated with preterm birth (Kallapur and Jobe 2006). In addition to infection, the most common sources of postnatal lung inflammation in ELGANs are hyperoxia and mechanical ventilation (Viscardi 2012). These exposures are often, to some extent, unavoidable as ELGANs will nearly always require some form of respiratory support (including the provision of supplemental oxygen and/or positive pressure ventilation) due to the low oxygen tension of fetal blood, even an FiO2 of 0.21, or 'room air', is a relatively hyperoxic state for the infant transitioning to the ex-utero environment (Perrone et al. 2016). The association of inflammation with lung injury and arrested lung development supports the hypothesis that perinatal inflammation may play a role in the pathogenesis of BPD (Balany and Bhandari 2015; Kalikkot Thekkeveedu et al. 2017).

The ELGAN study collected neonatal blood specimens in the first four postnatal weeks to measure inflammatory protein concentrations, which were used as biomarkers of systematic inflammation. The blood protein concentrations and their changes over time were then related to the risk of BPD in the ELGAN cohort.

The first study to examine this relationship measured 25 inflammatory proteins obtained from blood specimens sampled on postnatal days 1–3, 5–8, and 12–15 from >900 infants (Bose et al. 2011). Table 9.1 lists the name and function of each of the inflammatory proteins included in the analysis. Compared to infants who did not develop BPD, those who developed mild/moderate BPD tended to have higher concentrations of TNF-alpha on day 1, TNF-R2, MCP-1, and ICAM-1 on day 7, and IL-1b, IL-6, TNF-alpha, TNF-R1, IL-8, MCP-1, ICAM-1, and MMP-9 on day 14. Infants who developed severe BPD did not have elevated concentrations of any inflammatory protein on day 1. On day 7 day, however, they had elevated concentrations of TNF-R2, MCP-1, and ICAM-1 and on day 14 they had elevated concentrations of IL-6, TNF-alpha, TNF-R1, MCP-1, and ICAM-1, E-selectin1, and MMP-9. Infants who developed BPD had reduced concentrations of one chemokine, RANTES, on days 7 and 14 compared to infants without BPD, which suggests that this protein may be protective against inflammatory-mediated injury.

Including birth weight in time-oriented risk models did not alter the relationship between elevated protein concentrations and risk of BPD, suggesting the previously mentioned relationship of FGR and BPD is likely not mediated by systemic inflammation in the first two postnatal weeks. In contrast, mechanical ventilation reduced the association between elevated protein concentrations and BPD risk on days 7 and 14, implicating mechanical ventilation's role in systemic inflammation.

Table 9.1 Inflammatory proteins examined in the ELGAN study

Inflammatory protein	Function
IL-1β (Interleukin-1β)	Activates lymphocytes
IL-6 (Interleukin-6)	↑ cytokine production
IL-6R	Receptor for IL-6
TNF-α (Tumor Necrosis Factor-α)	Activates macrophages and T lymphocytes
TNF-R1 and TNF-R2	Receptors for TNF-α
IL-8 (Interleukin-8; CXCL8)	Chemotactic factor for neutrophils
MCP-1 (Monocyte Chemotactic Protein-1; CCL2)	Chemotactic factor for monocytes/lymphocytes
MCP-4 (Monocyte Chemotactic Protein-4; CCL13)	Chemotactic factor for monocytes/lymphocytes
MIP-1β (Macrophage Inflammatory Protein-1β; CCL4)	Chemotactic factor for monocytes/lymphocytes
RANTES (regulated upon activation, normal T-cell expressed, and secreted; CCL5)	Chemotactic factor for T cells, eosinophils, and basophils
I-TAC (Interferon-inducible T cell alpha-chemoattractant; CXCL11)	Chemotactic factor for activated T cells
ICAM-1 (Intercellular Adhesion Molecule-1; CD54)	↑ adhesion and migration of neutrophils
ICAM-3 (CD50)	↑ adhesion and migration of neutrophils
VCAM-1 (Vascular Cell Adhesion Molecule-1; CD106)	↑ adhesion of lymphocytes to vascular endothelium
E-selectin (CD62E)	↑ adhesion of neutrophils to endothelium
MMP-1 (Matrix Metalloproteinase-1)	Protease – breaks down collagen in extracellular matrix
MMP-9	Protease – breaks down collagen in extracellular matrix
CRP (C-reactive Protein)	Acute-phase protein; activates complement system
Serum Amyloid A	Apolipoprotein; acute-phase protein
MPO (Myeloperoxidase)	Microbicidal enzyme produces by neutrophils
VEGF (Vascular Endothelial Growth Factor)	Promotes angiogenesis and alveolarization
VEGF-R1 and VEGF-R2	Receptors for VEGF
IGFBP-1 (Insulin Growth Factor Binding Protein-1)	Regulates lung fibroblast proliferation

Two other studies provided additional details about the relationship between respiratory support and early systemic inflammation in ELGANs (Leviton et al. 2011; Bose et al. 2013). Compared to ELGANs receiving fewer than 7 days of mechanical ventilation, infants ventilated for 14 days had elevated day-14 blood concentrations of IL-1β, TNF-α, IL-8, MCP-1, ICAM-1, and MMP-9 and lower levels of RANTES, MIP-1β, MMP-1, and vascular endothelial growth factor (VEGF) (Bose et al. 2013). Therefore, a longer duration of exposure to mechanical ventilation in the first two postnatal weeks is associated with elevated markers of systemic inflammation and decreased levels of proteins suspected to be anti-inflammation (RANTES) or capable of protecting against injury or promoting lung repair (VEGF) (Yun et al. 2016). Another ELGAN study report documented that elevated day-14 concentrations of RANTES and VEGF were associated with reduced risk of EPPD and PD, while elevated concentrations of IL-8 and ICAM-1 were associated with increased risk of EPPD (Laughon et al. 2011a).

In summary, these findings suggest that elevated blood concentrations of a variety of pro-inflammatory cytokines, adhesion molecules, and proteases in the first weeks of life are associated with the development of BPD. A study from the Neonatal Research Network found that extremely low birth weight infants who developed BPD or died had a distinct pattern of cytokine elevation in early life reflecting an impaired transition from innate to adaptive immunity (Ambalavanan et al. 2009). These results imply that inflammatory proteins may be utilized as early markers of BPD risk. Furthermore, management strategies and therapeutic agents that reduce early inflammation may play an important role in preventing BPD.

FETAL GROWTH RESTRICTION IS ASSOCIATED WITH SYSTEMIC INFLAMMATION

Following the important finding that FGR is strongly associated with BPD, ELGAN investigators were interested in exploring mechanisms by which FGR led to BPD. As mentioned previously, several mechanisms for this association have been proposed, including reduced fetal alveolar growth, abnormal fetal programming, chronic fetal hypoxia, and an imbalance in pro- and anti-angiogenic factors (Jobe and Ikegami 1998; Ambalavanan et al. 2008; Alejandre Alcazar et al. 2011; Kovo et al. 2013). ELGAN investigators used data from blood protein measurements to explore whether systemic inflammation, which is also associated with the development of BPD, may mediate the relationship between FGR and BPD.

In the ELGAN cohort, infants with severe FGR (Z-score <−2) were not at increased risk of systemic inflammation shortly after birth, but were more likely than children whose growth was within the normal range to have elevated blood CRP, IL-1β, IL-6, TNF-α, IL-8, MCP-4, ICAM-1, ICAM-3, E-SEL, MMP-9, VEGF-R2, and/or IGFBP-1 concentrations by day 14 (McElrath et al. 2013). On days 21 and 28, infants with severe FGR had elevated concentrations of CRP, IL-1β, IL-8, ICAM-1, and thyroid-stimulating hormone (TSH). Furthermore, infants with less severe FGR (birthweight Z-score between −2 and −1) had elevated concentrations of IL-8, TNF-α, TNF-R2, ICAM-1, and MMP-9. A similar pattern of elevated protein blood concentrations was detected in infants delivered extremely preterm for maternal (pre-eclampsia) indications (a common correlate of FGR) or fetal indications (often for failure to grow in utero).

The observed 'late' elevation in inflammatory markers in growth-restricted infants has several possible explanations. One explanation postulates that abnormal fetal programming can have later deleterious effects (e.g. increased risks for hypertension, insulin resistance, and obesity) (Longo et al. 2013). This explanation is supported by evidence that epigenetic mechanisms can regulate inflammation (Jaeckle Santos et al. 2014; Visentin et al. 2014; Neu and Pammi 2018). Another explanation postulates that continued pro-inflammatory exposures, such as mechanical ventilation, contribute to elevated inflammatory protein concentrations at day 28.

EARLY BLOOD GAS VALUES AND BPD

As a potential strategy to prevent BPD, several studies prior to the ELGAN study examined to what extent permissive hypercapnia (higher levels of partial pressure of arterial carbon dioxide [PCO_2]) reduced ventilator-associated lung injury (Carlo et al. 2002; Kamper et al. 2004; Miller and Carlo 2007). In an effort to understand the association of early blood gas abnormalities with BPD risk, ELGAN study investigators evaluated the potential contribution of the highest and lowest quartiles of partial pressure of arterial oxygen (PO_2) and PCO_2 on blood gases obtained during the first three postnatal days to BPD (Sriram et al. 2014).

Newborns who had hypoxemia (lowest PO_2 quartile) were at increased risk of both mild/moderate BPD and severe BPD. In contrast, newborns who had hypocapnea (lowest PCO_2 quartile) were at reduced risk of non-ventilator-dependent BPD, while those who had hypercapnea (highest PCO_2 quartile) were at increased risk of severe BPD. After adjusting for ≥14 days of mechanical ventilation, the associations of hypoxemia and hypercapnea with BPD risk were reduced or eliminated, but the lowered BPD risk among infants with hypocapnea did not change.

In light of the finding that ≥2 days of acidemia in the first three postnatal days was associated with elevated markers of systemic inflammation in the first two postnatal weeks (Leviton et al. 2011), these hypoxemia and hypercapnea findings suggest that perhaps the need for mechanical ventilation accounts for what was found. As previously mentioned, mechanical ventilation is associated with early systemic inflammation, which is itself a risk factor for BPD (Bose et al. 2011, 2013). Therefore, the hypoxemia and hypercapnea findings can be viewed as supporting the concept that prolonged mechanical ventilation, resulting in systemic inflammation, is likely to be an intermediary factor relating early blood gas derangements to BPD risk.

NEURODEVELOPMENTAL OUTCOMES OF ELGANS WITH BPD

ELGANs with BPD appear to be at increased risk for cognitive deficits (Singer et al. 1997; Hughes et al. 1999; Lewis et al. 2002), language impairment (Singer et al. 2001; Gray et al. 2004), and motor delay compared to their peers without BPD (Hack et al. 2000; Majnemer et al. 2000). These deficits are more pronounced in infants exposed to prolonged mechanical ventilation (Short et al. 2007; Zhang et al. 2018).

The ELGAN study has contributed to our knowledge of the association of BPD with developmental delay and cerebral palsy (CP) at 2 years of age (Laughon et al. 2009b; Van Marter et al. 2011), and measures of cognitive, language, and executive functions, academic achievement, social skills, and quality of life scores at 10 years of age (Sriram et al. 2018). Understanding the relationship between BPD and neurodevelopmental outcomes is challenging. First, BPD and developmental delay share risk factors that the extremely preterm may be exposed to in early life, including prolonged mechanical ventilation (Short et al. 2007; Zhang et al. 2018), pneumothorax (Laptook et al. 2005), necrotizing enterocolitis (Vohr et al. 2000; Allendorf et al. 2018), and cerebral white matter injury (Wood et al. 2005; Leviton et al. 2010). These risk factors might mediate the relationship between prematurity and the outcomes of developmental delay and BPD. In addition, exposure to treatments for the prevention of BPD, specifically postnatal steroids, have been shown to increase the risk of CP (Shinwell et al. 2000; O'Shea et al. 2007; Kobaly et al. 2008). The ELGAN study investigators used several methods in their study design and data analysis to account for these complex associations.

In the first study, investigators included ELGANs (n = 915) assessed at 2 years of age with the Bayley Scales of Infant Development – 2nd Edition (Bayley 1993) (BSID-II) and, when necessary, the parent-reported Vineland Adaptive Behavior Scales (VABS) (Laughon et al. 2009b). To avoid attributing deficits of perception and cognition to motor impairments, we excluded children who had any motor impairment. The BSID-II evaluations were performed by certified examiners who were blinded to the details of the child's medical history. A significant developmental delay was defined as an MDI or PDI score <70 (i.e. >2 standard deviations below the mean standardized score) and severe delay as a score <55 (>3 standard deviations below the mean). Investigators tested the hypothesis that antecedents of BPD, in contrast to the diagnosis of BPD itself, are associated with childhood developmental delay.

After adjusting for confounding variables (i.e. FGR, higher SNAP-IIs, mechanical ventilation in the first postnatal month, late bacteremia, necrotizing enterocolitis, pneumothorax, and retinopathy of pre-maturity), BPD, regardless of severity, was not associated with an increased risk of developmental delay at 2 years of age. However, antecedents of BPD were clearly associated with a higher risk of developmental delay, which suggests that brain injury may occur as a result of exposure to these antecedents rather than being a consequence of BPD.

A second study examined the relationship of BPD with CP diagnosis at 2 years of age in ELGANs (Van Marter et al. 2011). Of the 120 children with CP, approximately half had quadriparesis (four limb), one-third had diparesis (leg dominant), and one-fifth had hemiparesis. Children with a history of BPD were more likely than their peers without BPD to have CP. In children with a history of ventilator-dependent BPD, the risk of quadriparesis or an inability to walk, even with assistance, was higher than in children with a history of BPD without mechanical ventilation. Children who had mechanical-ventilator-dependent BPD were at a six-fold elevated risk of quadriparesis and a four-fold risk of dipa-resis, but not at increased risk of hemiparesis. BPD without mechanical ventilation was not associated with any form of CP. The two forms of CP associated with ventilator-dependent BPD were the most commonly diagnosed phenotypes and reflect bilateral cerebral white matter injury, a relatively common finding on cranial imaging in ELGANs (Kuban et al. 2008).

Low birthweight infants given postnatal dexamethasone to facilitate extubation are at increased risk of CP (O'Shea et al. 1999). In contrast, those who receive hydrocortisone are not at increased risk of the composite of death or cerebral palsy, while still deriving pulmonary benefits (Doyle et al. 2014). The ability to draw inferences on the association of postnatal steroids and CP in the ELGAN study were limited as fewer than 3% of infants received postnatal dexamethasone. Infants who received hydrocorti-sone were at an increased risk of BPD and CP. However, as hydrocortisone is used for reasons other than the prevention of BPD, such as hypotension or adrenal insufficiency, this association may be confounded by indication, as infants who are critically ill are more likely to be treated with hydrocortisone.

At 10 years of age, ELGANs who had severe BPD had lower scores on assessments of executive func-tions, intelligence, academic achievement, and quality of life than children who had less severe BPD, who, in turn, had lower scores than their peers who had no BPD (Sriram et al. 2018). Nevertheless, approximately one-half of ELGANs with severe BPD had scores in the normal range for academic achievement. While previous studies have found an association with limited executive planning and academic achievement and a history of BPD in preterm infants (Singer et al. 1997; Lowe et al. 2013; Potharst et al. 2013; Wolfe et al. 2015; Taylor and Clark 2016; Cheong and Doyle 2018), the ELGAN Study is unique in describing this association as correlating with severity of BPD.

PULMONARY OUTCOMES OF ELGANS WITH BPD

Compared with individuals born at term, ELGANs more frequently report respiratory complaints of wheezing, asthma diagnoses, and use of medications for asthma in childhood (Palta et al. 2001; Anand et al. 2003; Doyle and Victorian Infant Collaborative Study Group 2006; Hennessy et al. 2008; Fawke et al. 2010; Teune et al. 2012; Cazzato et al. 2013; Vom Hove et al. 2014; Holsti et al. 2017). Despite variations in methods, most studies suggest that among those born extremely preterm, BPD is associ-ated with a greater risk of respiratory morbidities, including wheezing, lung function abnormalities, and use of bronchodilator medication (Palta et al. 2001; Anand et al. 2003; Doyle and Victorian Infant Collaborative Study Group 2006; Hennessy et al. 2008; Fawke et al. 2010; Teune et al. 2012; Cazzato et al. 2013; Vom Hove et al. 2014; Lodha et al. 2015). Among children enrolled in the National Institute of Child Health and Human Development Neonatal Research Network Very Low Birth Weight Infant

Registry, the likelihood of using pulmonary medications (bronchodilators and/or steroids) at 18–22 months increased with severity of BPD (Ehrenkranz et al. 2005).

While children born preterm, especially those who develop BPD, are at increased risk of recurrent wheezing in childhood, these symptoms are often unrelated to atopic status and therefore raise doubts over the applicability of the diagnosis of asthma in these children (Speer and Silverman 1998; Bhandari and Panitch 2006; Goncalves et al. 2016). It remains unclear whether the association of airway reactivity in children born extremely preterm is related to lung injury during the neonatal period or due to intrinsic factors related to prematurity. The ELGAN study investigators relied on parent-reported questionnaires of pulmonary health to examine risk factors for childhood asthma and whether BPD was an antecedent of asthma (Jackson et al. 2018). At the 12-month and 24-month follow-up visits, parents were asked whether their child was currently taking bronchodilator medication regularly or intermittently. At the 10-year visit, parents were asked about bronchodilator use and also whether their child had ever been given an asthma diagnosis by a health care provider since age 2 years. At each follow-up visit, maternal socioeconomic factors were assessed and growth parameters of the child were used to calculate weight gain velocity (grams/kilograms/day).

Fifty-two percent of the children assessed at age 10 years had a history of BPD and 38% reported receiving a diagnosis of childhood asthma. BPD was associated with bronchodilator use at 12 and 24 months of age, but not at 10 years of age. After adjusting for confounding variables, BPD, regardless of severity, was not associated with childhood asthma, while indicators/correlates of socioeconomic disadvantage and weight gain velocity between one and 10 years of age were associated with increased risk of asthma at age 10 years.

These findings suggest that long-term pulmonary dysfunctions in ELGANs are influenced more strongly by the limited socioeconomic resources available to the family and by excessive weight gain following NICU discharge than exposures in the neonatal period. This is consistent with previous studies demonstrating low socioeconomic status as a risk factor for asthma in term infants, attributed, in part, to higher prevalence of obesity and exposure to indoor allergens and environmental pollutants (Stevenson et al. 2001; von Mutius et al. 2001). The association of BPD with bronchodilator use in the first two years of life, but not at 10 years, suggests that early transient wheezing and childhood asthma may be two distinct entities with unique antecedents. Future studies on long-term pulmonary outcomes in ELGANs may be augmented by the use of pulmonary function tests and patient-reported outcomes as this population ages into adolescence and early adulthood.

CONCLUSION – FUTURE STUDIES

This chapter discussed important findings from the ELGAN study about BPD, as well as later wheezing and asthma. These findings have informed study design and analysis in other large cohorts of infants born premature. The strong association of FGR with BPD and the description of early patterns of lung disease, along with their complex relationships with systemic inflammation, have added to our understanding of mechanisms of BPD development. The recognition that severe BPD is an independent risk factor for cerebral palsy and neurocognitive dysfunction at 10 years of age, but not for childhood asthma, generates important hypotheses that can be examined in future studies.

Based on a pilot study more than a decade ago, ELGAN investigators reported that infants who developed BPD had distinct gene expression signatures involving chromatin remodeling and histone acetylation pathways. Since then, ELGAN investigators have shown that CpG hypermethylation levels at multiple sites in the placenta are associated with genes that encode proteins related to immune function, growth/transcription factor signaling and transport across cell membranes, placental microorganisms, and cognitive impairment at age 10 years (Martin et al. 2017; Tomlinson et al. 2017; Tilley et al. 2018). We hope that these techniques will be further leveraged to understand epigenetic changes that influence BPD risk in ELGANs.

REFERENCES

Alejandre Alcazar MA, Morty RE, Lendzian L et al. (2011) Inhibition of TGF-beta signaling and decreased apoptosis in IUGR-associated lung disease in rats. *PLoS One* **6**: e26371. doi: 10.1371/journal.pone.0026371.

Allendorf A, Dewitz R, Weber J, Bakthiar S, Schloesser R, Rolle U (2018) Necrotizing enterocolitis as a prognostic factor for the neurodevelopmental outcome of preterm infants – match control study after 2 years. *J Pediatr Surg* **53**: 1573–7. doi: 10.1016/j.jpedsurg.2018.01.006.

Ambalavanan N, Carlo WA (2004) Bronchopulmonary dysplasia: new insights. *Clin Perinatol* **31**: 613–28. doi: 10.1016/j.clp.2004.05.003.

Ambalavanan N, Carlo WA, D'Angio CT et al. (2009) Cytokines associated with bronchopulmonary dysplasia or death in extremely low birth weight infants. *Pediatrics* **123**: 1132–41. doi: 10.1542/peds.2008-0526.

Ambalavanan N, Nicola T, Hagood J et al. (2008) Transforming growth factor-beta signaling mediates hypoxia-induced pulmonary arterial remodeling and inhibition of alveolar development in newborn mouse lung. *Am J Physiol Lung Cell Mol Physiol* **295**: L86–95. doi: 10.1152/ajplung.00534.2007.

Anand D, Stevenson CJ, West CR, Pharoah PO (2003) Lung function and respiratory health in adolescents of very low birth weight. *Arch Dis Child* **88**: 135–8.

Balany J, Bhandari V (2015) Understanding the impact of infection, inflammation, and their persistence in the pathogenesis of bronchopulmonary dysplasia. *Front Med (Lausanne)* **2**: 90. doi: 10.3389/fmed.2015.00090.

Bayley N (1993) *Bayley Scales of Infant Development*. San Antonio, TX: Psychological Corporation.

Beam KS, Aliaga S, Ahlfeld SK, Cohen-Wolkowiez M, Smith PB, Laughon MM (2014) A systematic review of randomized controlled trials for the prevention of bronchopulmonary dysplasia in infants. *J Perinatol* **34**: 705–10. doi: 10.1038/jp.2014.126.

Bhandari A, Panitch HB (2006) Pulmonary outcomes in bronchopulmonary dysplasia. *Semin Perinatol* **30**: 219–26. doi: 10.1053/j.semperi.2006.05.009.

Bose C, Laughon M, Allred EN et al. (2011) Blood protein concentrations in the first two postnatal weeks that predict bronchopulmonary dysplasia among infants born before the 28th week of gestation. *Pediatr Res* **69**: 347–53. doi: 10.1203/PDR.0b013e31820a58f3.

Bose C, Van Marter LJ, Laughon M et al. (2009) Fetal growth restriction and chronic lung disease among infants born before the 28th week of gestation. *Pediatrics* **124**: e450–8. doi: 10.1542/peds.2008-3249.

Bose CL, Laughon MM, Allred EN et al. (2013) Systemic inflammation associated with mechanical ventilation among extremely preterm infants. *Cytokine* **61**: 315–22. doi: 10.1016/j.cyto.2012.10.014.

Carlo WA, Stark AR, Wright LL et al. (2002) Minimal ventilation to prevent bronchopulmonary dysplasia in extremely-low-birth-weight infants. *J Pediatr* **141**: 370–4.

Cazzato S, Ridolfi L, Bernardi F, Faldella G, Bertelli L (2013) Lung function outcome at school age in very low birth weight children. *Pediatr Pulmonol* **48**: 830–7. doi: 10.1002/ppul.22676.

Cheong JLY, Doyle LW (2018) An update on pulmonary and neurodevelopmental outcomes of bronchopulmonary dysplasia. *Semin Perinatol* **42**: 478–84.

Choi CW (2017) Chorioamnionitis: is a major player in the development of bronchopulmonary dysplasia? *Korean J Pediatr* **60**: 203–7. doi: 10.3345/kjp.2017.60.7.203.

Doyle LW, Halliday HL, Ehrenkranz RA, Davis PG, Sinclair JC (2014) An update on the impact of postnatal systemic corticosteroids on mortality and cerebral palsy in preterm infants: effect modification by risk of bronchopulmonary dysplasia. *J Pediatr* **165**: 1258–60. doi: 10.1016/j.jpeds.2014.07.049.

Doyle LW, Victorian Infant Collaborative Study Group (2006) Respiratory function at age 8–9 years in extremely low birthweight/very preterm children born in Victoria in 1991–1992. *Pediatr Pulmonol* **41**: 570–6. doi: 10.1002/ppul.20412.

Ehrenkranz RA, Walsh MC, Vohr BR et al. (2005) Validation of the National Institutes of Health consensus definition of bronchopulmonary dysplasia. *Pediatrics* **116**: 1353–60. doi: 10.1542/peds.2005-0249.

Eriksson L, Haglund B, Odlind V, Altman M, Ewald U, Kieler H (2015) Perinatal conditions related to growth restriction and inflammation are associated with an increased risk of bronchopulmonary dysplasia. *Acta Paediatr* **104**: 259–63. doi: 10.1111/apa.12888.

Fawke J, Lum S, Kirkby J, Hennessy E et al. (2010) Lung function and respiratory symptoms at 11 years in children born extremely preterm: the EPICure study. *Am J Respir Crit Care Med* **182**: 237–45. doi: 10.1164/rccm.200912-1806OC.

Garite TJ, Clark R, Thorp JA (2004) Intrauterine growth restriction increases morbidity and mortality among premature neonates. *Am J Obstet Gynecol* **191**: 481–7. doi: 10.1016/j.ajog.2004.01.036.

Goncalves C, Wandalsen G, Lanza F, Goulart AL, Sole D, Dos Santos A (2016) Repercussions of preterm birth on symptoms of asthma, allergic diseases and pulmonary function, 6–14 years later. *Allergol Immunopathol (Madr)* **44**: 489–96. doi: 10.1016/j.aller.2016.04.008.

Gray PH, O'Callaghan MJ, Rogers YM (2004) Psychoeducational outcome at school age of preterm infants with bronchopulmonary dysplasia. *J Paediatr Child Health* **40**: 114–20.

Hack M, Wilson-Costello D, Friedman H, Taylor GH, Schluchter M, Fanaroff AA (2000) Neurodevelopment and predictors of outcomes of children with birth weights of less than 1000 g: 1992–1995. *Arch Pediatr Adolesc Med* **154**: 725–31.

Hennessy EM, Bracewell MA, Wood N et al. (2008) Respiratory health in pre-school and school age children following extremely preterm birth. *Arch Dis Child* **93**: 1037–43. doi: 10.1136/adc.2008.140830.

Higgins RD, Jobe AH, Koso-Thomas M et al. (2018) Bronchopulmonary dysplasia: executive summary of a workshop. *J Pediatr* **197**: 300–8. doi: 10.1016/j.jpeds.2018.01.043.

Holsti A, Adamsson M, Hagglof B, Farooqi A, Serenius F (2017) Chronic conditions and health care needs of adolescents born at 23 to 25 weeks' gestation. *Pediatrics* **139**: e20162215. doi: 10.1542/peds.2016-2215.

Hughes CA, O'Gorman LA, Shyr Y, Schork MA, Bozynski ME, McCormick MC (1999) Cognitive performance at school age of very low birth weight infants with bronchopulmonary dysplasia. *J Dev Behav Pediatr* **20**: 1–8.

Jackson WM, O'Shea TM, Allred EN, Laughon MM, Gower WA, Leviton A (2018) Risk factors for chronic lung disease and asthma differ among children born extremely preterm. *Pediatr Pulmonol* **53**: 1533–40. doi: 10.1002/ppul.24148.

Jaeckle Santos LJ, Li C, Doulias PT, Ischiropoulos H, Worthen GS, Simmons RA (2014) Neutralizing Th2 inflammation in neonatal islets prevents beta-cell failure in adult IUGR rats. *Diabetes* **63**: 1672–84. doi: 10.2337/db13-1226.

Jobe AH (2011) The new bronchopulmonary dysplasia. *Curr Opin Pediatr* **23**: 167–72. doi: 10.1097/MOP.0b013e3283423e6b.

Jobe AH, Bancalari E (2001) Bronchopulmonary dysplasia. *Am J Respir Crit Care Med* **163**: 1723–9. doi: 10.1164/ajrccm.163.7.2011060.

Jobe AH, Ikegami M (1998) Mechanisms initiating lung injury in the preterm. *Early Hum Dev* **53**: 81–94.

Kalikkot Thekkeveedu R, Guaman MC, Shivanna B (2017) Bronchopulmonary dysplasia: a review of pathogenesis and pathophysiology. *Respir Med* **132**: 170–7. doi: 10.1016/j.rmed.2017.10.014.

Kallapur SG, Jobe AH (2006) Contribution of inflammation to lung injury and development. *Arch Dis Child Fetal Neonatal Ed* **91**: F132–5. doi: 10.1136/adc.2004.068544.

Kamper J, Feilberg Jorgensen N, Jonsbo F, Pedersen-Bjergaard L, Pryds O (2004) The Danish national study in infants with extremely low gestational age and birthweight (the ETFOL study): respiratory morbidity and outcome. *Acta Paediatr* **93**: 225–32.

Klevebro S, Lundgren P, Hammar U et al. (2016) Cohort study of growth patterns by gestational age in preterm infants developing morbidity. *BMJ Open* **6**: e012872. doi: 10.1136/bmjopen-2016-012872.

Kobaly K, Schluchter M, Minich N et al. (2008) Outcomes of extremely low birth weight (<1 kg) and extremely low gestational age (< 28 weeks) infants with bronchopulmonary dysplasia: effects of practice changes in 2000 to 2003. *Pediatrics* **121**: 73–81. doi: 10.1542/peds.2007-1444.

Kotecha SJ, Watkins WJ, Heron J, Henderson J, Dunstan FD, Kotecha S (2010) Spirometric lung function in school-age children: effect of intrauterine growth retardation and catch-up growth. *Am J Respir Crit Care Med* **181**: 969–74. doi: 10.1164/rccm.200906-0897OC.

Kovo M, Schreiber L, Bar J (2013) Placental vascular pathology as a mechanism of disease in pregnancy complications. *Thromb Res* **131**(Suppl 1): S18–21. doi: 10.1016/s0049-3848(13)70013-6.

Kuban KC, Allred EN, O'Shea M, Paneth N, Pagano M, Leviton A (2008) An algorithm for identifying and classifying cerebral palsy in young children. *J Pediatr* **153**: 466–72. doi: 10.1016/j.jpeds.2008.04.013.

Lacaze-Masmonteil T (2014) That chorioamnionitis is a risk factor for bronchopulmonary dysplasia – the case against. *Paediatr Respir Rev* **15**: 53–5. doi: 10.1016/j.prrv.2013.09.005.

Lal MK, Manktelow BN, Draper ES, Field DJ (2003) Chronic lung disease of prematurity and intrauterine growth retardation: a population-based study. *Pediatrics* **111**: 483–7.

Laptook AR, O'Shea TM, Shankaran S, Bhaskar B (2005) Adverse neurodevelopmental outcomes among extremely low birth weight infants with a normal head ultrasound: prevalence and antecedents. *Pediatrics* **115**: 673–80. doi: 10.1542/peds.2004-0667.

Laughon M, Allred EN, Bose C et al. (2009a) Patterns of respiratory disease during the first 2 postnatal weeks in extremely premature infants. *Pediatrics* **123**: 1124–31. doi: 10.1542/peds.2008-0862.

Laughon M, Bose C, Allred EN et al. (2011a) Patterns of blood protein concentrations of ELGANs classified by three patterns of respiratory disease in the first 2 postnatal weeks. *Pediatr Res* **70**: 292–6. doi: 10.1203/PDR.0b013e3182274f35.

Laughon M, Bose C, Allred EN et al. (2011b) Antecedents of chronic lung disease following three patterns of early respiratory disease in preterm infants. *Arch Dis Child Fetal Neonatal Ed* **96**: F114–20. doi: 10.1136/adc.2010.182865.

Laughon M, O'Shea MT, Allred EN et al. (2009b) Chronic lung disease and developmental delay at 2 years of age in children born before 28 weeks' gestation. *Pediatrics* **124**: 637–48. doi: 10.1542/peds.2008-2874.

Leviton A, Allred EN, Kuban KC et al. (2011) Blood protein concentrations in the first two postnatal weeks associated with early postnatal blood gas derangements among infants born before the 28th week of gestation. The ELGAN study. *Cytokine* **56**: 392–8. doi: 10.1016/j.cyto.2011.07.014.

Leviton A, Dammann O, Engelke S et al. (2010) The clustering of disorders in infants born before the 28th week of gestation. *Acta Paediatr* **99**: 1795–800. doi: 10.1111/j.1651-2227.2010.01973.x.

Lewis BA, Singer LT, Fulton S et al. (2002) Speech and language outcomes of children with bronchopulmonary dysplasia. *J Commun Disord* **35**: 393–406.

Lodha A, Ediger K, Rabi Y et al. (2015) Does chronic oxygen dependency in preterm infants with bronchopulmonary dysplasia at NICU discharge predict respiratory outcomes at 3 years of age? *J Perinatol* **35**: 530–6. doi: 10.1038/jp.2015.7.

Longo S, Bollani L, Decembrino L, Di Comite A, Angelini M, Stronati M (2013) Short-term and long-term sequelae in intrauterine growth retardation (IUGR). *J Matern Fetal Neonatal Med* **26**: 222–5. doi: 10.3109/14767058.2012.715006.

Lowe JR, Duncan AF, Bann CM et al. (2013) Early working memory as a racially and ethnically neutral measure of outcome in extremely preterm children at 18–22 months. *Early Hum Dev* **89**: 1055–61. doi: 10.1016/j.earlhumdev.2013.08.009.

Majnemer A, Riley P, Shevell M, Birnbaum R, Greenstone H, Coates AL (2000) Severe bronchopulmonary dysplasia increases risk for later neurological and motor sequelae in preterm survivors. *Dev Med Child Neurol* **42**: 53–60.

Martin E, Smeester L, Bommarito PA et al. (2017) Sexual epigenetic dimorphism in the human placenta: implications for susceptibility during the prenatal period. *Epigenomics* **9**: 267–78. doi: 10.2217/epi-2016-0132.

McElrath TF, Allred EN, Van Marte, L, Fichorova RN, Leviton A (2013) Perinatal systemic inflammatory responses of growth-restricted preterm newborns. *Acta Paediatr* **102**: e439–42. doi: 10.1111/apa.12339.

Metsala J, Kilkkinen A, Kaila M et al. (2008) Perinatal factors and the risk of asthma in childhood – a population-based register study in Finland. *Am J Epidemiol* **168**: 170–8. doi: 10.1093/aje/kwn105.

Miller JD, Carlo WA (2007) Safety and effectiveness of permissive hypercapnia in the preterm infant. *Curr Opin Pediatr* **19**: 142–4. doi: 10.1097/MOP.0b013e3280895e12.

Neu J, Pammi M (2018) Necrotizing enterocolitis: the intestinal microbiome, metabolome and inflammatory mediators. *Semin Fetal Neonatal Med* **6**: 400–5. doi: 10.1016/j.siny.2018.08.001.

Northway WH, Rosan RC, Porter DY (1967) Pulmonary disease following respirator therapy of hyaline-membrane disease. *New England Journal of Medicine* **276**: 357–68. doi: 10.1056/NEJM196702162760701.

O'Shea TM, Kothadia JM, Klinepeter KL et al. (1999) Randomized placebo-controlled trial of a 42-day tapering course of dexamethasone to reduce the duration of ventilator dependency in very low birth weight infants: outcome of study participants at 1-year adjusted age. *Pediatrics* **104**: 15–21.

O'Shea TM, Washburn LK, Nixon PA, Goldstein DJ (2007) Follow-up of a randomized, placebo-controlled trial of dexamethasone to decrease the duration of ventilator dependency in very low birth weight infants: neurodevelopmental outcomes at 4 to 11 years of age. *Pediatrics* **120**: 594–602. doi: 10.1542/peds.2007-0486.

Palta M, Sadek-Badawi M, Sheehy M et al. (2001) Respiratory symptoms at age 8 years in a cohort of very low birth weight children. *Am J Epidemiol* **154**: 521–9.

Panickar J, Scholefield H, Kumar Y, Pilling DW, Subhedar NV (2004) Atypical chronic lung disease in preterm infants. *J Perinat Med* **32**: 162–7. doi: 10.1515/jpm.2004.029.

Perrone S, Bracciali C, Di Virgilio N, Buonocore G (2016) Oxygen use in neonatal care: a two-edged sword. *Front Pediatr* **4**: 143. doi: 10.3389/fped.2016.00143.

Potharst ES, Van Wassenaer-Leemhuis AG, Houtzager BA et al. (2013) Perinatal risk factors for neurocognitive impairments in preschool children born very preterm. *Dev Med Child Neurol* **55**: 178–84. doi: 10.1111/dmcn.12018.

Reiss I, Landmann E, Heckmann M, Misselwitz B, Gortner L (2003) Increased risk of bronchopulmonary dysplasia and increased mortality in very preterm infants being small for gestational age. *Arch Gynecol Obstet* **269**: 40–4. doi: 10.1007/s00404-003-0486-9.

Richardson DK, Corcoran JD, Escobar GJ, Lee SK (2001) SNAP-II and SNAPPE-II: simplified newborn illness severity and mortality risk scores. *J Pediatr* **138**: 92–100.

Sasi A, Abraham V, Davies-Tuck M et al. (2015) Impact of intrauterine growth restriction on preterm lung disease. *Acta Paediatr* **104**: e552–6. doi: 10.1111/apa.13220.

Shennan AT, Dunn MS, Ohlsson A, Lennox K, Hoskins EM (1988) Abnormal pulmonary outcomes in premature infants: prediction from oxygen requirement in the neonatal period. *Pediatrics* **82**: 527–32.

Shinwell ES, Karplus M, Reich D et al. (2000) Early postnatal dexamethasone treatment and increased incidence of cerebral palsy. *Arch Dis Child Fetal Neonatal Ed* **83**: F177–81.

Short EJ, Kirchner HL, Asaad GR et al. (2007) Developmental sequelae in preterm infants having a diagnosis of bronchopulmonary dysplasia: analysis using a severity-based classification system. *Arch Pediatr Adolesc Med* **161**: 1082–7. doi: 10.1001/archpedi.161.11.1082.

Singer L, Yamashita T, Lilien L, Collin M, Baley J (1997) A longitudinal study of developmental outcome of infants with bronchopulmonary dysplasia and very low birth weight. *Pediatrics* **100**: 987–93.

Singer LT, Siegel AC, Lewis B, Hawkins S, Yamashita T, Baley J (2001) Preschool language outcomes of children with history of bronchopulmonary dysplasia and very low birth weight. *J Dev Behav Pediatr* **22**: 19–26.

Speer CP, Silverman M (1998) Issues relating to children born prematurely. *Eur Respir J Suppl* **27**: 13s–16s.

Sriram S, Condie J, Schreiber MD et al. (2014) Early blood gas predictors of bronchopulmonary dysplasia in extremely low gestational age newborns. *Int J Pediatr* **2014**: 210–18. doi: 10.1155/2014/210218.

Sriram S, Schreiber MD, Msall ME et al. (2018) Cognitive development and quality of life associated with BPD in 10-year-olds born preterm. *Pediatrics* **141**: e20172719. doi: 10.1542/peds.2017-2719.

Stevenson LA, Gergen PJ, Hoover DR, Rosenstreich D, Mannino DM, Matte TD (2001) Sociodemographic correlates of indoor allergen sensitivity among United States children. *J Allergy Clin Immunol* **108**: 747–52. doi: 10.1067/mai.2001.119410.

Stoll BJ, Hansen NI, Bell EF et al. (2015) Trends in care practices, morbidity, and mortality of extremely preterm neonates, 1993–2012. *JAMA* **314**: 1039–51. doi: 10.1001/jama.2015.10244.

Streubel AH, Donohue PK, Aucott SW (2008) The epidemiology of atypical chronic lung disease in extremely low birth weight infants. *J Perinatol* **28**: 141–8. doi: 10.1038/sj.jp.7211894.

Taylor HG, Clark CA (2016) Executive function in children born preterm: risk factors and implications for outcome. *Semin Perinatol* **40**: 520–9. doi: 10.1053/j.semperi.2016.09.004.

Teune MJ, Van Wassenaer AG, Van Buuren S, Mol BW, Opmeer BC, Dutch POPS Collaborative Study Group (2012) Perinatal risk-indicators for long-term respiratory morbidity among preterm or very low birth weight neonates. *Eur J Obstet Gynecol Reprod Biol* **163**: 134–41. doi: 10.1016/j.ejogrb.2012.04.015.

Thomas W, Speer CP (2014) Chorioamnionitis is essential in the evolution of bronchopulmonary dysplasia – the case in favour. *Paediatr Respir Rev* **15**: 49–52. doi: 10.1016/j.prrv.2013.09.004.

Tilley SK, Martin EM, Smeester L et al. (2018) Placental CpG methylation of infants born extremely preterm predicts cognitive impairment later in life. *PLoS One* **13**: e0193271. doi: 10.1371/journal.pone.0193271.

Tomlinson MS, Bommarito PA, Martin EM et al. (2017) Microorganisms in the human placenta are associated with altered CpG methylation of immune and inflammation-related genes. *PLoS One* **12**: e0188664. doi: 10.1371/journal.pone.0188664.

Torchin H, Ancel Py, Goffinet F et al. (2016) Placental complications and bronchopulmonary dysplasia: EPIPAGE-2 cohort study. *Pediatrics* **137**: e20152163. doi: 10.1542/peds.2015–2163.

Van Marter LJ, Kuban KC, Allred E et al. (2011) Does bronchopulmonary dysplasia contribute to the occurrence of cerebral palsy among infants born before 28 weeks of gestation? *Arch Dis Child Fetal Neonatal Ed* **96**: F20–9. doi: 10.1136/adc.2010.183012.

Viscardi RM (2012) Perinatal inflammation and lung injury. *Semin Fetal Neonatal Med* **17**: 30–5. doi: 10.1016/j.siny.2011.08.002.

Visentin S, Lapolla A, Londero AP et al. (2014) Adiponectin levels are reduced while markers of systemic inflammation and aortic remodelling are increased in intrauterine growth restricted mother-child couple. *Biomed Res Int* **2014**: 401–595. doi: 10.1155/2014/401595.

Vohr BR, Wright LL, Dusick AM et al. (2000) Neurodevelopmental and functional outcomes of extremely low birth weight infants in the National Institute of Child Health and Human Development Neonatal Research Network, 1993–1994. *Pediatrics* **105**: 1216–26.

Vom Hove M, Prenzel F, Uhlig HH, Robel-Tillig E (2014) Pulmonary outcome in former preterm, very low birth weight children with bronchopulmonary dysplasia: a case-control follow-up at school age. *J Pediatr* **164**: 40–5 e4. doi: 10.1016/j.jpeds.2013.07.045.

Von Mutius E, Schwartz J, Neas LM, Dockery D, Weiss ST (2001) Relation of body mass index to asthma and atopy in children: the National Health and Nutrition Examination Study III. *Thorax* **56**: 835–8.

Wolfe KR, Vannatta K, Nelin MA, Yeates KO (2015) Executive functions, social information processing, and social adjustment in young children born with very low birth weight. *Child Neuropsychol* **21**: 41–54. doi: 10.1080/09297049.2013.866217.

Wood NS, Costeloe K, Gibson AT, Hennessy EM, Marlow N, Wilkinson AR (2005) The EPICure study: associations and antecedents of neurological and developmental disability at 30 months of age following extremely preterm birth. *Arch Dis Child Fetal Neonatal Ed* **90**: F134–40.

Yun EJ, Lorizio W, Seedorf G, Abman SH, Vu TH (2016) VEGF and endothelium-derived retinoic acid regulate lung vascular and alveolar development. *Am J Physiol Lung Cell Mol Physiol* **310**: L287–98. doi: 10.1152/ajplung.00229.2015.

Zhang H, Dysart K, Kendrick DE et al. (2018) Prolonged respiratory support of any type impacts outcomes of extremely low birth weight infants. *Pediatr Pulmonol* **53**: 1447–1455. doi: 10.1002/ppul.24124.

Zysman-Colman Z, Tremblay GM, Bandeali S, Landry JS (2013) Bronchopulmonary dysplasia – trends over three decades. *Paediatr Child Health* **18**: 86–90.

PART III
Structural Brain Disorders

Chapter 10   Ultrasound   105

Chapter 11   Multispectral Quantitative MRI   115

Ultrasound

Genevieve Taylor and T Michael O'Shea

INTRODUCTION

Cranial ultrasonography is recommended by the American Academy of Neurology and the Child Neurology Society for routine screening of infants born before 30 weeks of gestation to identify intraventricular hemorrhage (IVH) and cerebral white matter abnormalities. Individuals born extremely preterm are at high risk for those brain disorders, and bedside cranial ultrasound is often the only feasible imaging technique for preterm infants in the first weeks of life due to their clinical instability. Cranial ultrasonography has been refined over the past 30 years, with increasing resolution and sensitivity (Levine et al. 1991; de Vries and Groenendaal 2002; de Vries et al. 2004; Govaert and De Vries 2010; Maller and Cohen 2017). A variety of classification schemes have been developed to guide prognostic studies of ultrasound abnormalities (Papile et al. 1983; Stewart et al. 1987; deVries et al. 1992; Paneth et al. 1994; Rademaker et al. 1994; Dammann and Leviton 1997; Paneth 1999; Bassan et al. 2006; Leviton et al. 2007). Although effective treatments are not available for either IVH or cerebral white matter abnormalities, per se, identification by cranial ultrasound allows for prognostication and identification of infants at highest risk of neurodevelopmental impairment, who may benefit from early intervention and planning of services.

In the ELGAN study of brain and related disorders among extremely low gestational age newborns, cranial ultrasound was the first brain-related outcome assessed in study participants. When developing procedures used to ascertain ultrasound outcomes, ELGAN study investigators drew from knowledge gained from the Neonatal Brain Hemorrhage Study (Nigel Paneth, principal investigator) and the Developmental Epidemiology Network (Alan Leviton, principal investigator). For example, these studies provided important insights regarding the timing of hemorrhages arising from the germinal matrix (Paneth et al. 1993), the typical extent of inter-reader disagreement about ultrasound abnormalities (Pinto-Martin et al. 1992), and the prevalences and rates of co-occurrence for IVH and cerebral white matter injury (Leviton and Gilles 1996; Kuban et al. 1999; Paneth 1999).

Based on estimates about the timing of occurrence of germinal matrix hemorrhage in very preterm infants, the ELGAN study focused on two sets of ultrasound scans collected in the first two weeks of life: scans obtained between the 1st and 4th days of life (n = 1123 infants) and scans obtained between the 5th and 14th days of life (n = 1302 infants). Based on estimates of the timing of appearance of indicators of cerebral white matter injury, that is, ventriculomegaly and intracerebral hypoechoic lesion (also referred to as echolucency), data were also collected on scans obtained between the 15th day of life and 40 weeks postmenstrual age (n = 1268 infants). All ultrasound data used in the ELGAN study were obtained as a part of clinical care for infant participants; no ultrasound scans were obtained solely for research purposes.

Based on prior research by ELGAN investigators (Kuban and Teele 1984; Pinto-Martin et al. 1992; O'Shea et al. 1993), extensive efforts were directed towards enhancing inter-rater reliability of ultrasound interpretations. The primary focuses of these efforts were cerebral white matter injury, as indicated by either ventriculomegaly or periventricular hypoechoic lesions, and IVH.

Prior work by ELGAN investigators provided prevalence estimates used to guide decisions about sample size. From prior studies, the projected incidence of a hypoechoic lesion was 8%. Using discharge data from the neonatal intensive care units at the 14 ELGAN enrollment sites, an enrollment rate of 90%, and a survival rate of 80%, we estimated that the ELGAN study would have sufficient power to identify a doubling of the risk of a hypoechoic lesion among infants with an inflammation-related protein level in the top quintile (as compared to infants in the lower four quintiles), even in halves of the sample characterized by the presence or absence of another risk factor or set of risk factors. The projected sample also provided sufficient power to see whether an inflammation-related protein level in the top quintile is associated with increased risk among infants with a blood level of a biomarker thought to have protective effects.

In this chapter we summarize published work based on brain ultrasound findings from the ELGAN study, including both studies of brain structural abnormalities as the outcome as well as studies of these abnormalities as the exposure. The strengths of these studies include the large multi-center sample, extensive efforts to enhance reliability of interpretations, and standardized and blinded assessment of developmental outcomes through 10 years of age.

INTER-RATER RELIABILITY OF CRANIAL ULTRASOUND INTERPRETATION

Prior studies on inter-rater reliability of cranial ultrasound in infants included very low birth weight infants as well as low birth weight infants, and groups that include preterm as well as small for gestational age infants born at term, some of whom were at relatively low risk of acquired brain lesions (Pinto et al. 1988; Pinto-Martin et al. 1992; O'Shea et al. 1993; Harris et al. 2005; Hintz et al. 2007a). In contrast, the ELGAN study focused on extremely low gestational age newborns, a group at high risk for IVH. The designers of the ELGAN study had gained experience with classifying neonatal brain ultrasound abnormalities in large prospectively studied cohorts of low birth weight (Pinto-Martin et al. 1992) and preterm neonates (Kuban et al. 1999). Among many important findings from these cohorts are three that are particularly relevant to the design of the ELGAN study; each was replicated in the ELGAN study (Kuban et al. 2007; O'Shea et al. 2012). First, the reliability (extent of inter-observer agreement) was higher for *observations* about brain ultrasound abnormalities than was the reliability about *diagnoses* (Pinto-Martin et al. 1992). Based on this finding, extensive pre-study efforts (described below) were directed towards maximizing inter-observer agreement about ultrasound findings (Kuban et al. 2007). Second, ultrasound indicators of white matter injury, particularly intracerebral echolucent lesions (also referred to as hypoechoic lesions) and enlargement of the cerebral ventricles (also referred to as ventriculomegaly), were more strongly associated with cerebral palsy than was intraventricular hemorrhage (Pinto-Martin et al. 1995). Based on this finding considerable investigator efforts were directed towards describing the location of echolucent lesions and the severity of ventriculomegaly in the ultrasounds obtained from ELGAN study participants. Third, ultrasound indicators of white matter injury, as just described, co-occurred with intraventricular hemorrhage much more frequently than would be expected by chance alone (Kuban et al. 1999). This finding informed the analysis plan for studies of the associations between ultrasound abnormalities and cerebral palsy.

Pre-study efforts to maximize inter-observer reliability of ultrasound interpretations involved 16 ultrasound readers at 14 centers. Each reader had at least 5 years of experience. They reviewed a manual and data collection form used in a previous study (the Developmental Epidemiology Network), and after incorporating suggested revisions, all readers agreed to the revised manual and data collection form. The manual and data collection form included templates of multiple levels of ventriculomegaly. The need for additional revision was assessed with scans that illustrated a variety of abnormalities that could be interpreted differently by experienced sonologists. These scans were distributed and served as discussion points for conference calls intended to develop strategies to minimize variation in interpretation. Potential sources of variation were identified, most of which had already been addressed in the manual. After training, at least two readers interpreted each cranial ultrasound using a standard form for recording observations and diagnoses. Observations were simple descriptive terms such as IVH, moderate or severe ventriculomegaly, and cerebral hypoechoic lesion or hyperechoic lesion. Diagnoses included early periventricular leukomalacia, cystic periventricular leukomalacia, periventricular hemorrhagic infarction, and 'other' white matter diagnoses. Each reader made diagnoses independently – uniform diagnostic criteria were omitted from the study design so that variability in the application of diagnostic labels could be measured (Westra et al. 2010). If readers disagreed on important observations, a third reader reviewed the ultrasound and provided a 'tie-breaker' interpretation (Kuban et al. 2007).

The rate of percent agreement positive ranged from 68% to 76% for ventriculomegaly, hypoechoic lesions, and IVH. Rates of negative agreement for these findings ranged from 92% to 97%, and kappa values ranged from 0.62 to 0.68. Considerably lower values of positive agreement (48%), negative agreement (84%), and kappa (0.32) were found for hyperechoic lesions (Kuban et al. 2007).

Inter-reader disagreement was greatest for the diagnosis of early periventricular leukomalacia (Westra et al. 2010). Three readers applied this label to more than one-fourth of the scans they read, while eight applied this diagnosis to 5% or fewer scans. Readers applied the diagnosis of periventricular hemorrhagic infarction to between 0% and 11% of scans. Among the diagnoses studied, inter-reader disagreement was lowest for cystic periventricular leukomalacia. Readers identified cystic periventricular leukomalacia in 1–9% of scans. While some experts regard cystic periventricular leukomalacia as a bilateral abnormality, in more than one-third of scans in which cystic periventricular leukomalacia was identified, the abnormality was a unilateral hypoechoic lesion. In summary, experienced readers differ greatly in their application of diagnostic labels for white matter lesions on cranial ultrasound, implying a lack of uniform diagnostic criteria.

PRENATAL FACTORS AND CRANIAL ULTRASOUND ABNORMALITIES

Maternal factors associated with an increased risk of ultrasound indicators of cerebral white matter injury (hypoechoic lesion and/or ventriculomegaly) were lack of antenatal steroids, preterm labor, premature rupture of fetal membranes, and cervical insufficiency. Maternal preeclampsia was associated with lower risk (McElrath et al. 2009). The recovery of multiple microorganisms from placenta was associated with an increased risk of ultrasound indicators of cerebral white matter injury (Leviton et al. 2010b). The recovery from the placenta of low-virulence microorganisms regarded as skin flora, such as *Corynebacterium* species and non-aureus *Staphylococcus* species, was associated with an increased risk of ultrasound indicators of cerebral white matter injury. However, the recovery of vaginal flora from the placenta was not associated with the risk of brain ultrasound abnormalities. Histologic findings indicative of placental inflammation were associated with increased risk of ventriculomegaly, whereas placenta infarct was associated with reduced risk (Leviton et al. 2010b).

NEONATAL FACTORS AND CRANIAL ULTRASOUND ABNORMALITIES

Among ELGAN study participants, recurrent blood gas derangements including hypoxemia, hypercapnia, and acidemia were associated with ventriculomegaly (including that which was accompanied or preceded by intraventricular hemorrhage and that which was not) (Leviton et al. 2010a). These multiple derangements are likely indicators of immaturity, vulnerability, and illness severity. Similarly, physiologic instability in the first 12 postnatal hours, represented by high SNAP-II or SNAPPE-II scores, was associated with IVH, moderate or severe ventriculomegaly, and echogenic white matter lesions. Markers of physiologic instability might be indicative of illness severity or underlying immaturity or vulnerability not captured by adjustment for gestational age and related factors (Dammann et al. 2010). Although hypotension had been posited, for many years, to be an important risk factor for preterm brain injury (Volpe 2001), in the ELGAN cohort, hypotension (defined by lowest mean arterial pressure in the lowest quartile for gestational age or treatment with a vasopressor) and blood pressure lability (defined as the upper quartile of the difference between each infant's lowest and highest MAP) in the first 24 hours were not associated with an increased risk of moderate/severe ventriculomegaly or hypoechoic lesions (Logan et al. 2011).

ELGAN study findings suggest that the risk profile of hypoechoic lesions with IVH is different from that of isolated hypoechoic lesions, consistent with the possibility that these entities have different casual pathways. Gestational age <25 weeks, high SNAP-II score, early recurrent or prolonged acidemia, analgesic exposure, and mechanical ventilation on the seventh postnatal day were associated with increased risk of hypoechoic lesions with IVH, but not isolated hypoechoic lesions (Logan et al. 2013).

Perinatal inflammation as a risk factor for preterm brain injury and developmental impairment was the primary focus of the ELGAN study. One of the approaches taken to explore the posited link between perinatal inflammation and adverse brain-related outcomes was to measure inflammation-related proteins in dried blood spots collected from ELGAN infants when blood was being drawn for clinically indicated laboratory studies. As detailed in the first chapter, inflammation-related protein biomarkers included cytokines, chemokines, adhesion molecules, matrix metalloproteinases, growth factors, angiogenic factors, and neurotrophins. In most ELGAN analyses infants were classified as having an elevated level of a biomarker if the level was in the highest quartile conditional on gestational age, postnatal age, and assay batch. Most infants contributed samples at five points in time: postnatal day 1 and around postnatal days 7, 14, 21, and 28. However, because clinical indications for laboratory testing diminished with advancing postnatal age, children who were 21 and 28 days old were less likely to have provided blood specimens than children who were younger. The result is the bias of 'not missing at random' (also known as non-ignorable non-response). Thus the most often used operational definition for 'sustained or recurrent elevation' of a biomarker was a level in the highest quartile on two or more days in the first 14 postnatal days.

Elevations of inflammation-related biomarkers in neonatal blood were associated with an increased risk of ultrasound findings indicative of white matter injury. Children who had ventriculomegaly were more likely than their peers to have a top quartile concentration of vascular endothelial growth factor receptor 1 (VEGF-R1), serum amyloid A (SAA), matrix metalloproteinase-9 (MMP-9), macrophage inflammatory protein-1β (MIP-1β), interleukin 8 (IL-8), and Regulated on Activation Normal T Cell Expressed and Secreted (RANTES). Those who had a hypoechoic lesion were more likely than others to have such elevated concentrations of vascular cell adhesion molecule 1 (VCAM-1), intracellular adhesion molecule 1 (ICAM-1), MIP-1β, and RANTES. Elevations of these proteins in blood co-occurred frequently, and no protein elevation was identified as clearly more important than any other (Leviton et al. 2011). Sustained or recurrent inflammation (defined above) was more strongly associated with white matter injury than was inflammation found on a single day. Ventriculomegaly and hypoechoic lesions were associated with elevated concentrations of inflammation-related biomarkers on postnatal day 1, which were much higher in newborns whose placenta showed histological indicators of inflammation, supporting the hypothesis that inflammation linked with white matter injury begins in utero.

Patterns of inflammation-related biomarker elevations suggested that IVH should be viewed as two entities – IVH without white matter abnormality and IVH with white matter abnormality (moderate to severe ventriculomegaly on late scan or hypoechoic lesions on any scan) (Leviton et al. 2012). IVH is known to co-occur with white matter injury more frequently than would be expected if their occurrences were independent of one anther (Kuban et al. 1999). Isolated IVH and IVH with white matter injury were both associated with increased inflammation, but IVH with white matter injury was associated with a stronger and more persistent inflammatory signal. IVH with white matter injury was associated with elevations of C-reactive protein and IL-8 on days 1, 7, and 14, and elevations of SAA and tumor necrosis factor-α (TNF-α) on two separate days in the first two postnatal weeks (Leviton et al. 2012).

CRANIAL ULTRASOUND ABNORMALITIES AND INFANT NEURODEVELOPMENTAL OUTCOMES

The ELGAN study provided a particularly rich source of data about the relationship between cranial ultrasound abnormalities and infant neurodevelopmental outcomes. The follow-up protocol at 24 months adjusted age included parents' completion of the Child Behavior Checklist, a standardized neurological assessment, with which infants could be classified as to the presence and subtype of cerebral palsy, and the Bayley Scales of Infant Development – Second Edition. At 10 years of age, assessments included intelligence testing, assessments of executive function, evaluations for epilepsy and autism, and parents' reports of communication and social functioning as well as symptoms of anxiety, depression, and attention deficit hyperactivity disorder. At both 24 months and 10 years, ELGAN participants were assessed by certified examiners who were not aware of the children's ultrasound findings. Analyses of relationships between cranial ultrasound findings and outcomes assessed at ten years of age are ongoing, so only studies involving outcomes assessed at 24 months adjusted age will be summarized here.

Among children without cranial ultrasound abnormalities, 23% had a low Mental Development Index (MDI) and 26% had low Psychomotor Development Index (PDI), with low scores defined as <70 (>2 standard deviations). Infants with moderate-to-severe ventriculomegaly and/or hypoechoic lesions, however, were three to five times more likely to have a low PDI and two to three times more likely to have a low MDI (O'Shea et al. 2008).

Infants with IVH, hypoechoic lesions, or ventriculomegaly were about three times more likely than children who had not had these ultrasound abnormalities to have microcephaly at 24 months' corrected age. These children were not microcephalic at birth, supporting the hypothesis that widespread white matter injury, indicated by ventriculomegaly and/or hypoechoic lesions, leads to reduced brain growth (Krishnamoorthy et al. 2011).

Isolated IVH was not associated with increased risk of cerebral palsy, microcephaly, or low scores on the Bayley Scales of Infant Development. Isolated IVH was associated with an increased risk of impaired visual fixation, but not other visual or hearing impairments (Kuban et al. 2009; O'Shea et al. 2012). In contrast, IVH with white matter injury (defined as ventriculomegaly, cerebral hyperechoic and hypoechoic lesions in this study) was strongly associated with cerebral palsy, microcephaly, Bayley Scales of Infant Development scores more than 3 standard deviations below the normative mean, visual impairment, and hearing impairment. However, infants with IVH plus white matter injury were not at greater risk for these outcomes than infants who had only white matter injury (O'Shea et al. 2012).

At 24 months adjusted age, cerebral palsy was the impairment most strongly associated with white matter injury on cranial ultrasound (Kuban et al. 2009; O'Shea et al. 2012). The prevalence of cerebral palsy was 6% for children with normal cranial ultrasounds. Infants with hypoechoic lesions were 24 times more likely than children who did not have hypoechoic lesions to be diagnosed with four-limb cerebral palsy (referred to in ELGAN study papers as quadriparesis) and 29 times more likely to be diagnosed with unilateral cerebral palsy (referred to in ELGAN study papers as hemiparesis). Infants with ventriculomegaly were 17 times more likely to be diagnosed with quadriparesis or hemiparesis than infants with normal cranial ultrasounds. In comparison to their peers who had normal ultrasound scans, those who had a history of hypoechoic lesions or ventriculomegaly were five to six times more likely to develop leg-dominated symmetric cerebral palsy (referred to in ELGAN study papers as diparesis) (Kuban et al. 2009). Nonetheless, in the ELGAN study, almost half the children with cerebral palsy had normal cranial ultrasounds (Kuban et al. 2009).

Bilateral cerebellar hemorrhages were strongly associated with microcephaly, low Bayley scores, and cerebral palsy. Among infants with bilateral cerebellar hemorrhage, almost 80% had microcephaly at 24 months, 30% had four-limb cerebral palsy, 30% had unilateral cerebral palsy, and 73% had low Bayley scores (Krishnamoorthy et al. 2011). These findings are limited by the small number of infants with cerebellar hemorrhage – only 14 were identified in the ELGAN cohort – and that mastoid views, which can more precisely evaluate the cerebellum, were not routinely obtained.

COMPARISONS WITH FINDINGS FROM OTHER EXTREMELY PRETERM COHORTS

Other investigators who have studied the reliability of interpretations of cranial ultrasounds concluded, as did the ELGAN study investigators, that even after training and consensus-building discussions, inter-reader agreement is higher for hypoechoic, as compared to hyperechoic, lesions, and is higher for lesions that are more strongly associated with neurodevelopmental impairment, as compared to lesions, such as isolated germinal matrix hemorrhage, which are only weakly associated with impairment (Pinto et al. 1988; Corbett et al. 1991; O'Shea et al. 1993; Hintz et al. 2007b; Hagmann et al. 2011). All of these studies point to the importance of focused efforts to enhance inter-reader reliability when conducting research studies that employ neonatal cranial ultrasound and the need for caution when counseling families about prognosis related to ultrasound lesions for which inter-reader reliability is low, such as germinal matrix hemorrhage and small intracerebral hyperechoic lesions.

Many of the ELGAN study findings about antecedents of cranial ultrasound abnormalities are novel, particularly those related to placenta characteristics (histology and microbiology) and those related to antecedents (e.g. preterm labor), correlates (e.g. high SNAP score), and biomarkers (e.g. levels of cytokines) of inflammation in neonatal blood. Consistent with these findings is the observation, in the EPIPAGE-2 cohort of infants born in France in 2011 at gestational age between 22 and 31 weeks, infants born to mothers with preterm labor and elevated C-reactive protein were at increased risk for intraventricular hemorrhage (Chevallier et al. 2017). The finding of increasing risk of cranial ultrasound abnormalities with decreasing gestational age has been reported previously in a study of the EPIPAGE-1 cohort of infants born in France in 1997, at 22–32 weeks of gestation. In that cohort, decreasing gestational age was associated with increasing risk of white matter damage, defined as cystic periventricular leukomalacia; echodensities persisting for more than 14 days without cyst formation; large unilateral parenchymal hyperdensity or large unilateral porencephalic cyst; and isolated ventricular dilatation with no associated IVH (Larroque et al. 2003). The ELGAN study investigators' observation that a mother's receipt of antenatal steroids was associated with a lower risk of cerebral white matter abnormality agrees with conclusions from a study of the EPICURE cohort (Costeloe et al. 2000).

Several of the ELGAN study findings about associations between specific neonatal cranial ultra-sound abnormalities and neurodevelopmental outcomes during infancy have been previously described in other cohorts of individuals born extremely preterm. In the EPICURE cohort, an abnormality on the final neonatal cranial ultrasound was associated with an increased risk of cerebral palsy (Wood et al. 2005). Similarly, in the EPIPAGE-1 cohort, severe cranial ultrasound abnormalities were associated with a lower developmental quotient at 2 years of age (Fily et al. 2006). As compared to infants with no cranial ultrasound abnormalities, infants with intraventricular hemorrhage accompanied by ventric-ular dilatation were about four times as likely, and infants with white matter abnormality (ventricular dilation, persistent echodensities, or cystic periventricular leukomalacia), about six times as likely, to develop cerebral palsy (Ancel et al. 2006). Consistent with findings from the ELGAN study, one-third of EPIPAGE-1 infants who developed cerebral palsy had no abnormality on neonatal cranial ultrasound. When the EPIPAGE cohort was assessed at 5 years of age, severe cranial ultrasound abnormalities (either intraventricular hemorrhage accompanied by ventricular dilatation or white matter abnormality) were associated with a higher likelihood of minor neuromotor dysfunctions (Arnaud et al. 2007), cerebral palsy (Beaino et al. 2010), and severe cognitive impairment (Beaino et al. 2011). Evaluation of the rela-tionship between cranial ultrasound abnormalities and neurodevelopmental outcome at school age are underway using data from the ELGAN study. In these studies, methodological aspects of the ELGAN study that could reduce the bias include extensive efforts to increase the validity of ultrasound interpre-tations and school-age cognitive and neuromotor assessments, as well as masking examiners to study participants' medical histories and cranial ultrasound findings.

SUMMARY

Reliable interpretation of cranial head ultrasound scans obtained in a large cohort of extremely low gesta-tional age newborns allowed for robust epidemiologic analysis of IVH and white matter injury, including their antecedents and associated outcomes. From the perspective of researchers interested in the epide-miology and prevention of neurodevelopmental impairments among individuals born preterm, probably the most important finding from the ELGAN study about cranial ultrasound findings is the strong association between elevations of inflammation-related proteins in neonatal blood collected in the first two postnatal weeks and ultrasound-defined evidence of cerebral white matter injury. Consistent with the concept that perinatal inflammation contributes to cerebral white matter injury are the ELGAN study findings that maternal treatment with antenatal steroids, which have anti-inflammatory effects, was associated with a lower risk, while correlates of intrauterine inflammation, including preterm delivery, preterm labor, premature rupture of the membranes, and microorganisms recovered from the placenta, were associated with a higher risk of ultrasound indicators of cerebral white matter injury. IVH, when not accompanied by ultrasound indicators of cerebral white matter injury, was not as strongly associated with inflammation as was cerebral white matter injury.

From the perspective of clinicians who care for infants born extremely preterm, probably the most important finding from the ELGAN study is that ultrasound indicators of cerebral white matter injury are strongly predictive of cerebral palsy, low scores on the Bayley Scales of Infant Development, and microcephaly at 24 months' adjusted age. The associations are strongest for unilateral cerebral palsy and symmetrical cerebral palsy affecting all four extremities. Despite the high positive predictive value of ultrasound for CP, sensitivity was low for CP and even lower for other developmental impairments. Cranial ultrasound indicators of cerebral white matter injury were not identified in almost half of the

ELGAN study participants who developed cerebral palsy, and the sensitivity of these ultrasound indicators was less than 20% for identification of infants who subsequently had low scores on the Bayley Scales of Infant Development Mental Developmental Index. These limitations of ultrasound for prediction of neurodevelopmental impairments were the basis for the ELGAN study's goal of longitudinal follow-up of study participants using validated assessment of neurodevelopment and constitute a compelling rationale for further study of neonatal brain magnetic resonance imaging to improve detection of white matter and cerebellum lesions not detected with ultrasound (Woodward et al. 2006; Hintz et al. 2018), as well as long-term developmental surveillance of survivors of extremely preterm birth.

REFERENCES

Ancel PY, Livinec F, Larroque B et al. (2006) Cerebral palsy among very preterm children in relation to gestational age and neonatal ultrasound abnormalities: the EPIPAGE cohort study. *Pediatrics* **117**: 828–35.

Arnaud C, Daubisse-Marliac L, White-Koning M et al. (2007) Prevalence and associated factors of minor neuromotor dysfunctions at age 5 years in prematurely born children: the EPIPAGE study. *Arch Pediatr Adolesc Med* **161**: 1053–61.

Bassan H, Limperopoulos C, Visconti K et al. (2006) Ultrasonographic severity scoring of periventricular hemorrhagic infarction in relation to neurological outcome. *Annals of Neurology* **60**: S158–9.

Beaino G, Khoshnood B, Kaminski M et al. (2011) Predictors of the risk of cognitive deficiency in very preterm infants: the EPIPAGE prospective cohort. *Acta Paediatr* **100**: 370–8.

Beaino G, Khoshnood B, Kaminski M et al. (2010) Predictors of cerebral palsy in very preterm infants: the EPIPAGE prospective population-based cohort study. *Dev Med Child Neurol* **52**: e119–25.

Chevallier M, Debillon T, Pierrat V et al. (2017) Leading causes of preterm delivery as risk factors for intraventricular hemorrhage in very preterm infants: results of the EPIPAGE 2 cohort study. *Am J Obstet Gynecol* **216**: 518 e1–518 e12.

Corbett S, Rosenfeld C, Laptook A et al. (1991) Intraoberver and interobserver reliability in assessment of neonatal cranial ultrasounds. *Early Hum Dev* **27**: 9–17.

Costeloe K, Hennessy E, Gibson AT, Marlow N, Wilkinson AR (2000) The EPICure study: outcomes to discharge from hospital for infants born at the threshold of viability. *Pediatrics* **106**: 659–71.

Dammann O, Leviton A (1997) Duration of transient hyperechoic images of white matter in very-low-birthweight infants: a proposed classification. *Dev Med Child Neurol* **39**: 2–5.

Dammann O, Naples M, Bednarek F et al. (2010) SNAP-II and SNAPPE-II and the risk of structural and functional brain disorders in extremely low gestational age newborns: the ELGAN study. *Neonatology* **97**: 71–82.

De Vries LS, Groenendaal F (2002) Neuroimaging in the preterm infant. *Mental Retardation and Developmental Disabilities Research Reviews* **8**: 273–80.

De Vries LS, Van Haastert ILC, Rademaker KJ, Koopman C, Groenedaal F (2004) Ultrasound abnormalities preceding cerebral palsy in high-risk preterm infants. *Journal of Pediatrics* **144**: 815–20.

Devries LS, Eken P, Dubowitz LMS (1992) The spectrum of leukomalacia using cranial ultrasound. *Behavioural Brain Research* **49**: 1–6.

Levine IL, Williams JL, Fawer C-L (eds) (1991) *Ultrasound of the Infant Brain.* London: Mac Keith Press.

Fily A, Pierrat V, Delporte V, Breart G, Truffert P (2006) Factors associated with neurodevelopmental outcome at 2 years after very preterm birth: the population-based Nord-Pas-de-Calais EPIPAGE cohort. *Pediatrics* **117**: 357–66.

Govaert P, De Vries LS (2010) *An Atlas of Neonatal Brain Sonography* (2nd edn). London: Mac Keith Press.

Hagmann C, Halbherr M, Koller B et al. (2011) Interobserver variability in assessment of cranial ultrasound in very preterm infants. *Journal of Neuradiology* **38**: 291–97.

Harris DL, Teele RL, Bloomfield FH, Harding JE (2005) Does variation in interpretation of ultrasonograms account for the variation in incidence of germinal matrix/intraventricular haemorrhage between newborn intensive care units in New Zealand? *Arch Dis Child Fetal Neonatal Ed* **90**: F494–9.

Hintz, SR, Slovis, T, Bulas D et al. (2007a) Interobserver reliability and accuracy of cranial ultrasound scanning interpretation in premature infants. *J Pediatr* **150**: 592–6, 596.e1–5.

Hintz SR, Slovis T, Bulas D et al. (2007b) Interobserver reliability and accuracy of cranial ultrasound scanning interpretation in premature infants. *Journal of Pediatrics* **150**: 592–6.

Hintz SR, Vohr BR, Bann CM et al. (2018) Preterm neuroimaging and school-age cognitive outcomes. *Pediatrics* **142**: e20174058.

Krishnamoorthy KS, Kuban KC, O'Shea TM, Westra SJ, Allred EN, Leviton A (2011) Early cranial ultrasound lesions predict microcephaly at age 2 years in preterm infants. *J. Child Neurol* **26**: 188–94.

Kuban K, Adler I, Allred E et al. (2007) Observer variability assessing US scans of the preterm brain: the ELGAN study. *Pediatr Radiol* **37**: 1201–8.

Kuban K, Sanocka U, Leviton A et al. (1999) White matter disorders of prematurity: association with intraventricular hemorrhage and ventriculomegaly. The Developmental Epidemiology Network. *J Pediatr* **134**: 539–46.

Kuban K, Teele RL (1984) Rationale for grading intracranial hemorrhage in premature-infants. *Pediatrics* **74**: 358–63.

Kuban KC, Allred EN, O'Shea TM et al. (2009) Cranial ultrasound lesions in the NICU predict cerebral palsy at age 2 years in children born at extremely low gestational age. *J Child Neurol* **24**: 63–72.

Larroque B, Marret S, Ancel PY et al. (2003) White matter damage and intraventricular hemorrhage in very preterm infants: The epipage study. *Journal of Pediatrics* **143**: 477–83.

Leviton A, Allred E, Dammann O et al. (2012) Systemic inflammation, intraventricular hemorrhage, and white matter injury. *J Child Neurol* Oct 30. doi: 10.1177/0883073812463068.

Leviton A, Allred E, Kuban KCK et al. (2010a) Early blood gas abnormalities and the preterm brain. *American Journal of Epidemiology* **172**: 907–16.

Leviton A, Gilles F (1996) Ventriculomegaly, delayed myelination, white matter hypoplasia, and 'periventricular' leukomalacia: how are they related? *Pediatr Neurol* **15**: 127–36.

Leviton A, Hecht J, Onderdonk A et al. (2010b) Microbiological and histologic characteristics of the extremely preterm infant's placenta predict white matter damage and later cerebral palsy. The ELGAN study. *Pediatric Research* **67**: 95–101.

Leviton A, Kuban K, O'Shea, T et al. (2011) The relationship between early concentrations of 25 blood proteins and cerebral white matter injury in preterm newborns. *Journal of Pediatrics* **158**: 897–903.

Leviton A, Kuban K, Paneth N (2007) Intraventricular haemorrhage grading scheme: time to abandon? *Acta Paediatrica* **96**: 1254–6.

Logan JW, O'Shea TM, Allred EN et al. (2011) Early postnatal hypotension is not associated with indicators of white matter damage or cerebral palsy in extremely low gestational age newborns. *J Perinatol* **31**: 524–34.

Logan JW, Westra SJ, Allred EN et al. (2013) Antecedents of perinatal cerebral white matter damage with and without intraventricular hemorrhage in very preterm newborns. *Pediatr Neurol* **49**: 88–96.

Maller VV, Cohen HL (2017) Neurosonography: assessing the premature infant. *Pediatr Radiol* **47**: 1031–45.

McElrath TF, Allred EN, Boggess KA et al. (2009) Maternal antenatal complications and the risk of neonatal cerebral white matter damage and later cerebral palsy in children born at an extremely low gestational age. *American Journal of Epidemiology* **170**: 819–28.

O'Shea TM, Allred EN, Kuban KCK et al. (2012) Intraventricular hemorrhage and developmental outcomes at 24 months of age in extremely preterm infants. *Journal of Child Neurology* **27**: 22–9.

O'Shea TM, Kuban KC, Allred EN et al. (2008) Neonatal cranial ultrasound lesions and developmental delays at 2 years of age among extremely low gestational age children. *Pediatrics* **122**: e662–9.

O'Shea TM, Volberg F, Dillard RG (1993) Reliability of interpretation of cranial ultrasound examinations of very low-birthweight neonates. *Dev Med Child Neurol* **35**: 97–101.

Paneth N (1999) Classifying brain damage in preterm infants. *J Pediatr* **134**: 527–9.

Paneth N, Pinto-Martin J, Gardiner J et al. (1993) Incidence and timing of germinal matrix intraventricular hemorrhage in low-birth-weight infants. *American Journal of Epidemiology* **137**: 1167–76.

Paneth N, Rudelli R, Kazam E, Monte W (1994) Prognosis. In: Paneth N, Rudelli R, Kazam E, Monte W (eds) *Brain Damage in the Preterm Infant* (1st edn) London: Cambridge University Press.

Papile LA, Munsickbruno G, Schaefer A (1983) Relationship of cerebral intraventricular hemorrhage and early-childhood neurologic handicaps. *Journal of Pediatrics* **103**: 273–7.

Pinto J, Paneth N, Kazam E et al. (1988) Interobserver variability in neonatal cranial ultrasonography. *Paediatr Perinat Epidemiol* **2**: 43–58.

Pinto-Martin J, Paneth N, Witomski T et al. (1992) The central New Jersey neonatal brain haemorrhage study: design of the study and reliability of ultrasound diagnosis. *Paediatr Perinat Epidemiol* **6**: 273–84.

Pinto-Martin JA, Riolo S, Cnaan A, Holzman C, Susser MW, Paneth N (1995) Cranial ultrasound prediction of disabling and nondisabling cerebral palsy at age two in a low birth weight population. *Pediatrics* **95**: 249–54.

Rademaker KJ, Groenendaal F, Jansen GH, Eken P, Devries LS (1994) Unilateral hemorrhagic parenchymal lesions in the preterm infant – shape, site and prognosis. *Acta Paediatrica* **83**: 602–8.

Stewart AL, Reynolds EO, Hope PL et al. (1987) Probability of neurodevelopmental disorders estimated from ultrasound appearance of brains of very preterm infants. *Dev Med Child Neurol* **29**: 3–11.

Volpe JJ (2001) Neurobiology of periventricular leukomalacia in the premature infant. *Pediatr Res* **50**: 553–62.

Westra S, Adler I, Batton D et al. (2010) Reader variability in the use of diagnostic terms to describe white matter lesions seen on cranial scans of severely premature infants: the ELGAN study. *J Clin Ultrasound* **38**: 409–19.

Wood NS, Costeloe K, Gibson AT, Hennessy EM, Marlow N, Wilkinson AR (2005) The EPICure study: associations and antecedents of neurological and developmental disability at 30 months of age following extremely preterm birth. *Archives of Disease in Childhood-Fetal and Neonatal Edition* **90**: 134–40.

Woodward LJ, Anderson PJ, Austin NC, Howard K, Inder TE (2006) Neonatal MRI to predict neurodevelopmental outcomes in preterm infants. *New England Journal of Medicine* **355**: 685–94.

Multispectral Quantitative MRI
Techniques and Preliminary Results

Hernán Jara and T Michael O'Shea

INTRODUCTION

In the past 16 years since the initiation of the ELGAN study in 2002, quantitative magnetic resonance imaging (qMRI) scanning technologies and companion computational algorithms have improved in speed, spatial resolution, anatomical coverage, numerical accuracy, and overall practicality. Moreover, several qMRI techniques using a single magnetic resonance imaging (MRI) acquisition have been developed that allow creating multiple spatially coregistered quantitative maps, each representing a different qMRI parameter, thus increasing use of multispectral (MS) qMRI as a more unified and informative imaging approach. MS-qMRI techniques simplify and enhance tissue identification and classification via automated or semi-automated segmentation algorithms, anatomic structural characterization via volumetrics, and the generation of parameter histograms, also known as qMRI spectrograms, and make possible new types of image contrast via Synthetic-MRI. MS-qMRI is rapidly transitioning from research laboratories to large-scale and multisite research initiatives. Importantly, many MS-qMRI pulse sequences are currently available across the major scanner platforms and prototypical MS-qMRI techniques are approaching inter-platform standardization leading to increased quantitative data consistency, thus reducing data harmonization difficulties.

For several reasons, MS-qMRI is exceptionally promising for detecting and characterizing the potentially altered (see Fig. 11.1) brain developmental pathways of preterm born individuals primarily:

1. Since MRI does not use ionizing radiation, it can be repeated longitudinally to characterize brain development.
2. By reporting on multispectral tissue information via separate qMRI channels that convey complementary information, qMRI parameters are descriptive of macroscopic structure as well as the voxel scale tissue information including hydration level, microkinetics, and molecular interactions of water, macromolecules, and lipids.
3. A wealth of qMRI information characterizing normal and abnormal brain developmental pathways of term born individuals is available for comparison.

In this chapter we will provide background information about MRI and MS-qMRI and review qMRI parameters as functions of age: normal brain development.

1. ELGAN study methods A: MRI acquisition protocols.
2. ELGAN study methods B: image processing.
3. ELGAN results: volumetry at 10 years (the second wave of ELGAN follow-up).

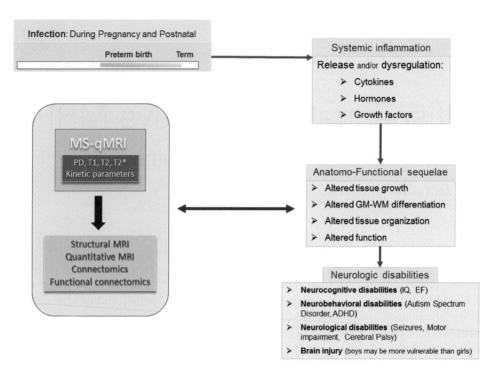

Figure 11.1 The ELGAN hypotheses and the MS-qMRI channels of information. A color version of this figure can be found in the color plate section.

4. Connectomics (from the completed second wave and the ongoing third wave of ELGAN follow-up).
5. Future research on the ELGAN-2 and ELGAN-3 MRI databases.

LIST OF ABBREVIATIONS

apparent diffusion coefficient (ADC)
diffusion tensor imaging (DTI)
gray matter (GM)
magnetic resonance imaging (MRI)
multispectral (MS)
quantitative magnetic resonance imaging (qMRI)
white matter (WM)
white matter tractography (WMT)

INTRODUCTORY THEORY

MR Imaging

MRI encompasses numerous experimental techniques known as MRI pulse sequences with which sectional images (slices) can be computer generated. Such MRI pulse sequences embody two complementary methods: first the nuclear magnetic resonance (NMR) induction method, which uses pulsed radio waves at the resonant frequency to interrogate the nuclear magnetism or magnetization of the imaging subject, and second, a spatial encoding method, which uses the so-called magnetic field gradients to tag the location in three-dimensional space of tissue. The result is the formation of tissue compartments, also known as volume elements or voxels. The great majority of MRI pulse sequences used in clinical practice are set up to probe the most abundant form of nuclear magnetization found in biological tissues, specifically that of the hydrogen nuclei (^{1}H-protons), hence the fundamental delineation of organs with MRI replicates the relative concentrations of protons among the tissues intersected by the imaging slice.

Principles of qMRI and MS-qMRI

An MS-qMRI technique consists of two complementary components that are designed as a matched pair, specifically a multi-contrast MRI pulse sequence and a multispectral processing algorithm. The former is used to generate the directly acquired images that are post-processed with the multispectral algorithm for generating the several qMRI parameter maps that are spatially coregistered.

MS-qMRI pulse sequences are special MRI pulse sequences that are optimized for the purpose of generating images suitable for qMRI processing. A very fruitful line of qMRI techniques stem from the *principle of differential weighting* with which a given qMRI parameter is mapped from images that are directly acquired under identical experimental conditions in all respects (i.e. spatial resolution, coverage), except for the degree of weighting to the specific qMRI parameter targeted for mapping. In other words, the only difference between two differentially weighted images is the value of the pulse sequence parameter that controls the degree of weighting of the targeted qMRI parameter. Accordingly, the most useful MS-qMRI pulse sequences can efficiently generate high quality 'differentially-weighted data sets' using short and therefore clinically useful scan times.

The principles of MS-qMRI can be summarized as follows: (1) weighting reversal with pixel value calibration for quantifying the 1H proton density, (2) differential weighting for quantifying the liquid pool qMRI parameters, and (3) differential weighting for the semisolid pool parameters. We draw a distinction between the principles of differential weighting for the liquid pool versus the semisolid pool because the qMRI parameters of the liquid pool can be determined individually and the parameters of the semisolid pool are calculated simultaneously as a group from a set of magnetization transfer weighted images.

MRI METRICS AS FUNCTIONS OF ADVANCING BRAIN DEVELOPMENT

The biological state of gray matter (GM) and white matter (WM) changes throughout the human lifespan and is highly complex. Advanced MRI offers a wide array of measurable parameters that can be used to describe biological properties of the tissue. Structural MRI (sMRI) reports metrics that are representative of groups of related voxels forming tissue or organ segments. At a finer spatial scale MS-qMRI metrics report information at the single voxel level. Typical sMRI metrics include segmental volumes, spatial distributions, surfaces, and volume shapes. The MS-qMRI metrics include: (a) measures of tissue hydration via ^{1}H-proton density of mobile water, (b) measures of microscopic and microvascular motion (e.g. water diffusion and blood perfusion parameters), and (c) measures of 1H-proton interactions with the microscopic magnetic environment, as reported by the relaxation times of the longitudinal magnetization (T_1) and the transverse magnetization (T_2 and T_2^*). In the following sections, we review sMRI and qMRI studies of age-related changes in brain tissue.

Structural MRI

SEQUENTIAL SUBJECT-BY-SUBJECT VS VOXEL-BASED-MORPHOMETRY PROCESSING PIPELINES

Sequential subject-by-subject processing pipelines consist of generating structural measures on individual subjects and then performing statistical analyses of the full cohort. These pipelines can be automated to a high degree and are preferred for analyzing cohorts with relatively high neuro-heterogeneity, as was the case in the ELGAN cohort at 10 years of age, when compared to an age matched cohort of full term born typically developing children.

Voxel-based morphometry is a fundamentally different neuroimaging analysis technique for detecting local differences in brain anatomy; it uses the approach of statistical parametric mapping (Ashburner and Friston 2000; Good et al. 2001). The voxel-based morphometry image processing protocol begins with registering every brain to a common template thus reducing most of the large differences in brain anatomy among subjects. Second, the brain images are smoothed so that each voxel represents the average of itself and its neighbors. Finally, the image volume is compared across brains at every voxel. Voxel-based morphometry can be sensitive to various artifacts, including misalignment of brain structures, misclassification of tissue types, differences in folding patterns and in cortical thickness.

Specific sMRI and qMRI Parameters as Functions of Advancing Age

The age dependencies of brain tissue volumes and qMRI parameters are illustrated in the following sections using approximate phenomenological mathematical expressions gained or developed from the literature. These functions of age are based on different cohorts of 'normal' subjects studied with various MRI technologies that have not yet been fully standardized; presented results must therefore be regarded as approximate age tendencies. Four distinct periods of brain structure have been defined: (1) maturation from birth to 2 years, (2) development from 2 to 20 years of age, (3) adulthood from 20 to 55 years, and (4) a very long senescence period from 55 to end of life, which can extend up to approximately 122 years.

VOLUMETRY

As shown in the idealized graphs in Figure 11.2A (Blatter et al. 1995; Courchesne et al. 2000; Ge et al. 2002; Saito et al. 2009; Watanabe et al. 2012), the total intracranial volume increases rapidly from birth to approximately 8 years of age and remains approximately constant thereafter. The total volume of brain matter (equal to WM+GM) of the combined cerebrum and cerebellum, also increases rapidly and peaks in early adolescence; it decreases gradually and approximately linearly during adulthood and quadratically during senescence. The volumetric age dependencies of males and females are very similar with smaller adult intracranial volume by about 150 cm^3.

PROTON DENSITY (MOBILE WATER)

Proton density is difficult to map accurately because a qMRI technique based on the principle of differential weighting has not yet been devised. Therefore, proton density maps are modulated by receiver coil sensitivity profile and in addition require the use of a calibration tissue/substance. For internal calibration intraventricular cerebrospinal fluid is commonly used as proton density reference, whereas external calibration typically involves a vial with water attached to the subject's forehead. Nevertheless, for brain tissue in general and WM in particular, an alternative and indirect approach is available, based on the empirical relationship proposed by Fatouros and Marmarou (1999). This proton density -T1 relationship has been assumed here as valid for all ages: as shown in the graph of Figure 11.2B, the MR-visible proton density of WM decreases rapidly from birth to approximately 2 years of age and continues to

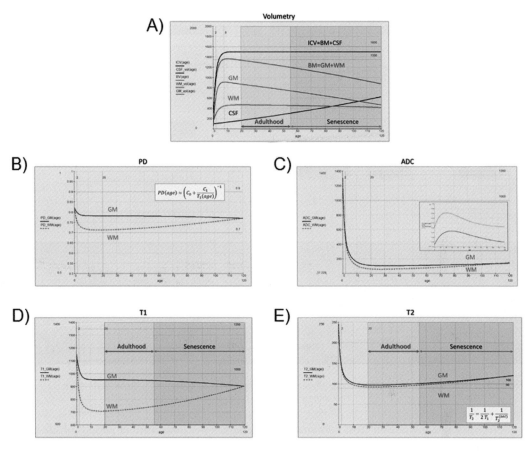

Figure 11.2   Brain qMRI parameters as functions of advancing age. A color version of this figure can be found in the color plate section.

decrease until early adulthood. During adulthood and senescence the WM-to-GM proton density difference decreases monotonically.

DIFFUSION MRI

MR-derived diffusion metrics are generated with diffusion-weighted pulse sequences using the *pulsed-field gradient* method, which includes balanced magnetic field gradient pulses (see Fig. 11.3, left panel). Pulsed-field gradient diffusion-encoding with balanced gradient pulses was initially conceived (Stejskal and Tanner 1965) for diffusion NMR of whole samples, later applied (Le Bihan and Breton 1985; Merboldt et al. 1985; Taylor and Bushell 1985) to mapping the diffusion coefficients along several directions, and for mapping high order mathematical constructs, starting with the diffusion tensor. Further processing of these high order diffusion constructs allows white matter tractography (WMT) techniques via diffusion tensor imaging (DTI). In total, diffusion MRI encompasses generating isotropic diffusion coefficients, apparent diffusion coefficients (ADC) that include the effects of perfusion for living tissue, the diffusion tensor, and high order diffusion constructs with which more accurate WM tractograms can be created. From the diffusion tensor, several scalar parameters can be derived, prominent among which is the fractional anisotropy.

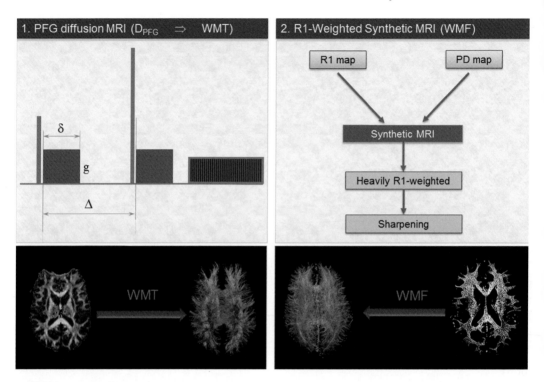

Figure 11.3   dMRI-WMT and WMF. A color version of this figure can be found in the color plate section.

A recent single-institution cross-sectional study demonstrated four distinct periods of life based on the age dependence of the peak ADC values of brain tissue (WM+GM), as derived from sequential patient-by-patient histogram analysis (Watanabe et al. 2012). It was shown that the peak value of the whole brain ADC can be accurately modeled as the sum of two decaying exponentials plus a constant term and a linearly increasing term. The two decaying exponential terms model the very fast ADC drop from birth to 2 years of age (maturation period) and the slower ADC decrease from 2 to 20 years (developmental period). The constant term is dominant between the ages of 20 and 60, and the positive linear term models the very gradual ADC increase observed during senescence.

The literature reporting WM age dependencies of DTI-derived parameters is extensive (Shimony et al. 1999; Chun et al. 2000; Pfefferbaum et al. 2000; Mukherjee et al. 2001; Abe et al. 2002; Moseley 2002; Barnea-Goraly et al. 2005; Zhang et al. 2005; Sullivan and Pfefferbaum 2006; Provenzale et al. 2007; Abe et al. 2008; Westlye et al. 2010) and an exhaustive listing is beyond the scope of this chapter. A recent DTI study showed that 12 white matter tracts followed similar general fractional anisotropy age dependent trajectories (Lebel et al. 2012). Fractional anisotropy increased from childhood to adulthood, reached a peak in early to mid-adulthood, and then decreased during later adulthood at a rate slower than the initial increases. Such peak fractional anisotropy value ages are fiber specific (see Fig. 11.2C: peak age for fractional anisotropy of the corpus callosum genu is approximately 10 years younger than that of the anterior limb). In contrast, the mean diffusivity age trends (not shown) are opposite, decreasing initially, reaching a minimum, and then increasing at a slower rate.

PERFUSION

Reported age-dependent qMRI measures of the normal brain perfusion are relatively scarce primarily because of risks associated with the current clinical MRI standard, which involves an injection of a gadolinium based contrast agent. Hence, the MR perfusion technique of choice for longitudinal studies and research in general with healthy volunteers, as well as with vulnerable populations, has been arterial spin labeling, which provides noninvasive measures of cerebral blood flow (Parkes et al. 2004; Biagi et al. 2007; Wang et al. 2008; Asllani et al. 2009; van Osch et al. 2009; Chen et al. 2011; Taki et al. 2011; Liu et al. 2012). Global cerebral blood flow measures as a function of age reveal (Biagi et al. 2007) a pronounced decrease in cerebral blood low for GM and WM at the onset of adulthood (e.g. 20 years of age) as well as linear decline in cerebral blood flow (with a slope of −0.38% per year) for cortical GM and relative cerebral blood flow stability for subcortical GM.

THE LONGITUDINAL MAGNETIZATION RELAXATION TIME (T1)

Among qMRI parameters, T1 is the clearest WM-to-GM discriminator because of the marked T1 shortening effects of myelin (see Figs 11.4 and 11.5). As shown in Figure 11.2D, at birth the T1s of WM and GM are very high and nearly equal. The T1 values of both tissues decrease with advancing age and begin to differentiate during maturation. WM-to-GM differentiation continues during the developmental period and peaks at about 20 years of age. During adulthood the WM-to-GM T1 difference is comparatively stable but decreases slowly. During adulthood and senescence, the T1s of WM and GM increase and decrease respectively. Interestingly, by extrapolating these T1 age curves, the GM curve crosses the WM curve at about 120 years of age (Fig. 11.2D). This coincides approximately with the reported ages of the oldest human beings.

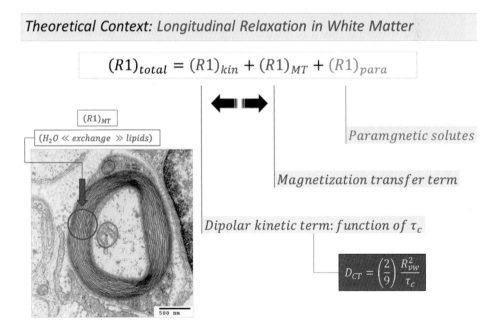

Theoretical Context: Longitudinal Relaxation in White Matter

$$(R1)_{total} = (R1)_{kin} + (R1)_{MT} + (R1)_{para}$$

$(R1)_{MT}$

$(H_2O \ll exchange \gg lipids)$

Paramgnetic solutes

Magnetization transfer term

Dipolar kinetic term: function of τ_c

$$D_{CT} = \left(\frac{2}{9}\right)\frac{R_{vw}^2}{\tau_c}$$

500 nm

Figure 11.4   The structure of myelin: Implications for qMRI. A color version of this figure can be found in the color plate section.

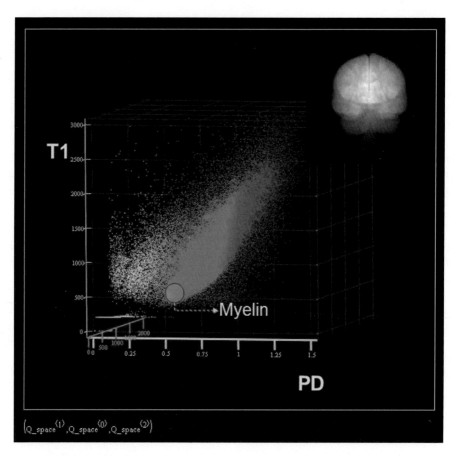

Figure 11.5   qMRI space of normal brain. A color version of this figure can be found in the color plate section.

THE TRANSVERSE MAGNETIZATION RELAXATION TIME (T2)

As shown in Figure 11.2E, the T2 versus age curves of healthy GM and WM also show four distinct periods of life (Ding et al. 2004; Saito et al. 2009): the maturation and developmental periods, during which T2 decreases exponentially and reaches minimum GM and WM T2 values at the onset of adulthood (20 years of age). T2 values remain comparatively stable during adulthood and slowly increase during senescence. The T2 differences between GM and WM are much smaller than for T1 because the T2 relaxation effects are dominated by the pure spin-spin dephasing interactions, the strength of which is much less myelin specific: see insert formula in Figure 11.2E.

ELGAN STUDY METHODS

Participants and Neurocognitive Measures

Among the 889 children enrolled and evaluated at 10 years, an *ELGAN-2 MRI sub-cohort* of 166 children (73 males and 93 females) ages 9–11 years (mean of 9.8 years) underwent cranial MRI evaluations at one of the 12 approved imaging centers after parents or legal guardians granted informed consent and children gave assent. Children were selected for the MRI subsample based on the level of circulating blood protein markers of inflammation in the first 2 weeks of life; approximately a third each had high, intermediate, and low inflammation values. Essentially all children with high inflammatory values were included in the MRI sample while the other two groups were a random sample of children with intermediate and low inflammatory exposure. Gestational age did not factor into the MRI selection decisions; the MRI sample had a modestly higher proportion of children from the oldest gestational age group (34% vs 28%) and a modestly lower proportion from the youngest gestational age group (21% vs 28%) compared to the overall sample. For these subjects, general cognitive ability (or IQ) was assessed with the School-Age Differential Ability Scales–II (DAS-II) Verbal and Nonverbal Reasoning scales (Elliot 2007) as reviewed in detail elsewhere (Joseph et al. 2016).

MRI Methods

The *ELGAN-ECHO-3 study* aims to recruit, at 15 years of age, at least 810 ELGAN participants and to obtain brain MRI on as many as possible. At this writing over 450 ELGAN participants have completed MRI at age 15, using a more comprehensive MS-qMRI protocol that includes dMRI, DTI, and resting state functional MRI. This protocol provides for volumetrics, MS-qMRI (proton density, T1, T2, and T2*), structural connectomics (WMT and white matter fibrography), and functional connectomics via default mode network rendering. Acquisition from MS-qMRI pulse sequences requires a scan time of slightly less than 8 minutes; pulse field gradient diffusion pulse sequences require about 10–12 minutes; and dynamic T2*-weighted pulse sequences require about 7 minutes. During functional scanning, participants are asked to close their eyes. MRI sequence details and details of image processing are provided in the Appendix.

ELGAN STUDY EARLY RESULTS

Comparative Volumetry at 10 Years (ELGAN-2)

The control group consisted of 61 full term (FT) born and typically developing children (30 males and 31 females) from the National Institutes of Health (NIH) MRI Study of Normal Brain Development (Evans 2006); the data were downloaded with permission from the National Database for Autism Research (NDAR) database (https://ndar.nih.gov/). The children had been scanned at 3T with a protocol that included a DE-TSE pulse sequence; they were selected to have a similar age and sex distribution as the ELGAN-2 MRI sub-cohort.

Marked differences were observed between ELGAN-2 and FT children. First, a much wider dispersion of the ELGAN volumes relative to FT children was observed, and was most pronounced for the larger segments from ICM, total brain, whole GM, cortical GM, and whole WM (p-value for variances <0.05). Such increased volumetric variability in the ELGAN cohort is further evidenced by the two-to-three-fold larger standard deviations. Second, the following ELGAN segments – boys and girls – were smaller relative to the FT children (from larger to smaller percent differences): cerebral WM (−25%), whole C&B (−15%), whole brain (−11%), C&B WM (−9%), and ICM (−6%). Third, two ELGAN segments were larger (p < 0.05) relative to FTs: dGM (males +18% and females +23%) and total cerebrospinal fluid (males +78% and females +27%). Fourth, whole GM and cortical GM volumes were smaller by about 3% but without achieving statistical significance (Alshamrani 2017).

White Matter Fibrography (WMF)

The network inventory of the human brain that accounts for the totality of neural elements including neurons, synapses, as well as the axonal interconnections is known as the connectome. Connectome realizations can be conceptualized at three progressively coarser neuro-structural spatial scales, from the

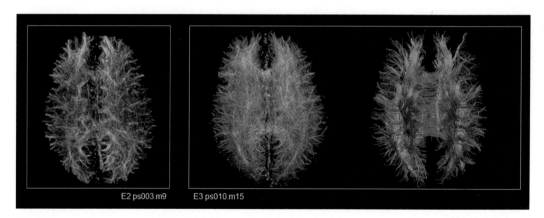

E2 ps003.m9   E3 ps010.m15

Figure 11.6   WMF: From E2 to E3 and MS-qMRI reports. A color version of this figure can be found in the color plate section.

microscale of individual neurons and synapses, to the mesoscale of mini columns of neurons and their connection patterns, to the macroscale of brain regions and pathways.

A microscopic rendition of the human brain connectome through imaging would entail creating a comprehensive three-dimensional map of its neural connection matrix as sampled at sub-cellular spatial resolution of voxels $\leq (1\mu m)^3$. The creation of such microscopic connectomes in vivo, while not currently possible, would have profound implications for understanding normal neurological function as well as for deciphering the complexities of neurologic disorders. Similarly, noninvasive in vivo connectome rendering at the mesoscale using voxels $\leq (50\mu m)^3$ is also currently out of reach.

Creating in vivo macroscopic connectome renditions at the coarser spatial resolution possible with current magnetic resonance imaging (MRI) technologies (voxels $\geq (500\mu m)^3$ could have far-reaching research and clinical implications provided that such connectome renditions are spatially accurate, reproducible, obtained with the short scan times needed for routine clinical workflow, and generated with standard configuration clinical equipment.

Diffusion-MRI white matter tractography (dMRI-WMT) is currently the only technique available for in vivo brain connectomics; we have developed a fundamentally different technique, white matter fibrography (WMF). WMF is a multi-step connectomics technique that includes two methods, specifically, MS-qMRI for creating a digital patient representation, and synthetic-MRI for virtual MRI scanning using simulated experimental conditions not easily achievable in vivo, specifically for generating synthetic images that are heavily weighted by the longitudinal relaxation rate ($R1 = 1/T1$). These images delineate the underlying architecture of WM and allow for the generation of structural connectome renditions. We illustrate with one example the organizational changes in the connectomes from the ELGAN-2 time point (10 years of age) to the ELGAN-3 time point (15 years of age), as shown in Figure 11.6.

FUTURE RESEARCH ON THE ELGAN-2 AND ELGAN-3 MRI DATABASES

In this chapter we have described the guiding imaging principles used for designing the MRI arms of the ELGAN-2 and ELGAN-3 studies at two special time points – 10 and 15 years of age – of the preterm brain development. Major emphasis has been on the implementation of MRI acquisition techniques that are quantitative, comprehensively informative, accurate, fast, and available across diverse imaging platforms as required by multisite research initiatives such as ELGAN. In addition, we have described the changes of brain qMRI parameters as functions of advancing age for healthy full term born individuals, in order to provide the (idealized) reference qMRI versus age patterns for future analyses of the ELGAN-2 and 3 databases.

We also have described key elements of the MS-qMRI image processing pipelines, which extend from macroscopic (volumetrics) measures, to voxel scale multispectral measures, to structural connectomics with two techniques (dMRI-WMT and WMF), and ending with functional connectomics via resting state functional MRI.

Early results of preliminary volumetric analyses point to a much increased volumetric variability of the extremely preterm brain tissues at age 10 relative to a comparable cohort of normally developing term born children. In addition, preliminary results are consistent with prior studies indicating that, on average, the brain of individuals born prematurely is reduced, primarily due to reduced WM volume.

Structural connectomics of the extremely preterm brain via WMF indicate very pronounced WM architectural changes from 10 to 15 years of age. These early observations suggest that between late childhood to adolescence, WM changes are predominantly in tissue quality – perhaps specialization – rather than tissue quantity by volume.

Summarizing, the ELGAN study MRI arms at ages 10 and 15 are generating MS-qMRI databases which, by virtue of being quantitative, have the potential of supporting a wide spectrum of research initiatives encompassing the original aims of the ELGAN studies and beyond.

APPENDIX: DETAILS OF THE MRI ACQUISITION PROTOCOLS AND IMAGE PROCESSING

MRI Acquisition

MS-qMRI Pulse Sequence: PD: T1: T2: and WMF

Dual-echo turbo spin echo (DE-TSE) consists of an excitation pulse followed by two turbo spin echo readouts and can be used to generate maps of PD and T2. Therefore, DE-TSE has two-fold multispectral and is one of the simplest, artifact resilient, fast, and most ubiquitous MS-qMRI pulse sequence.

Next in multispectrality is the Triple-TSE; this is a minimalistic triple weightings acquisition available in all platforms that achieves T1-weighting by magnetization saturation (short repetition time) and PD- and T2-weightings via a dual-echo TSE imaging. Key imaging parameters (Siemens Prisma 3T): voxel = $0.5 \times 0.5 \times 2$ mm^3, TEeff1, 2 = 12 ms and 102 ms, TR1, 2 = 0.5 s and 10 s, leading to a scan time of 7:34 minutes. The timing parameters vary slightly for different scanners.

Pulsed Field Gradient Diffusion Pulse Sequence: DTI and WMT

A diffusion weighted spin echo single-shot echoplanar imaging (DW-SE-sshEPI) acquisition, was implemented with 16 diffusion encoding directions and two b-values: 0 and 1000 s/mm^2. Key imaging parameter settings are: isotropic voxel = (1.5 mm)^3, TEeff = 89.2 ms, TR = 3230 ms, and multiband acceleration factor = 4 resulting in a scan time of 10–12 minutes depending on scanner.

Dynamic T2*-weighted Pulse Sequence: Default Mode Network (DMN)

Functional images are acquired using a gradient-echo planar imaging (EPI) sequence (TR = 2010 ms, TE = 36 ms, isotropic voxel = (2 mm)^3, 64 contiguous slices. A total of 270 EPI volumes are acquired with a total scan time of about 7 minutes depending on scanner.

Image Processing

MS-qMRI Algorithms

The directly acquired images of the mixed-TSE or tri-TSE acquisitions were used to create maps of the relaxation times and rates $R1,2 = 1/T1,2$, and the water-normalized proton density using in-house developed qMRI algorithms programmed in Python.

Brain Segmentation

The skull and extracranial tissues were removed using a dual clustering segmentation algorithm (Jara 2013). The skull stripped $R1$-weighted synthetic images, which show well-defined white matter structure, were processed with Fiji (Schindelin et al. 2012): first sharpened with the 'Unsharp mask' filter (radius = 1 and mask weight = 0.7).

DTI Processing

The ELGAN data set was processed using DSI Studio (http://dsi-studio.labslover.org), an open-source diffusion MRI analysis tool for connectome analysis. The source code is publicly available on the same website. A high angular resolution diffusion imaging (HARDI) scheme (Tuch et al. 2002) was used and the diffusion tensor was calculated on a pixel by pixel basis.

REFERENCES

Abe O, Aoki S, Hayashi N et al. (2002) Normal aging in the central nervous system: quantitative MR diffusion-tensor analysis. *Neurobiology of Aging* **23**: 433–41.

Abe O, Yamasue H, Aoki S et al. (2008) Aging in the CNS: comparison of gray/white matter volume and diffusion tensor data. *Neurobiology of Aging* **29**: 102–16.

Alshamrani KM (2017) *Whole-brain and segmental volumetry of extremely low gestational age newborn (ELGAN) children at ten years of age.* PhD thesis. University of Massachusetts Lowell.

Ashburner J, Friston K (2000) Voxel-based morphometry – the methods. *Neuroimage* **11**: 805–21.

Asllani I, Habeck C, Borogovac A, Brown TR, Brickman AM, Stern Y (2009) Separating function from structure in perfusion imaging of the aging brain. *Human Brain Mapping* **30**: 2927–35.

Barnea-Goraly N, Menon V, Eckert M et al. (2005) White matter development during childhood and adolescence: a cross-sectional diffusion tensor imaging study. *Cerebral Cortex* **15**: 1848.

Biagi L, Abbruzzese A, Bianchi M, Alsop D, Del Guerra A, Tosetti M (2007) Age dependence of cerebral perfusion assessed by magnetic resonance continuous arterial spin labeling. *Journal of Magnetic Resonance Imaging* **25**: 696–702.

Blatter DD, Bigler ED, Gale SD et al. (1995) Quantitative volumetric analysis of brain MR: normative database spanning 5 decades of life. *American Journal of Neuroradiology* **16**: 241–51.

Chen JJ, Rosas HD, Salat DH (2011) Age-associated reductions in cerebral blood flow are independent from regional atrophy. *Neuroimage* **55**: 468–78.

Chun T, Filippi C, Zimmerman R, Ulug A (2000) Diffusion changes in the aging human brain. *American Journal of Neuroradiology* **21**: 1078.

Courchesne E, Chisum HJ, Townsend J et al. (2000) Normal brain development and aging: quantitative analysis at in vivo MR imaging in healthy volunteers. *Radiology* **216**: 672.

Ding, XQ, Kucinski T, Wittkugel O et al. (2004) Normal brain maturation characterized with age-related T2 relaxation times: an attempt to develop a quantitative imaging measure for clinical use. *Investigative Radiology* **39**: 740.

Elliot C (2007) *Differential Ability Scales-II (DAS-II).* San Antonio, TX: Pearson.

Evans AC (2006) The NIH MRI study of normal brain development. *Neuroimage* **30**: 184–202.

Fatouros P, Marmarou A (1999) Use of magnetic resonance imaging for in vivo measurements of water content in human brain: method and normal values. *Journal of Neurosurgery* **90**: 109.

Ge Y, Grossman RI, Babb JS, Rabin ML, Mannon LJ, Kolson DL (2002) Age-related total gray matter and white matter changes in normal adult brain. Part I: volumetric MR imaging analysis. *American Journal of Neuroradiology* **23**: 13–27.

Good CD, Johnsrude IS, Ashburner J, Henson RNA, Friston KJ, Frackowiak RSJ (2001) A voxel-based morphometric study of ageing in 465 normal adult human brains. *Neuroimage* **14**: 21–36.

Jara H (2013) *Theory of Quantitative Magnetic Resonance Imaging.* Singapore: World Scientific Publishing Co. Pte. Ltd.

Joseph RM, O'Shea TM, Allred EN et al. (2016) Neurocognitive and academic outcomes at age 10 years of extremely preterm newborns. *Pediatrics* **137**: e20154343.

Le Bihan D, Breton E (1985) Imagerie de diffusion in vivo par résonance magnétique nucléaire = in vivo magnetic resonance imaging of diffusion. *CR Acad Sci Paris* **301**: 1109–12.

Lebel C, Gee M, Camicioli R, Wieler M, Martin W, Beaulieu C (2012) Diffusion tensor imaging of white matter tract evolution over the lifespan. *Neuroimage* **60**: 340–52.

Liu Y, Zhu X, Feinberg D et al. (2012) Arterial spin labeling MRI study of age and gender effects on brain perfusion hemodynamics. *Magnetic Resonance in Medicine* **68**: 912–22.

Merboldt KD, Hanicke W, Frahm J (1985) Self-diffusion NMR imaging using stimulated echoes. *Journal of Magnetic Resonance* **64**: 479–86.

Moseley M (2002) Diffusion tensor imaging and aging – a review. *NMR in Biomedicine* **15**: 553–60.

Mukherjee P, Miller J, Shimony J et al. (2001) Normal brain maturation during childhood: developmental trends characterized with diffusion-tensor MR imaging. *Radiology* **221**: 349.

Parkes LM, Rashid W, Chard DT, Tofts PS (2004) Normal cerebral perfusion measurements using arterial spin labeling: reproducibility, stability, and age and gender effects. *Magnetic Resonance in Medicine* **51**: 736–43.

Pfefferbaum A, Sullivan EV, Hedehus M, Lim KO, Adalsteinsson E, Moseley M (2000) Age related decline in brain white matter anisotropy measured with spatially corrected echo planar diffusion tensor imaging. *Magnetic Resonance in Medicine* **44**: 259–68.

Provenzale J, Liang L, Delong D, White L (2007) Diffusion tensor imaging assessment of brain white matter maturation during the first postnatal year. *American Journal of Roentgenology* **189**: 476.

Saito N, Sakai O, Ozonoff A, Jara H (2009) Relaxo-volumetric multispectral quantitative magnetic resonance imaging of the brain over the human lifespan: global and regional aging patterns. *Magn Reson Imaging* **27**: 895–906.

Schindelin J, Arganda-Carreras I, Frise E et al. (2012) Fiji: an open-source platform for biological-image analysis. *Nature Methods* **9**: 676.

Shimony JS, McKinstry RC, Akbudak E et al. (1999) Quantitative diffusion-tensor anisotropy brain MR imaging: normative human data and anatomic analysis1. *Radiology* **212**: 770.

Stejskal E, Tanner J (1965) Spin diffusion measurements: spin echoes in the presence of a time-dependent field gradient. *Journal of Chemical Physics* **42**: 288–92.

Sullivan EV, Pfefferbaum A (2006) Diffusion tensor imaging and aging. *Neuroscience & Biobehavioral Reviews* **30**: 749–61.

Taki Y, Hashizume H, Sassa Y et al. (2011) Correlation between gray matter density-adjusted brain perfusion and age using brain MR images of 202 healthy children. *Human Brain Mapping* **32**: 1973–85.

Taylor D, Bushell M (1985) The spatial mapping of translational diffusion coefficients by the NMR imaging technique. *Physics in Medicine and Biology* **30**: 345.

Tuch DS, Reese TG, Wiegell MR, Makris N, Belliveau JW, Wedeen VJ (2002) High angular resolution diffusion imaging reveals intravoxel white matter fiber heterogeneity. *Magnetic Resonance in Medicine* **48**: 577–82.

Van Osch MJP, Teeuwisse WM, Van Walderveen MAA, Hendrikse J, Kies DA, Van Buchem MA (2009) Can arterial spin labeling detect white matter perfusion signal? *Magnetic Resonance in Medicine* **62**: 165–73.

Wang Z, Fernández-Seara M, Alsop D et al. (2008) Assessment of functional development in normal infant brain using arterial spin labeled perfusion MRI. *Neuroimage* **39**: 973–8.

Watanabe M, Sakai O, Ozonoff A, Kussman S, Jara H (2012) Age-related apparent diffusion coefficient changes in the normal brain. *Radiology* **266**: 575–82.

Westlye LT, Walhovd KB, Dale AM et al. (2010) Life-span changes of the human brain white matter: diffusion tensor imaging (DTI) and volumetry. *Cerebral Cortex* **20**: 2055–68.

Zhang L, Thomas K, Davidson M, Casey B, Heier L, Ulug A (2005) MR quantitation of volume and diffusion changes in the developing brain. *American Journal of Neuroradiology* **26**: 45.

PART IV
Functional Brain Disorders

Chaprer 12 Cerebral Palsy among Children Born Extremely
Preterm   131

Chapter 13 Cognitive and Behavioral Functioning   145

Chapter 14 Autism, Social Impairment, and Social
Communication Deficits in Children Born
Prior to the 28th Week of Gestation   157

Chapter 15 Psychiatric and Behavioral Outcomes at
Age 2 and 10 Years in Individuals
Born Extremely Preterm   171

Chapter 16 Concluding Chapter   195

Cerebral Palsy among Children Born Extremely Preterm

The ELGAN Study

Stephanie Watkins and T Michael O'Shea

ASCERTAINMENT AND PREVALENCE OF CEREBRAL PALSY IN THE ELGAN STUDY

The diagnosis of cerebral palsy (CP) is challenging. CP is a group of clinical disorders that are heterogeneous with respect to the location, symmetry, and severity of the tone, posture, and movement abnormalities and functional impact. A majority of prematurely born children with CP have spasticity (Galea et al. 2018) referring to increased muscle tone (resistance to stretch of the muscle) with exaggerated tendon reflexes. Dyskinesia (difficulty performing voluntary movements) and ataxia (impaired coordination of movements) are not prominent in most prematurely born children with CP. Spastic forms of CP can be subtyped based on the topography of the predominant motor abnormality. Diparesis refers to involvement of both legs to a greater extent than the arms; quadriparesis to more or less equal involvement of arms and legs; and hemiparesis to involvement of the arm and leg on one side of the body.

There is no laboratory or radiographic diagnostic test; rather, CP is diagnosed based on clinical findings about which examiners do not always agree. The typical abnormalities of muscle tone, posture, and movement can be undetectable at birth and evolve over the first months to years of life; conversely abnormalities of tone may appear and then resolve during infancy. For these reasons, recent prospective studies, including the ELGAN study, have not ascertained CP before 24 months of age (Rouse et al. 2008; Juul et al. 2015).

Prior to classifying ELGAN study participants at 24 months corrected age, examiners completed a one-day training workshop that focused on videotaped examinations of child with normal and abnormal neurological findings. Trainees showed very high reliability compared to gold-standard child neurology assessments after watching the training video (Kuban et al. 2005). The standardized assessment included muscle tone in the upper and lower extremities; posture of the hand at rest; precision of the grasping of a small donut-shaped cereal; lateral protective reflexes and the parachute reflex; lower and upper extremity strength; deep tendon reflexes, sitting, and independent gait. Examiners were asked to remain unaware of the infant's medical history and brain ultrasound findings in an effort to maximize objectivity. Examiners were not asked to decide whether the study participant had CP or not; rather, a computer algorithm was applied to the individual examination items and based on the presence or absence of abnormalities and the location of the abnormalities, the child was classified as having or not having CP. If CP was present, the computer algorithm assigned a subtype (quadriparesis, hemiparesis, or diparesis). No effort was made to ascertain non-spastic forms of CP in these 2-year-olds in whom identification of dyskinetic forms is less reliable (Kuban et al. 2008). Of note, abnormalities of deep tendon reflexes were found not to contribute to the identification of CP in the ELGAN cohort and were not included in the algorithm used for case ascertainment.

Among 1056 children in the ELGAN cohort who were evaluated at about 24 months corrected age, 11.4% were classified as having CP based on the examination and algorithm described above. The most common CP subtype was quadriparesis (52%), followed by diparesis (31%), and then hemiparesis (17%). Of note, the proportion of cases of CP that were classified as quadriparesis using the ELGAN algorithm is higher than in other published studies of cohorts born prematurely (Tommiska et al. 2003; Marlow et al. 2005; Mikkola et al. 2005; Vohr et al. 2005; Robertson et al. 2007; Serenius et al. 2013).

In addition to ascertaining the presence or absence of CP in study participants, ELGAN investigators also evaluated the child's level of functional ability using the Gross Motor Function Classification System (GMFCS). The GMFCS defines five levels of functional limitation, with 1 being the mildest and 5 being the most severe (Palisano et al. 1997). This measure of disability was included because prior research indicated that ascertainment of CP is more reliable for 'disabling' CP, as compared to 'non-disabling' CP (Paneth et al. 2003). In the ELGAN cohort, moderate-to-severe functional limitation (GMFCS ≥ 2) was found in 76% of children with quadriparesis, 11% of children with hemiparesis, and 8% of children with diparesis. Performance on a standardized test of motor development, the Bayley Scales of Infant and Toddler Development-Second Edition Psychomotor Development Index (PDI) also differed across CP subtypes. Ninety-three percent of children with quadriparesis had PDI scores more than two standard deviations below the normative mean, whereas 63% of children with hemiparesis and 62% of those with diparesis had such low PDI scores (Kuban et al. 2008).

CO-MORBIDITIES AMONG ELGAN STUDY CHILDREN WITH CEREBRAL PALSY

As was the case for functional limitation, the prevalence of co-morbidities at 24 months of age varied across CP subtypes. Microcephaly, defined as head circumference more than 2 standard deviations below the mean for age, was present in 42% of children with quadriparesis, 21% of children with hemiparesis, and 8% of children with diparesis. On a standardized test of early cognitive function, the Bayley Scales of Infant and Toddler Development-Second Edition Mental Development Index (MDI), the proportions with MDI more than 2 standard deviations below the mean were 72% for quadriparesis, 58% for hemiparesis, and 34% for diparesis (Kuban et al. 2008). On the Modified Checklist for Autism in Toddlers (M-CHAT), a screening assessment for autism, the proportions with a positive screen for autism were 76% for quadriparesis, 44% for hemiparesis, and 30% for diparesis, although we recognize the limitations of the M-CHAT instrument in children with neurosensory disabilities (Luyster et al. 2011).

Slightly more than 75% of children classified as having CP at 24 months corrected age were evaluated again at 10 years of age (n = 93). Evaluations at 10 years included assessment of intelligence quotient (IQ) and executive function, as well as rigorous evaluation for autism spectrum disorder and epilepsy. Fully 68% of ELGAN children with CP had one or more additional neurodevelopmental impairment. Fifty-five percent had moderate-to-severe cognitive impairment; 20% had autism spectrum disorder, and 47% had epilepsy (Hirschberger et al. 2018).

PRENATAL RISK FACTORS FOR CEREBRAL PALSY IN THE ELGAN STUDY

The primary goal of the ELGAN study was to identify potentially modifiable risk factors for brain and related disorders among individuals born extremely preterm (O'Shea et al. 2009). To that end, data were collected about a large number of pre-, peri-, and post-natal factors, with a focus on biomarkers of inflammation and presumed initiators of inflammation, such as microorganisms and tissue injury. One of the strengths of the ELGAN study was the relatively large number of cases of CP, providing the investigators the opportunity to analyze exposure-outcome relationships separately for the three subtypes of spastic CP that were ascertained in the ELGAN study. In this section we summarize findings of analyses of the relationship between prenatal exposures and CP in the offspring.

Placental Microbiology and Histology

The methods used to identify microorganisms in the placentas obtained at the time of ELGAN study participants' deliveries have been described by Onderdonk et al. (2008a, 2008b). Associations between the presence of microorganisms and CP in the offspring were particularly evident for diparesis and were not observed for hemiparesis. The presence of any aerobe was associated with a four-fold increase in the odds of diparesis, and the presence of two or more species of bacteria was associated with a 5.2-fold increase in odds. Two exposures, any anaerobe and two or more species of bacteria, were associated with an approximate doubling of the odds of quadriparesis (Leviton et al. 2010b).

Prior to the enrollment of study participants, pathologists who identified histological abnormalities in the placentas obtained from ELGAN study infants participated in training sessions designed to enhance the reliability of histological findings (Hecht et al. 2008). Associations between placental histological findings and CP in the offspring were limited to diparesis. Inflammation of the chorionic plate (odds ratio: 2.3; 95% confidence limits: 1.1, 4.8) and inflammation of the chorion/decidua (odds ratio: 3.4; 95% confidence limits: 1.6, 7.4) were associated with an increased risk of diparesis. As compared to infants from whose placentas no microorganisms were recovered and no histological findings indicative of inflammation were seen, infants with microorganisms but no histological indications of inflammation were at highest risk of diparesis (odds ratio: 4.0; 95% confidence limits: 1.04, 16).

Pregnancy Complications

ELGAN investigators evaluated histological, microbiological, and clinical data from the pregnancies enrolled in the ELGAN study and concluded that pregnancy complications leading to extreme prematurity can be grouped broadly into disorders associated with intrauterine inflammation (preterm labor, prelabor preterm rupture of membranes, cervical incompetence, and placenta abruption) and disorders associated with aberrations of placentation (fetal growth restriction and preeclampsia) (McElrath et al. 2008). None of these pregnancy complications was associated with a significantly increased or decreased risk of CP as compared to infants born to mothers with preeclampsia.

Because maternal pre-pregnancy obesity has been associated with systemic inflammation (Leibowitz et al. 2012; van der Burg et al. 2013; van der Burg et al. 2016), ELGAN investigators studied its relationship to CP. Neither infants of overweight nor of obese women were at significantly increased risk of CP. Overweight was associated with risk ratios ranging between 1.1 for quadriparesis (95% CI = 0.5, 2.1) and 2.0 for hemiparesis (95% CI = 0.4, 9.8); obesity was associated with risk ratios ranging between 0.7 for diparesis (95% CI = 0.2, 2.5) to 2.5 for hemiparesis (95% CI = 0.4, 13) (van der Burg et al. 2018).

Maternal Medications

In randomized trials, antenatal treatment of mothers in preterm labor with magnesium sulfate decreased the risk of CP in the offspring (Rouse et al. 2008; Crowther et al. 2017). However, among ELGAN study participants this maternal treatment was only associated with a small reduction in risk of CP (McElrath et al. 2009). In addition to the non-random assignment of magnesium, the modest sample size might explain the difference between the findings from the ELGAN study and randomized trial results.

Because both infection and inflammation during pregnancy are associated with an increased risk of preterm birth and, in turn, an increased risk of white matter damage and subsequent CP (Dammann and Leviton 1997, 2004, 2007; Dammann et al. 2002; Dammann and O'Shea 2008) the ELGAN study investigated the association between maternal use of over-the-counter non-steroidal anti-inflammatory medications (the use of which presumably is associated somewhat with maternal infection and inflammation) and the risk of cerebral white matter damage and CP at age 2 years. In the ELGAN cohort, the use of aspirin and other NSAIDSs during pregnancy was associated with a two- to-three-fold increased risk of quadriparetic CP compared to women who were not exposed to these medications during pregnancy. Children who were exposed to other NSAIDs without physician indication had a 3.5-fold increased risk of diparetic CP (Tyler et al. 2012).

Causal pathways that could explain the association of NSAID exposure with CP include direct injury to the brain as well as injury by the inflammatory process accompanying the medical indication for the antenatal medication (Tyler et al. 2012). However, the association of NSAID and CP risk has not been found in other samples of EP children (Farrell et al. 1995; Marret et al. 2010). An example of the potential complexity of the NSAID – CP association is the finding, in preclinical models, that indomethacin (an NSAID) can decrease production of inflammatory prostaglandins (Ahmad et al. 2006; Takemiya et al. 2007, 2010, 2011), but also can decrease production of anti-inflammatory proteins (Kushima et al. 2009).

Comparisons with Findings from Other Extremely Preterm Cohorts

The prevalence of CP among surviving ELGAN participants (11.4%) is very similar to the prevalence found in the EXPRESS study of infants born before 27 weeks of gestation in Sweden (10.5%). As would be expected given the strong inverse relationship between gestational age and risk of CP, the prevalence of CP in ELGAN was higher than the prevalence found in the EPIPAGE study of infants born before 33 weeks of gestation and lower than the prevalence found in the EPICure study of infants born before 26 weeks of gestation (14%). In addition to the distribution of gestational age, factors contributing to these differences could include differences in maternal health conditions, prenatal and postnatal therapies, pregnancy complications, survival rates, follow-up rates, and criteria used to define CP.

In contrast to the finding from the ELGAN study that the indication for preterm delivery was not associated with the risk of CP, in the EPICure study of infants born in the United Kingdom before 26 weeks of gestation, chorioamnionitis was associated with a lower risk of CP, while in the EPIPAGE study of infants born in France before 33 weeks of gestation, preterm premature rupture of membranes with short latency, and prolonged preterm premature rupture of membranes, both of which are risk factors for chorioamnionitis, were associated with an increased risk for CP. In the EXPRESS study, of infants born before 27 weeks of gestation in Sweden, chorioamnionitis was not associated with neurosensory impairment at 2.5 years of age. (Data were not reported separately for CP.) In a recent meta-analysis, preterm histological chorioamnionitis, but not clinical chorioamnionitis, was associated with an increased risk of CP (Shi et al. 2017). In a study of 42 cases of CP among very low birth weight infants, placentas from infants with CP, as compared to placenta from infants without CP, were more likely to have chorionic plate thrombi or diffuse villous edema (Redline et al. 1998). This study was limited by aggregating all three subtypes of CP, precluding detection of subtype-specific associations. This is especially unfortunate in light of our finding that placental histological evidence of inflammation was associated with only one form of CP, diparesis. To our knowledge no other investigators have evaluated relationships between placental microorganisms and CP among extremely preterm infants.

NEONATAL RISK FACTORS FOR CEREBRAL PALSY IN THE ELGAN STUDY

Neonatal Attributes

At age 2 years, the rate of CP diagnosis was four times higher in infants born at 23 weeks than in infants born at 27 weeks (McElrath et al. 2009). Males were about twice as likely to develop CP as females (Kuban et al. 2016). Fetal growth restriction was not associated with the risk of CP in the ELGAN cohort (Streimish et al. 2012). Microcephaly at birth (a head circumference more than 2 standard deviations below the expected mean) was associated with an increased risk of CP only if the abnormally low head circumference persisted at 24 months of age (Kuban et al. 2009b). Physiological instability in the first 12 postnatal hours was assessed using the Score for Neonatal Acute Physiology (SNAP); higher SNAP scores indicate a higher degree of physiological instability. No statistically significant associations were found between high SNAP scores and the risk of CP in the ELGAN cohort (Dammann et al. 2010).

Blood Gas and Blood Pressure Abnormalities

When the ELGAN study was initiated some experts posited that physiologic instability of infants born extremely preterm can limit cerebral blood flow, leading to tissue hypoxia and damage (Volpe 2009). Thus data were collected about high and low values of oxygen, carbon dioxide, and pH on blood gas assays. Associations were found between high carbon dioxide and low pH and an increased risk of hemiparesis, particularly when the blood gas aberrations were found on multiple days. When interpreting this finding, we have argued that blood gas abnormalities may be indicators of brain and lung immaturity that is not captured by gestational age and thus leads to residual confounding. Hypocarbia on multiple days was associated with an increased risk of quadriparesis and diparesis (Leviton et al. 2010a), a finding also described in the Neonatal Brain Hemorrhage Study (Collins et al. 2001). This finding provides some support for the hypothesis that ischemia (due to hypocarbia-induced cerebral vasoconstriction) contributes to CP in the preterm newborn. On the other hand, hypotension, which could cause cerebral ischemia when auto-regulation is impaired, was not associated with the risk of CP in the ELGAN cohort (Logan et al. 2011).

Sepsis and Necrotizing Enterocolitis

Among infants born extremely preterm, sepsis and neonatal enterocolitis are prominent among neonatal morbidities as correlates, and probably initiators, of neonatal systemic inflammation (Leviton et al. 2012; Martin et al. 2013), a primary focus of the ELGAN study. Sepsis occurs in about 30–60% of neonates who develop necrotizing enterocolitis (Walsh et al. 1989; Salhab et al. 2004; Hintz et al. 2005; Soraisham et al. 2006). In the ELGAN cohort, infants with necrotizing enterocolitis without sepsis and infants with sepsis without necrotizing enterocolitis were not at increased risk for CP. However, necrotizing enterocolitis and sepsis was associated with an increased odds of diparetic CP (odds ratio: 8.4; 95% confidence limits: 1.9, 39).

Brain Ultrasound Abnormalities

Brain ultrasonography is a recommended screening test for extremely preterm infants (Ment et al. 2002); thus these assessments were collected on ELGAN participants as a component of clinical care, providing the opportunity to evaluate the extent to which neonatal cranial ultrasound abnormalities predict CP. Ninety-four percent of infants with developmental follow-up at two years of age had at least one ultrasound performed between 5 and 14 postnatal days of age, and 100% had at least one ultrasound scan performed between postnatal day 15 and the day on which the infant reached 40 weeks post-menstrual age (see Chapter 10) (O'Shea et al. 2012).

In the ELGAN cohort, intraventricular hemorrhage was associated with a statistically significant increase in the risk of quadriparesis (odds ratio: 5.1; 95% confidence limits 2.8, 9.6), diparesis (odds ratio: 2.3; 955 confidence limits 1.1, 5.0), and hemiparesis (odds ratio: 5.8; 95% confidence limits 2.1, 17) (Kuban et al. 2009a). However, among infants with intraventricular hemorrhage who did not have concomitant white matter injury (intracerebral echolucency and/or moderate-to-severe ventriculomegaly), no association was found between intraventricular hemorrhage and any form of CP (O'Shea et al. 2012). Thus while neonatal intraventricular hemorrhage was predictive of subsequent CP, this association can be explained by the frequent co-occurrence of hemorrhage with white matter injury.

White matter injury itself was associated with the strongest relative risks for CP in the ELGAN study. Infants with white matter lesions imaged on neonatal cranial ultrasound had 28 times the odds of quadriplegia if IVH was absent, 19 times the odds if present. For diplegia, the parallel odds ratios were 5.6 and 4.5, while for hemiplegia they were 5.6 and 15 (O'Shea et al. 2012). All odds ratios but the one for isolated white matter lesions and hemiplegia were statistically significant.

These observations are consistent with the premise that disrupted myelination of periventricular white matter tracts underlies spastic CP (Kuban and Leviton 1994). Progenitors of the cells that are necessary for myelination (oligodendrocytes) appear to be highly sensitive to injurious exposures, such as inflammation, which could explain the increased susceptibility to white matter injury among neonates born extremely preterm (Back et al. 2007).

As compared to ELGAN children with diparesis, those with quadriparesis and hemiparesis had less favorable overall neurodevelopment at age 2 years (Kuban et al. 2008) implying that white matter lesions are not only predictive of CP but also of more serious functional impairment among ELGAN children with CP. Also notable is the observation that 43% of children with CP had a normal neonatal brain ultrasound. This finding agrees with another large multicenter cohort study (Laptook et al. 2005), and suggests that brain ultrasonography did not detect all of the white matter injury present in the ELGAN cohort.

Cerebellar hemorrhage was not frequently detected in the ELGAN cohort, perhaps because mastoid fontanelle views were not routinely used (Steggerda et al. 2009). Among the four infants with ultrasonographically diagnosed unilateral cerebellar hemorrhage, none had CP; among the ten with bilateral cerebellar hemorrhage, 60% had CP (Kuban et al. 2009a).

Neonatal Chronic Lung Disease

Infants born preterm often require respiratory support due to disruption in alveolarization leading to neonatal chronic lung disease (Coalson 2003). Bronchopulmonary dysplasia (BPD), a neonatal chronic lung disease in survivors of preterm birth and treatment with mechanical ventilation was first described in 1967 (Northway et al. 1967). BPD is the most prevalent adverse outcome among infants born less than 30 weeks gestation (Jobe 2016). In large cohorts, approximately 40% of infants born extremely preterm were diagnosed with BPD (Stoll et al. 2010; Lapcharoensap et al. 2015).

A variety of definitions of BPD have been used in epidemiologic studies (Bancalari et al. 1979; Kraybill et al. 1987; Palta et al. 1998; Marshall et al. 1999); in the years when the ELGAN cohort was recruited the receipt of supplemental oxygen at 36 weeks post-menstrual age was a frequently used definition and was used when evaluating the relationship of neonatal chronic lung disease to the neuro-developmental outcomes of ELGAN study participants (Laughon et al. 2009; Van Marter et al. 2010). In addition, BPD was characterized as severe if mechanical ventilation was needed at 36 weeks post-menstrual age. A limitation of the ELGAN study is that sufficient details of respiratory therapies were not collected to allow classification with regard to the stages of BPD that have been proposed by a recent group of experts (Higgins et al. 2018).

In the ELGAN study, 51% of infants who were alive at 36 weeks post-menstrual age were classified as having BPD at 36 weeks, including 93 infants (9%) with severe BPD (requirement for mechanical ventilation at 36 weeks post-menstrual age). When adjusting for variables associated with BPD and CP, oxygen supplementation at 36 weeks post-menstrual age was not associated with risk of CP (Van Marter et al. 2010). In contrast, infants with severe BPD were nearly six times more likely to develop quad-riparesis and four times more likely to develop diparesis as compared to children who did not receive either supplemental oxygen or mechanical ventilation at 36 weeks post-menstrual age. Severe BPD was not associated with the risk of hemiparesis. In a meta-analysis of 11 studies of the association of BPD and CP (including the ELGAN study analysis), BPD was associated with an increased risk of CP, and the strength of association was strongest for severe BPD. However, most studies did not have uniform diagnostic criteria for BPD or CP, some studies did not adjust for potential confounders, and results were not reported for subtypes of CP (Gou et al. 2018).

Protein Biomarkers

As the ELGAN study was being designed, a report from the California CP Registry described the measurement of inflammation-related cytokines, such as tumor necrosis factor-alpha, in archived dried blood spots collected from neonates for the purpose of newborn screening for inborn errors of metabolism. Blood spots were retrieved from storage for a sample of children with CP and from a control group, and levels of protein biomarkers of inflammation were measured using novel immune-affinity chromatographic methods. Levels of multiple inflammation biomarkers were higher in the neonatal blood of children born at term who subsequently developed CP, as compared to controls without CP (Nelson et al. 1998). Based on these exciting findings, scavenged blood was obtained from ELGAN study neonates at various times when blood was being collected for clinical indications. Measurements were then made of inflammation-related proteins, as well as proteins that might play a role in 'endogenous protection' against brain injury (Dammann and Leviton 1999). By protocol, dried blood spots were stored for later protein analysis at five time intervals: the first postnatal day and on days 7, 14, 21, and 28, if available. Elevations were defined as levels in the highest quartile, conditional on postnatal day of the sample, gestational age at birth, and 'batch' of measurements. 'Persistent or sustained' elevations were defined as elevations on two or more days 1 week apart.

As was the case for multiple outcomes studied in the ELGAN cohort, single-day elevations of inflammation-related proteins were not associated with an increased risk of CP (Kuban et al. 2014). In contrast, persistent or sustained elevations of interleukin-8 and macrophage chemotactic protein-1 were associated with an increased risk of quadriparesis. Persistent or sustained elevations of tumor necrosis factor-alpha, tumor necrosis factor-alpha receptor-1, interleukin-8, and intracellular adhesion molecule-1 were associated with an increased risk of diparesis, while persistent or sustained elevations of interleukin-6, interleukin-8, E-selectin, and insulin-like growth factor binding protein-1 were associated with an increased risk of hemiparesis (Kuban et al. 2014). Further analysis of a subset of the protein biomarkers that were consistently associated with adverse neurodevelopmental outcomes in the ELGAN cohort (interleukin-6, tumor necrosis factor-a, tumor necrosis factor-a-receptor-1, interleukin-8, intercellular adhesion molecule-1, E-selectin, C-reactive protein, serum amyloid A, and insulin-like growth factor binding protein-1), indicated that neonates with four or more persistent or sustained elevations of proteins in this subset had an increased risk of diparesis (odds ratio: 3.0; 95% confidence limits: 1.3, 7.1) and an increased risk of hemiparesis (odds ratio: 4.2; 95% confidence limits: 1.3, 14), but not an increased risk of quadriparesis (Kuban et al. 2014).

Comparisons with Findings from Other Extremely Preterm Cohorts

Sepsis has been studied in multiple studies of preterm infants, including one focused on extremely preterm infants. In the largest of these studies, extremely low birth weight infants with clinical infection (presumed sepsis with negative blood culture), sepsis, sepsis plus necrotizing enterocolitis, and meningitis with or without sepsis were all associated with elevated risk of CP (Stoll et al. 2004). Among extremely low birth weight infants, necrotizing enterocolitis was a risk factor for CP only when surgical intervention was required (Hintz et al. 2005). Both early (presumed due to vertical transmission of maternal infection) and late onset (presumed due to postnatal acquisition) sepsis were associated with an increased risk of CP in the EPIPAGE study of infants born at 22–32 weeks of gestation (Mitha et al. 2013). In the study of the sample most similar to ELGAN, of infants born 24–27 weeks of gestation, proven sepsis, but not suspected sepsis, was associated with an increased risk of CP, and this increased risk was found only for gram-positive infections and not for gram-negative infections (Schlapbach et al. 2011).

With regard to the association of BPD with an increased risk of CP, in a cohort of extremely low birth weight infants, the risk of quadriparesis and diparesis was increased among infants with BPD, but no association was found with hemiparesis. These subtype-specific associations are the same as those identified in the ELGAN study (Natarajan et al. 2012). A strength of this study of extremely low birth weight infants is that the validity of the diagnosis of BPD was improved by using a physiological definition of BPD. In a study of infants born before 30 weeks of gestation, BPD was not associated with CP, but the power to detect associations with CP was limited by the inclusion of only 14 cases of CP (Malavolti et al. 2018). Further, in a meta-analysis of 11 studies, including ELGAN, both BPD and severe BPD were associated with increased risk of CP (Gou et al. 2018).

A large number of studies of preterm infants have reported associations between a variety of ultrasound abnormalities and CP. Among studies completed prior to the ELGAN study, the most informative was the Neonatal Brain Hemorrhage Study (NBH), which identified an increased risk of CP among low birth weight infants whose brain ultrasound showed evidence of white matter injury, as indicated by parenchymal echodensities/lucencies or ventricular enlargement (Pinto-Martin et al. 1995). The primary limitation of that study, as compared to the ELGAN study, was that many study infants did not undergo ultrasounds after the first two weeks of life, which is likely to have led to under-ascertainment of white matter injury.

Focusing on studies of infants similar to those in the ELGAN study, white matter injury was identified as a risk factor for CP in the EPICure study of infants born before 26 weeks of gestation (Wood et al. 2005) and the Neonatal Research Network study of infants born before 28 weeks of gestation (Hintz et al. 2015). While ELGAN reaffirmed the strong association of white matter injury to CP in the NBH, ELGAN was uniquely able to distinguish a gradient of associations between white matter injury and CP, from very large for quadriparesis to quite large for hemiparesis, to more moderately large for diparesis.

Prior to the completion of biomarkers measurements in the ELGAN study, the relationship of inflammation-related proteins to the risk of CP has been studied in at least two other cohorts of infants born prematurely. In a case-control study that included 62 cases of CP and 107 controls born before 32 weeks of gestation, dried blood spots that were drawn, on average, 2.4 days after birth, were the source of measurements of numerous inflammation-related proteins including cytokines, chemokines, and vascular endothelial growth factor. None of these proteins were elevated in cases as compared to controls and none differed across subtypes of CP (diparesis, quadriparesis, hemiparesis) (Nelson et al. 2003). In contrast, in a cohort study of 1067 infants with extremely low birth weight (n = 102 cases of CP), interleukin-8 was higher on multiple days during the first three postnatal months among infants who subsequently developed CP (Carlo et al. 2011). The added values of the ELGAN study include the analysis of persistent or sustained elevations, as compared to single-day elevations, and the consideration of associations between inflammation-related proteins and subtypes of CP (Kuban et al. 2014).

SUMMARY

A primary goal of the ELGAN study was to identify potentially modifiable risk factors for neurodevelopmental impairments. Among the disorders that disproportionately affect individuals born extremely preterm, CP is the disorder that is most strongly associated with extremely preterm birth. An important contribution of the ELGAN study was the development of a teaching tool, in the form of a training workshop and training video, which incorporated a uniform approach to identifying and classifying abnormalities of tone, posture, primitive reflexes, and muscle strength and, based on these abnormalities, a consistent algorithmic approach to classifying infants with regard to the presence and type of CP. This approach is currently being used in at least two large multi-center randomized trials to identify CP as a component of the primary outcome for these trials.

The ELGAN study detected no associations between clinical diagnoses in the mother and subsequent CP. However several aspects of placental pathology and microbiology, which could serve as biomarkers of perinatal infection and/or inflammation, were associated with the risk of CP. Among neonatal brain ultrasound abnormalities, those most strongly associated with CP are intracerebral echolucency and moderate-to-severe ventriculomegaly, both evidence of damage to white matter. One indirect indicator of brain ischemia, systemic hypotension, was not associated with an increased risk of CP, whereas another indirect indicator, persistent hypocarbia, was. Also consistently associated with CP were neonatal morbidities associated with neonatal systemic inflammation, and protein biomarkers of inflammation. These indicators of inflammation were associated with an increased risk of hemiparesis and diparesis, but not quadriparesis.

REFERENCES

Ahmad AS, Saleem S, Ahmad M, Dore S (2006) Prostaglandin EP1 receptor contributes to excitotoxicity and focal ischemic brain damage. *Toxicol Sci* **89**: 265–70.

Back SA, Riddle A, McClure MM (2007) Maturation-dependent vulnerability of perinatal white matter in premature birth. *Stroke* **38**: 724–30.

Bancalari E, Abdenour GE, Feller R, Gannon J (1979) Bronchopulmonary dysplasia: clinical presentation. *J Pediatr* **95**: 819–23.

Cans C (2000) Surveillance of cerebral palsy in Europe: a collaboration of cerebral palsy surveys and registers. *Develop Med Child Neurol* **42**: 816–24.

Carlo WA, McDonald SA, Tyson JE et al. (2011) Cytokines and neurodevelopmental outcomes in extremely low birth weight infants. *Journal of Pediatrics* **159**: 919–U77.

Coalson JJ (2003) Pathology of new bronchopulmonary dysplasia. *Semin Neonatol* **8**: 73–81.

Collins MP, Lorenz JM, Jetton JR, Paneth N (2001) Hypocapnia and other ventilation-related risk factors for cerebral palsy in low birth weight infants. *Pediatr Res* **50**: 712–9.

Crowther CA, Middleton PF, Voysey M et al. (2017) Assessing the neuroprotective benefits for babies of antenatal magnesium sulphate: an individual participant data meta-analysis. *PLoS Med* **14**: e1002398.

Dammann O, Kuban KCK, Leviton A (2002) Perinatal infection, fetal inflammatory response, white matter damage, and cognitive limitations in children born preterm. *Mental Retardation and Developmental Disabilities Research Reviews* **8**: 46–50.

Dammann O, Leviton A (1997) Maternal intrauterine infection, cytokines, and brain damage in the preterm newborn. *Pediatr Res* **42**: 1–8.

Dammann O, Leviton A (1999) Brain damage in preterm newborns: might enhancement of developmentally regulated endogenous protection open a door for prevention? *Pediatrics* **104**: 541–50.

Dammann O, Leviton A (2004) Inflammatory brain damage in preterm newborns – dry numbers, wet lab, and causal inferences. *Early Human Development* **79**: 1–15.

Dammann O, Leviton A (2007) Perinatal brain damage causation. *Developmental Neuroscience* **29**: 280–8.

Dammann O, Naples M, Bednarek F et al. (2010) SNAP-II and SNAPPE-II and the risk of structural and functional brain disorders in extremely low gestational age newborns: the ELGAN study. *Neonatology* **97**: 71–82.

Dammann O, O'Shea TM (2008) Cytokines and perinatal brain damage. *Clinics in Perinatology* **35**: 643–63.

Farrell B, Heineman J, Handoll H et al. (1995) Low dose aspirin in pregnancy and early childhood development: follow up of the collaborative low dose aspirin study in pregnancy. CLASP collaborative group. *Br J Obstet Gynaecol* **102**: 861–8.

Galea C, McIntyre S, Smithers-Sheedy H et al. (2018) Cerebral palsy trends in Australia (1995–2009): a population-based observational study. *Dev Med Child Neurol* **61**: 186–93.

Gou X, Yang L, Pan L, Xiao D (2018) Association between bronchopulmonary dysplasia and cerebral palsy in children: a meta-analysis. *BMJ Open* **8**: e020735.

Hecht JL, Allred EN, Kliman HJ et al. (2008) Histological characteristics of singleton placentas delivered before the 28th week of gestation. *Pathology* **40**: 372–6.

Higgins RD, Jobe AH, Koso-Thomas M et al. (2018) Bronchopulmonary dysplasia: executive summary of a workshop. *J Pediatr* **197**: 300–8.

Hintz SR, Barnes PD, Bulas D et al. (2015) Neuroimaging and neurodevelopmental outcome in extremely preterm infants. *Pediatrics* **135**: e32–42.

Hintz SR, Kendrick DE, Stoll BJ et al. (2005) Neurodevelopmental and growth outcomes of extremely low birth weight infants after necrotizing enterocolitis. *Pediatrics* **115**: 696–703.

Hirschberger RG, Kuban KCK, O'Shea TM et al. (2018) Co-occurrence and severity of neurodevelopmental burden (cognitive impairment, cerebral palsy, autism spectrum disorder, and epilepsy) at age ten years in children born extremely preterm. *Pediatr Neurol* **79**: 45–52.

Jobe AH (2016) Mechanisms of lung injury and bronchopulmonary dysplasia. *Am J Perinatol* **33**: 1076–8.

Juul SE, Mayock DE, Comstock BA, Heagerty PJ (2015) Neuroprotective potential of erythropoietin in neonates; design of a randomized trial. *Matern Health Neonatol Perinatol* **1**: 27.

Kraybill EN, Bose CL, Dercole J (1987) Chronic lung-disease in infants with very-low-birth-weight – a population-based study. *American Journal of Diseases of Children* **141**: 784–8.

Kuban K, Adler I, Allred E et al. (2007) Observer variability assessing US scans of the preterm brain: the ELGAN study. *Pediatr Radiol* **37**: 1201–8.

Kuban K, Allred E, O'Shea TM, Paneth N, Pagano M, for the ELGAN Study Cerebral Palsy-Algorithm Group (2008) An algorithm for identifying and classifying cerebral palsy in young children. *Journal of Pediatrics* **153**: 466–72.

Kuban K, Sanocka U, Leviton A et al. (1999) White matter disorders of prematurity: association with intraventricular hemorrhage and ventriculomegaly. The Developmental Epidemiology Network. *J Pediatr* **134**: 539–46.

Kuban KC, Allred EN, O'Shea TM et al. (2009a) Cranial ultrasound lesions in the NICU predict cerebral palsy at age 2 years in children born at extremely low gestational age. *J Child Neurol* **24**: 63–72.

Kuban KC, Allred EN, O'Shea TM et al. (2009b) Developmental correlates of head circumference at birth and two years in a cohort of extremely low gestational age newborns. *J Pediatr* **155**: 344–9 e1–3.

Kuban KC, Joseph RM, O'Shea TM et al. (2016) Girls and boys born before 28 weeks gestation: risks of cognitive, behavioral, and neurologic outcomes at age 10 years. *J Pediatr* **173**: 69–75 e1.

Kuban KC, Leviton A (1994) Cerebral palsy. *N Engl J Med* **330**: 188–95.

Kuban KC, O'Shea TM, Allred EN (2015) The breadth and type of systemic inflammation and the risk of adverse neurological outcomes in extremely low gestation newborns. *Pediatr Neurol* **52**: 42–8.

Kuban KC, O'Shea TM, Allred EN et al. (2014) Systemic inflammation and cerebral palsy risk in extremely preterm infants. *J Child Neurol* **29**: 1692–8.

Kuban KCK, O'Shea M, Allred E et al. (2005) Video and CD-ROM as a training tool for performing neurologic examinations of 1-year-old children in a multicenter epidemiologic study. *Journal of Child Neurology* **20**: 829–31.

Kushima K, Sakuma S, Furusawa S, Fujiwara M (2009) Prenatal administration of indomethacin modulates Th2 cytokines in juvenile rats. *Toxicol Lett* **185**: 32–7.

Lapcharoensap W, Gage SC, Kan P et al. (2015) Hospital variation and risk factors for bronchopulmonary dysplasia in a population-based cohort. *JAMA Pediatr* **169**: e143676.

Laptook A, O'Shea T, Shankaran S, Bhaskar B, NICHD Neonatal Network (2005) Adverse neurodevelopmental outcomes among extremely low birth weight infants with a normal head ultrasound: prevalence and antecedents. *Pediatrics* **115**: 673–80.

Laughon M, O'Shea TM, Allred EN et al. (2009) Chronic lung disease and the risk of developmental delay at two years of age in children born before 28 weeks postmenstrual age. *Pediatrics* **124**: 637–48.

Leibowitz KL, Moore RH, Ahima RS et al. (2012) Maternal obesity associated with inflammation in their children. *World Journal of Pediatrics* **8**: 76–9.

Leviton A, Allred E, Kuban KCK et al. (2010a) Early blood gas abnormalities and the preterm brain. *American Journal of Epidemiology* **172**: 907–16.

Leviton A, Hecht J, Onderdonk A et al. (2010b) Microbiological and histologic characteristics of the extremely preterm infant's placenta predict white matter damage and later cerebral palsy. The ELGAN study. *Pediatric Research* **67**: 95–101.

Leviton A, O'Shea TM, Bednarek FJ, Allred EN, Fichorova RN, Dammann O (2012) Systemic responses of preterm newborns with presumed or documented bacteraemia. *Acta Paediatrica* **101**: 355–9.

Logan JW, O'Shea TM, Allred EN et al. (2011) Early postnatal hypotension is not associated with indicators of white matter damage or cerebral palsy in extremely low gestational age newborns. *J Perinatol* **31**: 524–34.

Luyster R, Kuban K, O'Shea T et al. (2011) The Modified Checklist for Autism in Toddlers (M-CHAT) in extremely low gestational age newborns: individual items associated with cognitive, motor, vision, and hearing limitations. *Journal of Developmental and Behavioral Pediatrics* **25**: 366–76.

Malavolti AM, Bassler D, Arlettaz-Mieth R, Faldella G, Latal B, Natalucci G (2018) Bronchopulmonary dysplasia-impact of severity and timing of diagnosis on neurodevelopment of preterm infants: a retrospective cohort study. *BMJ Paediatr Open* **2**: e000165.

Marlow N, Wolke D, Bracewell MA, Samara M, EPICure Study Group (2005) Neurologic and developmental disability at six years of age after extremely preterm birth. *N Engl J Med* **352**: 9–19.

Marret S, Marchand L, Kaminski M et al. (2010) Prenatal low-dose aspirin and neurobehavioral outcomes of children born very preterm. *Pediatrics* **125**: e29–34.

Marshall DD, Kotelchuck M, Young TE, Bose CL, Kruyer, L, O'Shea TM (1999) Risk factors for chronic lung disease in the surfactant era: a North Carolina population-based study of very low birth weight infants. *Pediatrics* **104**: 1345–50.

Martin CR, Bellomy M, Allred EN, Fichorova RN, Leviton A (2013) Systemic inflammation associated with severe intestinal injury in extremely low gestational age newborns. *Fetal and Pediatric Pathology* **32**: 222–34.

Martin CR, Dammann O, Allred EN et al. (2010) Neurodevelopment of extremely preterm infants who had necrotizing enterocolitis with or without late bacteremia. *Journal of Pediatrics* **157**: 751–6.

Martin JA, Osterman MJ, Kirmeyer SE, Gregory EC (2015) Measuring gestational age in vital statistics data: transitioning to the obstetric estimate. *Natl Vital Stat Rep* **64**: 1 20.

McElrath TF, Allred EN, Boggess KA et al. (2009) Maternal antenatal complications and the risk of neonatal cerebral white matter damage and later cerebral palsy in children born at an extremely low gestational age. *American Journal of Epidemiology* **170**: 819–28.

McElrath TF, Hecht JL, Onderdonk A et al. (2008) Pregnancy disorders that lead to delivery before the 28th week of gestation: an epidemiologic approach to classification. *Am J Epidemiol* **168**: 980–9.

Ment LR, Bada HS, Barnes P et al. (2002) Practice parameter: neuroimaging of the neonate – report of the Quality Standards Subcommittee of the American Academy of Neurology and the Practice Committee of the Child Neurology Society. *Neurology* **58**: 1726–38.

Mikkola K, Ritari N, Tommiska V et al. (2005) Neurodevelopmental outcome at 5 years of age of a national cohort of extremely low birth weight infants who were born in 1996–1997. *Pediatrics* **116**: 1391–400.

Mitha A, Foix-L'Helias L, Arnaud C et al. (2013) Neonatal infection and 5-year neurodevelopmental outcome of very preterm infants. *Pediatrics* **132**: e372–80.

Natarajan G, Pappas A, Shankaran S et al. (2012) Outcomes of extremely low birth weight infants with broncho-pulmonary dysplasia: impact of the physiologic definition. *Early Hum Dev* **88**: 509–15.

Nelson KB, Dambrosia JM, Grether JK, Phillips TM (1998) Neonatal cytokines and coagulation factors in children with cerebral palsy. *Ann Neurol* **44**: 665–75.

Nelson KB, Grether JK, Dambrosia JM et al. (2003) Neonatal cytokines and cerebral palsy in very preterm infants. *Pediatric Research* **53**: 600–7.

Northway WH Jr, Rosan RC, Porter DY (1967) Pulmonary disease following respirator therapy of hyaline-membrane disease. Bronchopulmonary dysplasia. *N Engl J Med* **276**: 357–68.

O'Shea TM, Allred EN, Dammann O (2009) The ELGAN study of the brain and related disorders in extremely low gestational age newborns. *Early Human Development* **85**: 719–25.

O'Shea TM, Allred EN, Kuban KCK et al. (2012) Intraventricular hemorrhage and developmental outcomes at 24 months of age in extremely preterm infants. *Journal of Child Neurology* **27**: 22–9.

Onderdonk AB, Delaney ML, Dubois AM, Allred EN, Leviton A (2008a) Detection of bacteria in placental tissues obtained from extremely low gestational age neonates. *American Journal of Obstetrics and Gynecology* **198**: e1–e7.

Onderdonk AB, Hecht JL, McElrath TF, Delaney ML, Allred EN, Leviton A (2008b) Colonization of second-trimester placenta parenchyma. *American Journal of Obstetrics and Gynecology* **199**: 52.e1–52.e10.

Palisano R, Rosenbaum P, Walter S, Russell D, Wood E, Galuppi B (1997) Development and reliability of a system to classify gross motor function in children with cerebral palsy. *Dev Med Child Neurol* **39**: 214–23.

Palta M, Sadek M, Barnet JH et al. (1998) Evaluation of criteria for chronic lung disease in surviving very low birth weight infants. Newborn Lung Project. *J Pediatr* **132**: 57–63.

Paneth N, Qiu H, Rosenbaum P et al. (2003) Reliability of classification of cerebral palsy in low-birthweight children in four countries. *Developmental Medicine and Child Neurology* **45**: 628–33.

Pinto-Martin J, Paneth N, Witomski T et al. (1992) The central New Jersey neonatal brain haemorrhage study: design of the study and reliability of ultrasound diagnosis. *Paediatr Perinat Epidemiol* **6**: 273–84.

Pinto-Martin JA, Riolo S, Cnaan A et al. (1995) Cranial ultrasound prediction of disabling and nondisabling cerebral palsy at age two in a low birth weight population. *Pediatrics* **95**: 249–54.

Redline RW, Wilson-Costello D, Borawski E, Fanaroff AA, Hack M (1998) Placental lesions associated with neurologic impairment and cerebral palsy in very low-birth-weight infants. *Arch Pathol Lab Med* **122**: 1091–8.

Robertson CMT, Watt MJ, Yasui Y (2007) Changes in the prevalence of cerebral palsy for children born very prematurely within a population-based program over 30 years. *Jama-Journal of the American Medical Association* **297**: 2733–40.

Rosenbaum P, Paneth N, Leviton A et al. (2007) A report: the definition and classification of cerebral palsy April 2006. *Dev Med Child Neurol Suppl* **109**: 8–14.

Rouse DJ, Hirtz DG, Thom E et al. (2008) A randomized, controlled trial of magnesium sulfate for the prevention of cerebral palsy. *New England Journal of Medicine* **359**: 895–905.

Salhab WA, Perlman JM, Silver L, Sue Broyles R (2004) Necrotizing enterocolitis and neurodevelopmental outcome in extremely low birth weight infants <1000 g. *J Perinatol* **24**: 534–40.

Shi Z, Ma L, Bajaj M et al. (2017) Chorioamnionitis in the development of cerebral palsy: a meta-analysis and systematic review. *Pediatrics* **139**: E20163781.

Schlapbach LJ, Aebischer M, Adams M et al. (2011) Impact of sepsis on neurodevelopmental outcome in a Swiss national cohort of extremely premature infants. *Pediatrics* **128**: e348–57.

Serenius F, Kallen K, Blennow M et al. (2013) Neurodevelopmental outcome in extremely preterm infants at 2.5 years after active perinatal care in Sweden. *Jama-Journal of the American Medical Association* **309**: 1810–20.

Soraisham AS, Amin HJ, Al-Hindi MY, Singhal N, Sauve RS (2006) Does necrotising enterocolitis impact the neurodevelopmental and growth outcomes in preterm infants with birthweight < or =1250 g? *J Paediatr Child Health* **42**: 499–504.

Steggerda SJ, Leijser LM, Wiggers-De Bruine FT, Van Der Grond J, Walther FJ, Van Wezel-Meijler G (2009) Cerebellar injury in preterm infants: incidence and findings on US and MR images. *Radiology* **252**: 190–9.

Stoll BJ, Hansen NI, Adams-Chapman I et al. (2004) Neurodevelopmental and growth impairment among extremely low-birth-weight infants with neonatal infection. *Jama-Journal of the American Medical Association* **292**: 2357–65.

Stoll BJ, Hansen NI, Bell EF et al. (2010) Neonatal outcomes of extremely preterm infants from the NICHD neonatal research network. *Pediatrics* **126**: 443–56.

Streimish IG, Ehrenkranz RA, Allred EN et al. (2012) Birth weight- and fetal weight-growth restriction: impact on neurodevelopment. *Early Human Development* **88**: 765–71.

Takemiya T, Matsumura K, Sugiura H et al. (2010) Endothelial microsomal prostaglandin E synthase-1 exacerbates neuronal loss induced by kainate. *J Neurosci Res* **88**: 381–90.

Takemiya T, Matsumura K, Sugiura H et al. (2011) Endothelial microsomal prostaglandin E synthase-1 facilitates neurotoxicity by elevating astrocytic Ca2+ levels. *Neurochem Int* **58**: 489–96.

Takemiya T, Matsumura K, Yamagata K (2007) Roles of prostaglandin synthesis in excitotoxic brain diseases. *Neurochem Int* **51**: 112–20.

Tommiska V, Heinonen K, Kero P et al. (2003) A national two year follow up study of extremely low birthweight infants born in 1996–1997. *Arch Dis Child Fetal Neonatal Ed* **88**: F29–35.

Tyler CP, Paneth N, Allred EN et al. (2012) Brain damage in preterm newborns and maternal medication: the ELGAN study. *Am J Obstet Gynecol* **207**: 192–9.

Van Der Burg JW, Allred EN, McElrath TF et al. (2013) Is maternal obesity associated with sustained inflammation in extremely low gestational age newborns? *Early Hum Dev* **89**: 949–55.

Van Der Burg JW, O'Shea TM, Kuban K et al. (2018) Are extremely low gestational age newborns born to obese women at increased risk of cerebral palsy at 2 years? *J Child Neurol* **33**: 216–24.

Van Der Burg JW, Sen S, Chomitz VR, Seidell JC, Leviton A, Dammann O (2016) The role of systemic inflammation linking maternal BMI to neurodevelopment in children. *Pediatr Res* **79**: 3–12.

Van Marter, Kuban KC, Allred E et al. (2010) Does bronchopulmonary dysplasia contribute to the occurrence of cerebral palsy among infants born before 28 weeks gestation? *Arch Dis Child Fetal Neonatal Ed* **96**: F20–9.

Vohr BR, Msall ME, Wilson D, Wright LL, McDonald S, Poole WK (2005) Spectrum of gross motor function in extremely low birth weight children with cerebral palsy at 18 months of age. *Pediatrics* **116**: 123–9.

Volpe JJ (2009) Brain injury in premature infants: a complex amalgam of destructive and developmental disturbances. *Lancet Neurology* **8**: 110–24.

Walsh MC, Kliegman RM, Hack M (1989) Severity of necrotizing enterocolitis: influence on outcome at 2 years of age. *Pediatrics* **84**: 808–14.

Wood NS, Costeloe K, Gibson AT, Hennessy EM, Marlow N, Wilkinson AR (2005) The EPICure study: associations and antecedents of neurological and developmental disability at 30 months of age following extremely preterm birth. *Archives of Disease in Childhood-Fetal and Neonatal Edition* **90**: 134–40.

Cognitive and Behavioral Functioning

Lauren Bush, Megan N Scott, and Scott J Hunter

INTRODUCTION

Accumulated research to date has highlighted that cognitive and behavioral development is an area of particular risk for infants born extremely prematurely and at low birth weight. As discussed in preceding chapters, the ELGAN project has emphasized an array of concerns regarding specific, diagnosable developmental disorders, but a significant focus of the ELGAN study was also on cognitive and behavioral developmental outcomes per se, in an effort to best define areas of functioning that most require support and intervention in regard to adaptive and educational opportunity. As discussed recently by Jaekel and Scott (2018), this emphasis on neurocognitive functioning across current research projects addressing extreme prematurity has led to a substantially stronger understanding of the risks that exist for affected children as they develop, across both a broader, and simultaneously more focused set of potential outcome variables affecting outcome and opportunity. This has led to a more informed ability to engage, understand, and then address these factors with families, in an effort to promote greater resilience in extremely preterm (EP) infants.

Research utilizing current neuropsychological methodologies for understanding cognitive and behavioral development has indicated that delivery at any period earlier than full term promotes vulnerability for several neurological insults, particularly among developing cortical structures and brain networks, that can lead to poor neurodevelopmental outcomes (MacKay et al. 2010; Quigley et al. 2012; Jaekel and Scott 2018). These potential alterations in neural organization, discussed both in this chapter and others in this book, can influence skill development in areas such as attention, information processing speed, and executive functioning, and in the coordination of behavioral and regulatory capacities.

This chapter focuses specifically on cognitive and behavioral outcomes. Because cognitive and behavioral regulation are intimately related, and presentation of diagnoses within the neurodevelopmental realm are a reflection of these challenges, we discuss both broad and more specific considerations regarding neurodevelopment and potential outcomes, and their relationship with defined developmental diagnoses.

AGE 2 OUTCOMES

Cognitive Development

Several studies have examined general cognitive development in a sample of toddlers born EP (Anderson and Doyle 2003; Stoelhorst et al. 2003; Johnson et al. 2008; De Jesus et al. 2013; Ribeiro et al. 2017; Luu and Nuyt 2018; Adams-Chapman et al. 2018).

Focusing exclusively on children born <28 weeks gestation has the potential to identify patterns of findings that may be unique to this particular subgroup, thus joining ELGAN to other large studies that investigate early emerging cognitive skills.

At 24 months' corrected age, participants in the ELGAN study completed a developmental assessment comprised of the Bayley Scales of Infant Development-Second Edition (BSID-II) and the Gross Motor Function Classification System, an assessment of gross motor functioning for children with cerebral palsy (CP). Consistent with the broader literature, toddlers in the ELGAN study cohort demonstrated delays across developmental domains at significantly higher rates than in the general population (O'Shea et al. 2009). These delays were more severe for boys relative to girls, as ELGAN boys were more likely to score 3 or more standard deviations below the normative mean than girls (O'Shea et al. 2012a).

This increased risk for developmental delay among extremely preterm infants is attributable to a number of different factors (O'Shea et al. 2008, 2009, 2013; Kuban et al. 2009), including especially ultrasound-detected white matter damage (O'Shea et al. 2009); neonatal inflammation (O'Shea et al. 2013) and microcephaly at 2 years of age, but not at birth (Kuban et al. 2009). The presence of moderate/severe ventriculomegaly and echolucent lesions were strongly associated with risk of lower developmental scores on the BSID-II at age 2, and slightly more strongly associated with increased risk of CP (O'Shea et al. 2008). Variations in weight gain from 7–28 days did not affect cognitive outcomes at age 2. Low weight at age 2 did contribute to lower cognitive scores at age 2, but when children with CP were excluded, no association was found (Belfort et al. 2016).

Behavior and Emotion Regulation

Premature birth is also associated with a range of behavior and emotion problems that begin early in development (Wolf et al. 2002; Delobel-Ayoub et al. 2009; Spittle et al. 2009; Arpi and Ferrari 2013). The most common challenges reported include poor behavioral and emotional self-regulation skills, emotional and social communication challenges, and problems with attention (Wolf et al. 2002; Spittle et al. 2009; Arpi and Ferrari 2013). In line with this broader literature, children within the ELGAN cohort show similar behavior and emotion challenges at age 2 (Boyd et al. 2013). Using the BSID-II Behavioral Rating Scale (BRS), Boyd et al. (2013) found that 31% of children scored within the questionable (i.e. 11–25th percentiles) or non-optimal ranges (i.e. less than 11th percentile) on a scale of Emotion Regulation, while 27% scored within these same ranges on a scale of Orientation/Engagement. The effects of these findings were strongest among boys and children with co-occurring cognitive and motor problems. They were also associated with lower gestational age, birth weight, head circumference, and a range of maternal demographic factors (e.g. race, education, socioeconomic status) (Boyd et al. 2013).

AGE 10 OUTCOMES

General Cognitive Ability

At 10 years of age, over 870 children from the original ELGAN cohort participated in extensive follow-up testing that included cognitive, behavioral, and neurologic assessment. General cognitive ability was assessed using the Differential Ability Scale-II (DAS-II) Verbal and Nonverbal Reasoning scales. Consistent with the broader literature examining global cognitive abilities in this population (Saigal et al. 2000; Bhutta et al. 2002; Hack et al. 2002; Anderson et al. 2003; Saigal et al. 2007; Lohaugen et al. 2010; Johnson et al. 2016; Cheong et al. 2017), more than half of the children in the ELGAN study showed moderate to severe neurocognitive deficits at age 10 (Joseph et al. 2016). Indeed, a non-normal distribution of DAS-II scores was observed in this sample, such that verbal and nonverbal cognitive scores shifted significantly toward lower values compared to the normal distribution than is expected in the general population (Joseph et al. 2016; Kuban et al. 2016). This pattern was moderated by gestational age, as the distribution of scores tended to shift further downward with decreasing gestational ages (Joseph et al. 2016). For example, children born at 23–24 weeks were at the highest risk of scoring more than 2 standard deviations below normative age expectations (Joseph et al. 2016). Moreover, and consistent with what is observed at 2 years of age, boys showed more striking difficulties compared to girls at age 10 (Kuban et al. 2016), though it is necessary to consider the fact that boys were also more likely than girls to be born at earlier gestational ages (Kuban et al. 2016).

Although a range of cognitive difficulties exist across development in children born extremely preterm, it is important to understand how these challenges manifest over time and the ways in which early developmental testing can predict later cognitive outcomes (O'Shea et al. 2018). O'Shea et al. (2018) investigated these relationships, finding that among children identified as having cognitive impairment at age 2 on the BSID-II (i.e. scoring 3 or more standard deviations below the mean, <55), more than half no longer met criteria for cognitive impairment on the DAS-II at age 10. This finding may therefore suggest that among infants born extremely preterm, cognitive impairment may either not persist throughout the school age years and/or may be grossly overestimated early in development (O'Shea et al. 2018). Additional research aimed at identifying the mechanisms and factors that influence this relationship will be important for informing future assessment and intervention efforts with this population.

A number of risk factors that contribute to patterns of lower cognitive test scores and increased rates of cognitive impairment have been identified. These include bronchopulmonary dysplasia (BPD) (Sriram et al. 2018), lower gestational ages (a relationship that may be mediated by a greater risk for bacteremia) (Joseph et al. 2016; Bright et al. 2017), CpG methylation levels of critical genes associated with normal development (Meakin et al. 2018; Tilley et al. 2018), and maternal education and socioeconomic status (Joseph et al. 2018). Elevations of neurotrophic proteins (proteins that support neuronal survival/function) during the first 2 weeks of life are associated with a reduced risk of cognitive impairment at age 10 (Kuban et al. 2018), potentially representing an important protective factor. The role of body mass index (BMI) has also been considered in relation to cognitive functioning in this group, though no significant relationships have emerged (Linthavong et al. 2018).

Attention and Executive Functioning

Significant attention and executive functioning deficits are observed in children born extremely preterm, a finding that is well-documented in the literature (Atkinson and Braddick 2007; van de Weijer-Bergsma et al. 2008; Aarnoudse-Moens et al. 2009; Frye et al. 2009; Mulder et al. 2009; Hallin and Stjernqvist 2011; Luu et al. 2011; Scott et al. 2012) and persists across the ELGAN sample (Joseph et al. 2016; Scott et al. 2017; Korzeniewski et al. 2017a; Leviton et al. 2018c). As part of the ELGAN study, a range of attention and executive functions were assessed at age 10 using subtests from the Differential Ability Scales, Second Edition (DAS-II; i.e. Recall of Digits Backward and Recall of Sequential Order) and the NEPSY-II: A Developmental Neuropsychological Assessment, Second Edition (i.e. Auditory Attention and Auditory Response Set, Inhibition and Inhibition Switching, Animal Sorting, and Inhibition Naming). Together, these subtests provide comprehensive information across domains of executive functions, including verbal working memory, auditory attention, set switching, simple and complex inhibition, concept generation, mental flexibility, and speed of processing.

As was the case for general cognition, a distribution of downward shifted scores was observed across all executive functioning tasks, though this pattern of performance was most striking for measures of inhibition, set maintenance, shifting, mental flexibility, and processing speed (Joseph et al. 2016). Indeed, across these specific domains, 51–69% of scores were greater than 1 standard deviation below the population mean (Joseph et al. 2016), with executive control and processing speed representing the most significant areas of weakness. Children born severely or less severely growth restricted demonstrated additional difficulties on the DAS-II Working Memory subtest (Korzeniewski et al. 2017a), the NEPSY-II Auditory Response subtest (Korzeniewski et al. 2017a), and the NEPSY-II Inhibition-Inhibition and Inhibition-Switching subtests (Leviton et al. 2018c) compared to children born with higher birth weights. Additional variability in executive function across the ELGAN sample emerged based on results of a latent profile analysis (LPA), in which subgroups of children were identified on the basis of general cognitive scores and performance across executive functioning tasks (Heeren et al. 2017). Results of this LPA suggested four distinct cognitive functioning profiles: 'normal', 'low normal', 'moderately impaired', and 'severely impaired' (Heeren et al. 2017). Interestingly, although children in both the 'normal' and 'low normal' group showed minimal impairment across domains, children in the 'low normal' group and not the 'normal' group showed a specific set of impairments in sustained attention, concept generation, and inhibition. In contrast, children in the 'moderate' and 'severe' groups showed more global deficits across all cognitive and executive functioning tasks. Additionally, executive dysfunction and general cognitive impairment exist at higher rates among children with co-occurring attention problems (i.e. those who meet criteria for attention deficit hyperactivity disorder [ADHD]; Scott et al. 2017).

Similar to the risk factors identified for poorer general cognitive skills, BPD has also been linked to greater attention and executive functioning difficulties (Sriram et al. 2018). Socioeconomic disadvantage (Leviton et al. 2018c), newborn immaturity/vulnerability (Leviton et al. 2018c), inflammation (Leviton et al. 2018c), fetal growth restriction (Leviton et al. 2018c), and high concentrations of inflammatory proteins (IL-8, TNF-α, and ICAM-1) (Leviton et al. 2018d) have also been found to increase the risk for executive dysfunction in this population. Moreover, ADHD symptoms, based on parent, teacher, and/or physician report, have been linked to a range of maternal factors (e.g. age, obesity, smoking) (van der Burg et al. 2017; Leviton et al. 2018a), birth-related events (e.g. magnesium administered at delivery for seizure prophylaxis, *Mycoplasma* sp. in the placenta) (Leviton et al. 2018a), low gestational age and birth weight (Leviton et al. 2018a), and demographic factors (e.g. male, singleton) (Leviton et al. 2018a).

Academic Achievement

Academic skills are impaired across subjects for children in the ELGAN study (Joseph et al. 2016; Akshoomoff et al. 2017; Korzeniewski et al. 2017a), which is not surprising given the extent of known cognitive and executive functioning weaknesses. However, this finding remains highly consistent with what has been reported in the broader prematurity literature (Hack et al. 2002; Wocadlo and Rieger 2007; Aarnoudse-Moens et al. 2011; Johnson et al. 2011; D'Onofrio et al. 2013; Jaekel and Wolke 2014; Kelly 2016; Twilhaar et al. 2018) and persists above and beyond the impact of other factors (e.g. birth weight, sex, maternal IQ, and socioeconomic indicators). Indeed, children in the ELGAN study scored significantly below normative age/grade expectations across domains of the Wechsler Individual Achievement Test-III (WIAT-III), which included measures of word recognition, decoding, spelling, and math-related computational skills. These lower academic scores occurred at significantly higher rates than in the general population (Joseph et al. 2016). Importantly, although a broad range of academic challenges has been noted, Akshoomoff et al. (2017) found that children in the ELGAN study were at an additional and increased risk for experiencing specific difficulty in math, indicating that math learning disabilities occurred at higher rates relative to reading disabilities in this cohort. This finding parallels a number of other studies that have also reported increased difficulties in mathematics among children born prematurely (Taylor et al. 2009; Simms et al. 2013; Lee et al. 2017), a finding that, in part, may be related to executive functioning weaknesses (Tatsuoka et al. 2016). Risk factors for experiencing increased academic difficulties include fetal growth restriction and inflammation (though this is specific to reading only and reading/math combined learning disabilities) (Leviton et al. 2018b), socioeconomic disadvantage (Leviton et al. 2018b), newborn immaturity/vulnerability (Leviton et al. 2018b), and symptoms of ADHD (Scott et al. 2017).

Language Ability

Expressive and receptive language skills were assessed as part of the ELGAN study using the Oral and Written Language Scales (OWLS), a test that measures semantic, morphologic, syntactic, and pragmatic language comprehension and production. Nineteen percent of children in the ELGAN sample scored more than 2 standard deviations below the mean on both expressive and receptive language domains, while 20–30% scored between 1 and 2 standard deviations below the mean (Joseph et al. 2016). Although prior studies have similarly highlighted language difficulties in this population (Largo et al. 1990; Wolke 1999; Wolke et al. 2008), these weaknesses are generally best understood in the context of the more global cognitive delays that are associated with extreme prematurity (Wolke et al. 2008).

Gross Motor, Fine Motor, and Visual Perceptual Skills

At 10 years of age, only 1.9% of children in the ELGAN sample were identified as having severe gross motor impairment, defined as having a Gross Motor Function Classification Score of 5 (Joseph et al. 2016). In contrast, a higher proportion of children showed deficits in their fine motor abilities. As part of this study, fine motor skills were assessed using the NEPSY-II Visuomotor Precision subtest. Twenty-one percent of children in the ELGAN study scored more than 2 standard deviations below the mean, while 35% scored within 1 and 2 standard deviations below the mean (Joseph et al. 2016). Similarly, visual perceptual skills represented an area of difficulty for a large portion of children in the study. Visual perception was tested using the NEPSY-II Arrows and Geometric Puzzles subtests, which represent measures of perception of line orientation and mental rotation of complex visual-spatial figures, respectively. Seventeen percent of children demonstrated performance that was greater than 2 standard deviations below the mean on the Geometric Puzzles subtest, while 26% scored in this range on the Arrows subtest (Joseph et al. 2016). Fine motor and visual perceptual skills may be worse in ELGAN children who are left-hand dominant (Burnett et al. 2018) and children who present with co-morbid ADHD (Scott et al. 2017). Overall, the findings on fine motor and visuo-perceptual skills are consistent with what has been reported in the preterm literature more broadly, as these tend to be areas of relative weakness above and beyond general cognitive abilities in this population (Geldof et al. 2012; Bos et al. 2013; Lee et al. 2017).

Behavior and Emotion Regulation

Behavior and emotion regulation challenges occur at higher rates in extremely premature children relative to the general population (Farooqi et al. 2007; Johnson et al. 2011; D'Onofrio et al. 2013). Consistent with this, a portion of children in the ELGAN study continue to show social impairment, attention problems, and emotional challenges throughout the school-age years (Korzeniewski et al. 2017b). Importantly, more than one third of children in the ELGAN sample have at least one neurodevelopmental burden, such as cognitive impairment (IQ < 70), autism spectrum disorder (ASD), cerebral palsy, or epilepsy (Hirschberger et al. 2018). Of these children, over 40% present with more than one co-occurring neurodevelopmental condition (Hirschberger et al. 2018), likely exacerbating many of the behavioral, social, and emotional challenges that are observed.

THE ROLE OF CO-MORBID ADHD ON NEUROPSYCHOLOGICAL OUTCOMES IN ELGANS

As is discussed in more detail in another chapter, the extremely preterm population is at significantly higher risk for a diagnosis of attention deficit hyperactivity disorder (ADHD) (Anderson et al. 2011; Scott et al. 2012; Franz et al. 2018). In fact, children born extremely preterm demonstrate attentional and social problems by early school age (ages 5 and 6 years) (Sykes et al. 1997; Clark et al. 2008; Spittle et al. 2009; Scott et al. 2012). Despite the well-established findings of higher rates of ADHD in extremely preterm children compared to the general population, little is known about the neurocognitive limitations that accompany ADHD in these high-risk children beyond academic outcomes. Several studies have indicated early attention problems in low birth weight and very low birth weight children are associated with poor academic outcomes in early and late adolescence even when controlling for IQ and socio-demographic variables (Breslau et al. 2009; Jaekel et al. 2013). Taylor et al. (2019) recently demonstrated that parent-reported ADHD symptoms in kindergarten were predictive of slower academic attainment or progress in word reading and mathematics across the first 3 years of school.

Using the battery described above, the neurocognitive correlates of ADHD symptoms in children with extreme prematurity were examined as part of the ELGAN study (Scott et al. 2017). This examination yielded important findings that add to our understanding of this high-risk population. For these analyses, children were classified as having significant ADHD symptoms based on several sources of information, whether parent or teacher ratings on the Child Symptom Inventory-4 (CSI-4) were above the norm-based cut-off scores and parent report of a history of a diagnosis of ADHD (Sprafkin et al. 2002; Gadow and Sprafkin 2002). Participants were classified as demonstrating significant ADHD symptoms if they met criteria in any two of these three contexts.

In general, children classified as having significant ADHD symptoms performed more poorly than the normative sample across measures of intellectual functioning, executive function, and academic achievement, with the median score on all assessments falling approximately 1 standard deviation below the mean (Scott et al. 2017). Importantly, this pattern of performance was consistently 0.25 to 0.75 standard deviations below the scores attained by children in the ELGAN cohort who were not reported to have significant ADHD symptoms. When examining IQ alone, the ELGAN group with significant ADHD symptoms demonstrated a downward shift in the distribution of IQ scores compared to the general population and this shift was much more prominent than that seen when examining the ELGAN group as a whole. Specifically, 23% of the ELGAN participants with significant ADHD symptoms performed 2 standard deviations below the mean compared to 12% of those without ADHD symptoms (Scott et al. 2017). A similar pattern was demonstrated across other assessments of neurocognitive functioning with the pattern of doubling of the frequency of scores at or lower than 2 standard deviations below the mean compared to ELGAN participants without significant ADHD symptoms in the areas of receptive language (OWLS Listening Comprehension), expressive language (OWLS Oral Expression), academic achievement (WIAT-III), and working memory (Scott et al. 2017). These differences were more modest on assessments of sustained attention, inhibition, cognitive flexibility, concept formation, fine motor functioning and visual perceptual skills with the multiple of increased frequency of significant impairment (<-2 Z) between the two groups ranging from 1.4 to 1.8 (Scott et al. 2017).

Even when restricting the sample to children whose IQ ≥ 70 and to those whose IQ ≥ 85, children classified as ADHD were more likely than their ELGAN peers to have specific deficits in a number of areas although the severity of these deficits was less significant than when including the entire sample. Specifically, this group was more likely to demonstrate challenges on the DAS-II Working Memory and NEPSY-II Auditory Response. These difficulties across tasks requiring sustained and dual attention, working memory capacity, inhibitory control, and cognitive flexibility were also present even after adjusting for important sociodemographic and medical variables (Scott et al. 2017). These results support previous findings of deficits in working memory and cognitive flexibility in preterm children with ADHD symptoms while also identifying inhibitory control as an area of challenge, which is a unique contribution to the literature (Shum et al. 2008). Finally, deficits on NEPSY-II Visuomotor Precision persisted when examining those whose IQ ≥ 70, but was no longer significant when limiting the sample to those whose IQ ≥ 85.

Importantly, the findings of poorer academic achievement on the WIAT-III in the areas of reading, spelling, and mathematics persisted even when examining the subsample of children whose IQ was ≥70 and whose IQ ≥ 85. These findings inform our understanding of the impact of attention and executive function deficits on learning and academic development among children born extremely preterm and highlight the need for research and development of multifaceted interventions and supports in the academic setting for this high risk population.

THE ROLE OF CO-MORBID ASD ON NEUROPSYCHOLOGICAL OUTCOMES

Children born extremely preterm are at an increased risk for experiencing co-morbid ASD and related symptomatology (Hack et al. 2009; Johnson et al. 2010a, 2010b; Moore et al. 2012; Dudova et al. 2014), which further complicates the neuropsychological profile of this unique subgroup. Indeed, Johnson et al. (2010a) found that in a sample of children born less than 26 weeks' gestation, children with co-occurring ASD were more likely to have lower general cognitive skills and greater difficulties across reading and math compared to children without ASD. The odds of cognitive impairment are also significantly higher among this particular subgroup (Johnson et al. 2010b). To further explore the relationship between ASD and neuropsychological outcomes in children born extremely preterm, participants in the ELGAN study were administered a hierarchical series of well-validated ASD-related measures. First, parents were instructed to complete the Social Communication Questionnaire (SCQ), a parent-report questionnaire that served as the initial screen for ASD symptoms. For children who screened positive on this measure, an in-depth parent interview, the Autism Diagnostic Interview-Revised (ADI-R), was administered by a trained clinician in order to further assess ASD symptomatology. If children met criteria for autism or ASD based on the ADI-R, they were then assessed using the Autism Diagnostic Observation Schedule, Second Edition (ADOS-2), a gold standard diagnostic measure used to evaluate a range of social and communicative behaviors. Based on these rigorous and empirically-supported criteria, approximately 7% of the sample ultimately met diagnostic criteria for ASD (Joseph et al. 2017; Hirschberger et al. 2018).

Consistent with other study samples (Johnson et al. 2010a, 2010b), participants with ASD in the ELGAN sample were more likely to have verbal and nonverbal cognitive abilities that fell within the intellectually disabled range (i.e. IQ scores below 70) compared to children without ASD (Joseph et al. 2017; Hirschberger et al. 2018). In fact, 40% of the sample with ASD had verbal and nonverbal scores that fell within the cognitively impaired range, while 60% had either verbal or nonverbal (or both) fall within this range (Joseph et al. 2017). Of note, the prevalence rates for co-morbid ASD and intellectual disability did not differ in the ELGAN sample from what is reported in the broader population of individuals with ASD (Joseph et al. 2017). However, based on findings from Joseph et al. (2017), 46% of the children with ASD who had verbal and nonverbal scores below 70 failed to obtain a basal score on the IQ measure, suggesting nonverbal mental ages of only 3 and a half years or younger. This cognitive profile was further impacted by impairments in executive functioning, such that children who met the threshold for cognitive and executive function impairments together had seven times the risk of being diagnosed with ASD compared to children without this same degree of gross neurocognitive impairment (Hirschberger et al. 2018).

Finally, above and beyond meeting diagnostic threshold for an ASD, children in the ELGAN cohort who showed increased social impairments more generally were also at an increased risk for experiencing deficits across neuropsychological domains relative to their peers with developmentally normal social behaviors (Korzeniewski et al. 2017). This included increased difficulties in attention, executive function, language, communication, behavior, and emotional functioning (Korzeniewski et al. 2017).

Overall, it is clear that the presence of ASD in children born extremely preterm exacerbates the range of neurocognitive deficits that are generally observed in this group. However, additional research in this area is needed to further delineate the profile of strengths and weaknesses and inform future assessment and intervention efforts within this particular subgroup, as these individuals may benefit from additional supports and accommodations that their peers without ASD do not require.

CONCLUSION AND FUTURE DIRECTIONS

Children born extremely preterm and at extremely low birth weight face significant potential for neurocognitive and behavioral challenges throughout development. Attentional and social difficulties are commonly identified across both the ELGAN project and other research that is simultaneously taking place. This highlights the vulnerability of specific neural systems that guide engagement, focus, vigilance, and executive aspects of both learning and adaptive/social functioning. Together, these findings reiterate the need for continued research tracking the potential dose related effects of low gestational age on brain development, particularly as these individuals begin to transition into adulthood when executive capacities are known to further develop and unfold.

The clinical implications of the ELGAN findings – that ELGANs are at substantial risk for deficits in cognitive development – are important to recognize and address. Challenges with the acquisition of attention, regulation, processing speed, and executive functioning cannot fail to make an impact on academic achievement, affecting both early foundational academics and later functioning, as skills are integrated for handling more demanding learning goals. Findings from ELGAN provide guidance in shaping practical recommendations both for regular neuropsychological assessments and for interventions with therapists and academic skills resources, so as to support appropriate accommodation and treatment to enhance development and promote resilience. As findings are updated with ongoing longitudinal investigations, further enhancements to consultation and intervention are expected to be helpful for families and the youth born extremely prematurely. ELGAN's findings can also serve as a basis for developing trials to assess the value of proposed intervention strategies.

REFERENCES

Aarnoudse-Moens CS, Oosterlaan J, Duivenvoorden HJ, van Goudoever JB, Weisglas-Kuperus N (2011) Development of preschool and academic skills in children born very preterm. *J Pediatr* **158**: 51–6.

Aarnoudse-Moens CS, Smidts DP, Oosterlaan J, Duivenvoorden HJ, Weisglas-Kuperus N (2009) Executive function in very preterm children at early school age. *J Abnorm Child Psychol* **37**: 981–93.

Adams-Chapman I, Heyne RJ, DeMauro SB et al. (2018) Neurodevelopmental impairment among extremely preterm infants in the neonatal research network. *Pediatrics* **141**: pii: e20173091.

Akshoomoff N, Joseph RM, Taylor HG et al. (2017) Academic achievement deficits and their neuropsychological correlates in children born extremely preterm. *J Dev Behav Pediatr* **38**: 627–37.

Anderson P, Doyle LW, Victorian Infant Collaborative Study Group (2003) Neurobehavioral outcomes of school-age children born extremely low birth weight or very preterm in the 1990s. *JAMA* **289**: 3264–72.

Anderson PJ, De Luca CR, Hutchinson E et al. (2011) Attention problems in a representative sample of extremely preterm/extremely low birth weight children. *Dev Neuropsychol* **36**: 57–73.

Arpi E, Ferrari F (2013) Preterm birth and behaviour problems in infants and preschool-age children: a review of the recent literature. *Dev Med Child Neurol* **55**: 788–96.

Atkinson J, Braddick O (2007) Visual and visuocognitive development in children born very prematurely. *Prog Brain Res* **164**: 123–49.

Belfort MB, Kuban KC, O'Shea TM et al. (2016) Weight status in the first 2 years of life and neurodevelopmental impairment in extremely low gestational age newborns. *J Pediatr* **168**: 30–5 e32.

Bhutta AT, Cleves MA, Casey PH, Cradock MM, Anand KJ (2002) Cognitive and behavioral outcomes of school-aged children who were born preterm: a meta-analysis. *JAMA* **288**: 728–37.

Bos AF, Van Braeckel KN, Hitzert MM, Tanis JC, Roze E (2013) Development of fine motor skills in preterm infants. *Dev Med Child Neurol* **55**: 1–4.

Boyd LAC, Msall ME, O'Shea TM et al. (2013) Social–emotional delays at 2 years in extremely low gestational age survivors: correlates of impaired orientation/engagement and emotional regulation. *Early Hum Dev* **89**: 925–30.

Breslau J, Miller E, Breslau N, Bohnert K, Lucia V, Schweitzer J (2009) The impact of early behavior disturbances on academic achievement in high school. *Pediatrics* **123**: 1472–6.

Bright HR, Babata K, Allred EN et al. (2017) Neurocognitive outcomes at 10 years of age in extremely preterm newborns with late-onset bacteremia. *J Pediatr* **187**: 43–9 e41.

Burnett AC, Anderson PJ, Joseph RM et al. (2018) Hand preference and cognitive, motor, and behavioral functioning in 10-year-old extremely preterm children. *J Pediatr* **195**: 279–82 e273.

Carrow-Woolfolk E (1996) *Oral and Written Language Skills: Written Expression Scale Manual*. Circle Pines, MN: American Guidance Service.

Cheong JLY, Anderson PJ, Burnett AC (2017) Changing neurodevelopment at 8 years in children born extremely preterm since the 1990s. *Pediatrics* **139**: e20164086. doi: 10.1542/peds.2016-4086.

Clark CA, Woodward LJ, Horwood LJ, Moor S (2008) Development of emotional and behavioral regulation in children born extremely preterm and very preterm: biological and social influences. *Child Development* **79**: 1444–62.

D'Onofrio BM, Class QA, Rickert ME et al. (2013) Preterm birth and mortality and morbidity: a population-based quasi-experimental study. *JAMA Psychiatry* **70**: 1231–40.

De Jesus LC, Pappas A, Shankaran S et al. (2013) Outcomes of small for gestational age infants born at <27 weeks' gestation. *J Pediatr* **163**: 55–60 e51–53.

Delobel-Ayoub M, Arnaud C, White-Koning M et al. (2009) Behavioral problems and cognitive performance at 5 years of age after very preterm birth: the EPIPAGE Study. *Pediatrics* **123**: 1485–92.

Dudova I, Kasparova M, Markova D et al. (2014) Screening for autism in preterm children with extremely low and very low birth weight. *Neuropsychiatr Dis Treat* **10**: 277–82.

Elliott CD (2007) *Differential Ability Scales* (2nd edn) San Antonio, TX: The Psychological Corporation.

Farooqi A, Hagglof B, Sedin G, Gothefors L, Serenius F (2007) Mental health and social competencies of 10- to 12-year-old children born at 23 to 25 weeks of gestation in the 1990s: a Swedish national prospective follow-up study. *Pediatrics* **120**: 118–33.

Franz AP, Bolat GU, Bolat H et al. (2018) Attention-deficit/hyperactivity disorder and very preterm/very low birth weight: a meta-analysis. *Pediatrics* **141**: e20171645.

Frye RE, Landry SH, Swank PR, Smith KE (2009) Executive dysfunction in poor readers born prematurely at high risk. *Dev Neuropsychol* **34**: 254–71.

Gadow KD, Sprafkin JN (2002) *Child Symptom Inventory 4: Screening and Norms Manual*. Stony Brook, NY: Checkmate Plus.

Geldof CJ, van Wassenaer AG, de Kieviet JF, Kok JH, Oosterlaan J (2012) Visual perception and visual-motor integration in very preterm and/or very low birth weight children: a meta-analysis. *Res Dev Disabil* **33**: 726–36.

Hack M, Flannery DJ, Schluchter M et al. (2002) Outcomes in young adulthood for very-low-birth-weight infants. *N Engl J Med* **346**: 149–57.

Hack M, Taylor HG, Schluchter M et al. (2009) Behavioral outcomes of extremely low birth weight children at age 8 years. *J Dev Behav Pediatr* **30**: 122–30.

Hallin AL, Stjernqvist K (2011) Adolescents born extremely preterm: behavioral outcomes and quality of life. *Scand J Psychol* **52**: 251–6.

Heeren T, Joseph RM, Allred EN et al. (2017) Cognitive functioning at the age of 10 years among children born extremely preterm: a latent profile approach. *Pediatr Res* **82**: 614–9.

Hirschberger RG, Kuban KCK, O'Shea TM et al. (2018) Co-occurrence and severity of neurodevelopmental burden (cognitive impairment, cerebral palsy, autism spectrum disorder, and epilepsy) at age ten years in children born extremely preterm. *Pediatr Neurol* **79**: 45–52.

Jaekel J, Scott M (2018) Preterm and low-birth-weight birth. In: Donders J, Hunter SJ (eds), *Neuropsychological Conditions across the Lifespan.* Cambridge, UK: Cambridge University Press, pp. 2–23.

Jaekel J, Wolke D, Bartmann P (2013) Poor attention rather than hyperactivity/impulsivity predicts academic achievement in very preterm and full-term adolescents. *Psychological Medicine* **43**: 183–96.

Jaekel J, Wolke D (2014) Preterm birth and dyscalculia. *J Pediatr* **164**: 1327–32.

Johnson S, Hollis C, Kochhar P et al. (2010a) Autism spectrum disorders in extremely preterm children. *J Pediatr* **156**: 525–31 e522.

Johnson S, Hollis C, Kochhar P et al. (2010b) Psychiatric disorders in extremely preterm children: longitudinal finding at age 11 years in the EPICure study. *J Am Acad Child Adolesc Psychiatry* **49**: 453–63 e451.

Johnson S, Strauss V, Gilmore C et al. (2016) Learning disabilities among extremely preterm children without neurosensory impairment: comorbidity, neuropsychological profiles and scholastic outcomes. *Early Hum Dev* **103**: 69–75.

Johnson S, Wolke D, Hennessy E, Marlow N (2011) Educational outcomes in extremely preterm children: neuropsychological correlates and predictors of attainment. *Dev Neuropsychol* **36**: 74–95.

Johnson S, Wolke D, Marlow N, Preterm Infant Parenting Study G (2008) Developmental assessment of preterm infants at 2 years: validity of parent reports. *Dev Med Child Neurol* **50**: 58–62.

Joseph RM, O'Shea TM, Allred EN et al. (2016) Neurocognitive and academic outcomes at age 10 years of extremely preterm newborns. *Pediatrics* **137**(4): e20154343. doi: 10.1542/peds.2015-4343.

Joseph RM, O'Shea TM, Allred EN et al. (2017) Prevalence and associated features of autism spectrum disorder in extremely low gestational age newborns at age 10 years. *Autism Res* **10**: 224–32.

Joseph RM, O'Shea TM, Allred EN, Heeren T, Kuban KK (2018) Maternal educational status at birth, maternal educational advancement, and neurocognitive outcomes at age 10 years among children born extremely preterm. *Pediatr Res* **83**: 767–77.

Kelly MM (2016) Educational implications of preterm birth: a national sample of 8- to 11-year-old children born prematurely and their full-term peers. *J Pediatr Health Care* **30**: 464–70.

Korkman M, Kirk U, Kemp S (2007) *NEPSY-Second Edition (NEPSY-II).* San Antonio, TX: The Psychological Corporation.

Korzeniewski SJ, Allred EN, Joseph RM et al. (2017a) Neurodevelopment at age 10 years of children born <28 weeks with fetal growth restriction. *Pediatrics* **140**: e20170697. https://doi.org/10.1542/peds.2017-0697.

Korzeniewski SJ, Joseph RM, Kim SH et al. (2017b) Social responsiveness scale assessment of the preterm behavioral phenotype in 10-year-olds born extremely preterm. *J Dev Behav Pediatr* **38**: 697–705.

Kuban KC, Allred EN, O'Shea TM et al. (2009) Developmental correlates of head circumference at birth and two years in a cohort of extremely low gestational age newborns. *J Pediatr* **155**: 344–9 e341–343.

Kuban KC, Joseph RM, O'Shea TM et al. (2016) Girls and boys born before 28 weeks gestation: risks of cognitive, behavioral, and neurologic outcomes at age 10 years. *J Pediatr* **173**: 69–75 e61.

Kuban KCK, Heeren T, O'Shea TM et al. (2018) Among children born extremely preterm a higher level of circulating neurotrophins is associated with lower risk of cognitive impairment at school age. *J Pediatr* **201**: 40–8 e44.

Largo RH, Molinari L, Kundu S, Lipp A, Duc G (1990) Intellectual outcome, speech and school performance in high risk preterm children with birth weight appropriate for gestational age. *Eur J Pediatr* **149**: 845–50.

Lee M, Pascoe JM, McNicholas CI (2017) Reading, mathematics and fine motor skills at 5 years of age in us children who were extremely premature at birth. *Matern Child Health J* **21**: 199–207.

Leviton A, Hooper SR, Hunter SJ et al. (2018a) Antecedents of screening positive for attention deficit hyperactivity disorder in ten-year-old children born extremely preterm. *Pediatr Neurol* **81**: 25–30.

Leviton A, Joseph RM, Allred EN, O'Shea TM, Kuban KKC (2018b) Antenatal and neonatal antecedents of learning limitations in 10-year-old children born extremely preterm. *Early Hum Dev* **118**: 8–14.

Leviton A, Joseph RM, Allred EN et al. (2018c) Antenatal and neonatal antecedents of executive dysfunctions in extremely preterm children. *J Child Neurol* 33: 198–208.

Leviton A, Joseph RM, Fichorova RN et al. (2018d) Executive dysfunction early postnatal biomarkers among children born extremely preterm. *J Neuroimmune Pharmacol* 14: 188–99.

Linthavong O, O'Shea TM, Allred E et al. (2018) Neurocognitive and health correlates of overweight and obesity among ten-year-old children born extremely preterm. *J Pediatr* 200: 84–90 e84.

Lohaugen GC, Gramstad A, Evensen KA et al. (2010) Cognitive profile in young adults born preterm at very low birthweight. *Dev Med Child Neurol* 52: 1133–8.

Lord C, Rutter M, Le Couteur A (1994) Autism diagnostic interview-revised: a revised version of a diagnostic interview for caregivers of individuals with possible pervasive developmental disorders. *J Autism Dev Disord* 24: 659–85.

Lord C, Rutter M, DiLavore P, Risi S, Gotham K, Bishop S (2012) *Autism Diagnostic Observation Schedule–2 (ADOS-2)*. Los Angeles, CA: Western Psychological Corporation.

Luu TM, Ment L, Allan W, Schneider K, Vohr BR (2011) Executive and memory function in adolescents born very preterm. *Pediatrics* 127: e639–46.

Luu TM, Nuyt AM (2018) Cognitive trajectories from infancy to early adulthood in the EPICure cohort: time to refocus research on how to break the 'natural limits' of brain plasticity. *Arch Dis Child Fetal Neonatal Ed* 103: F399–F400.

MacKay DF, Smith GCS, Dobbie R, Pell JP (2010). Gestational age at delivery and special education need: Retrospective cohort study of 407,503 school children. *PLoS Medicine* 7: e1000289.

Meakin CJ, Martin EM, Santos HP, Jr et al. (2018) Placental CpG methylation of HPA-axis genes is associated with cognitive impairment at age 10 among children born extremely preterm. *Horm Behav* 101: 29–35.

Moore T, Johnson S, Hennessy E, Marlow N (2012) Screening for autism in extremely preterm infants: problems in interpretation. *Dev Med Child Neurol* 54: 514–20.

Mulder H, Pitchford NJ, Hagger MS, Marlow N (2009) Development of executive function and attention in preterm children: a systematic review. *Dev Neuropsychol* 34: 393–421.

O'Shea TM, Allred EN, Dammann O et al. (2009) The ELGAN study of the brain and related disorders in extremely low gestational age newborns. *Early Hum Dev* 85: 719–25.

O'Shea TM, Allred EN, Kuban KC et al. (2012a) Elevated concentrations of inflammation-related proteins in postnatal blood predict severe developmental delay at 2 years of age in extremely preterm infants. *J Pediatr* 160: 395–401 e394.

O'Shea TM, Allred EN, Kuban KC et al. (2012b) Intraventricular hemorrhage and developmental outcomes at 24 months of age in extremely preterm infants. *J Child Neurol* 27: 22–9.

O'Shea TM, Joseph RM, Allred EN et al. (2018) Accuracy of the Bayley-II mental development index at 2 years as a predictor of cognitive impairment at school age among children born extremely preterm. *J Perinatol* 38: 908–16.

O'Shea TM, Kuban KC, Allred EN et al. (2008) Neonatal cranial ultrasound lesions and developmental delays at 2 years of age among extremely low gestational age children. *Pediatrics* 122: e662–9.

O'Shea TM, Shah B, Allred EN et al. (2013) Inflammation-initiating illnesses, inflammation-related proteins, and cognitive impairment in extremely preterm infants. *Brain Behav Immun* 29: 104–112.

Quigley M, Poulsen G, Boule EM et al. (2012). Early term and late preterm birth is associated with poorer school performance at age 5 years: a cohort study. *Archives of Disease in Childhood – Fetal and Neonatal Edition* 97: F167–F73. doi: 10.1136/archdischild-2011-3400888.

Ribeiro CD, Pachelli MR, Amaral NC, Lamonica DA (2017) Development skills of children born premature with low and very low birth weight. *Codas* 29: e20160058.

Rutter M, Bailey A, Lord C (2003) *The Social Communication Questionnaire*. Los Angeles, CA: Western Psychological Services.

Saigal S, Hoult LA, Streiner DL, Stoskopf BL, Rosenbaum PL (2000) School difficulties at adolescence in a regional cohort of children who were extremely low birth weight. *Pediatrics* 105: 325–31.

Saigal S, Stoskopf B, Boyle M et al. (2007) Comparison of current health, functional limitations, and health care use of young adults who were born with extremely low birth weight and normal birth weight. *Pediatrics* 119: e562–73.

Scott MN, Hunter SJ, Joseph RM et al. (2017) Neurocognitive correlates of attention-deficit hyperactivity disorder symptoms in children born at extremely low gestational age. *J Dev Behav Pediatr* **38**: 249–59.

Scott MN, Taylor HG, Fristad MA et al. (2012) Behavior disorders in extremely preterm/extremely low birth weight children in kindergarten. *J Dev Behav Pediatr* **33**: 202–13.

Shum D, Neulinger K, O'Callaghan M, Mohay H (2008) Attentional problems in children born very preterm or with extremely low birth weight at 7–9 years. *Arch Clin Neuropsychol* **23**: 103–12.

Simms V, Cragg L, Gilmore C, Marlow N, Johnson S (2013) Mathematics difficulties in children born very preterm: current research and future directions. *Arch Dis Child Fetal Neonatal Ed* **98**: F457–63.

Spittle AJ, Treyvaud K, Doyle LW et al. (2009) Early emergence of behavior and social-emotional problems in very preterm infants. *J Am Acad Child Adolesc Psychiatry* **48**: 909–18.

Sprafkin J, Gadow KD, Salisbury H, Schneider J, Loney J (2002) Further evidence of reliability and validity of the Child Symptom Inventory-4: Parent checklist in clinically referred boys. *J Clin Child Adolesc Psychol* **31**: 513–24.

Sriram S, Schreiber MD, Msall ME et al. (2018) Cognitive development and quality of life associated with BPD in 10-year-olds born preterm. *Pediatrics* **141**: e20172719. doi: https://doi.org/10.1542/peds.2017-2719.

Stoelhorst GM, Rijken M, Martens SE et al. (2003) Developmental outcome at 18 and 24 months of age in very preterm children: a cohort study from 1996 to 1997. *Early Hum Dev* **72**: 83–95.

Sykes DH, Hoy EA, Bill JM, McClure BG, Halliday HL, Reid MM (1997) Behavioural adjustment in school of very low birthweight children. *J Clin Child Adolesc Psychol* **38**: 315–25.

Tatsuoka C, McGowan B, Yamada T et al. (2016) Effects of extreme prematurity on numerical skills and executive function in kindergarten children: an application of partially ordered classification modeling. *Learn Individ Differ* **49**: 332–40.

Taylor HG, Orchinik L, Fristad MA (2019) Associations of attention deficit hyperactivity disorder (ADHD) at school entry with early academic progress in children born prematurely and full-term controls. *Learn Individ Differ* **69**: 1–10.

Taylor HG, Espy KA, Anderson PJ (2009) Mathematics deficiencies in children with very low birth weight or very preterm birth. *Dev Disabil Res Rev* **15**: 52–9.

Tilley SK, Martin EM, Smeester L et al. (2018) Placental CpG methylation of infants born extremely preterm predicts cognitive impairment later in life. *PLoS One* **13**: e0193271.

Twilhaar ES, de Kieviet JF, Aarnoudse-Moens CS, van Elburg RM, Oosterlaan J (2018) Academic performance of children born preterm: a meta-analysis and meta-regression. *Arch Dis Child Fetal Neonatal Ed* **103**: F322–30.

van de Weijer-Bergsma E, Wijnroks L, Jongmans MJ (2008) Attention development in infants and preschool children born preterm: a review. *Infant Behav Dev* **31**: 333–51.

van der Burg JW, Jensen ET, van de Bor M et al. (2017) Maternal obesity and attention-related symptoms in the preterm offspring. *Early Hum Dev* **115**: 9–15.

Wechsler D (2009) *The Wechsler Individual Achievement Test-III*. San Antonio, TX: Pearson Assessment.

Wocadlo C, Rieger I (2007) Phonology, rapid naming and academic achievement in very preterm children at eight years of age. *Early Hum Dev* **83**: 367–77.

Wolf MJ, Koldewijn K, Beelen A et al. (2002) Neurobehavioral and developmental profile of very low birthweight preterm infants in early infancy. *Acta Paediatr* **91**: 930–8.

Wolke D (1999) Language problems in neonatal at risk children: towards an understanding of developmental mechanisms. *Acta Paediatr* **88**: 488–90.

Wolke D, Samara M, Bracewell M, Marlow N, Group EPS (2008) Specific language difficulties and school achievement in children born at 25 weeks of gestation or less. *J Pediatr* **152**: 256–62.

Autism, Social Impairment, and Social Communication Deficits in Children Born Prior to the 28th Week of Gestation

Steven J Korzeniewski

INTRODUCTION

Social cognition is one of the six core domains of neurocognitive function, and refers to the ability to sense, process, interpret, and appropriately respond to others (Happe and Conway 2016). Social impairment is a key feature of autism spectrum disorders (ASD), but social communication deficits are also documented in children and adults who do not have the full range of characteristics of autism (Corradi-Dell'Acqua et al. 2016; Happe and Conway 2016; Lipscombe et al. 2016). Social impairment and social communication problems can limit lifetime opportunities and achievement (Ritchie and Bora 2015).

In this chapter, I summarize and put in perspective the ELGAN study's experience studying three entities – children screening positive for an ASD with the Modified-Checklist for Autism in Toddlers (M-CHAT) (Robins et al. 2001) at 24 months (Kuban et al. 2009; Luyster et al. 2011; Kim et al. 2016), children diagnosed with ASD at age 10 years defined with the Social Communication Questionnaire (SCQ) (Rutter et al. 2003a), Autism Diagnostic Interview–Revised (ADI-R) (Rutter et al. 2003b) and the Autism Diagnostic Observation Schedule, Second Version (ADOS-2) (Lord et al. 2012; Joseph et al. 2017a, 2017b; Korzeniewski et al. 2017a, 2018) and children with social impairment at age 10 defined by a high score on the Social Responsiveness Scale (SRS) (Constantino and Gruber 2005) (total score ≥65) (Korzeniewski et al. 2017b, 2018).

THE ELGAN STUDY

The Modified-Checklist for Autism in Toddlers (M-CHAT) at 24 Months

The ELGAN study first used the M-CHAT to test the hypothesis that children born extremely preterm are more likely to screen positive at age 2 years, while exploring the possibility that motor, vision, hearing and cognitive impairments might explain an increased tendency to screen positive (Kuban et al. 2009). Of the 1200 children who survived to 24 months' corrected age, 988 had a complete developmental assessment. Of these, the M-CHAT screen positive rate was 16%, more than three-fold higher than expected based on general population norms. Even when excluding children with cognitive impairment, the M-CHAT screen positive rate was 10%, nearly twice the expected rate.

Four of the six M-CHAT 'critical items' were commonly affected by presence and severity of concurrent impairments (motor, cognitive, vision, and hearing) (Luyster et al. 2011). These results prompted the inference that impaired sensory or motor function among children born at extremely low gestational ages might give rise to false positive M-CHAT screening determinations. Indeed, in light of ASD diagnoses made at age 10 years, sensorimotor and cognitive impairments, as well as socioeconomic deprivation, and emotional/behavioral dysregulation appeared to contribute significantly to M-CHAT misclassifications (Kim et al. 2016).

The M-CHAT at 24 months had a sensitivity of 52%, a specificity of 84%, a positive predictive value (PPV) of 20%, and a negative predictive value (NPV) of 96% for the identification of rigorously defined ASD made at age 10 years. The likelihood ratio for ASD (i.e. the 52% sensitivity divided by the 16% false positive rate) generated by a positive M-CHAT was just 3.25, meaning that a child was just a little more than three times more likely to have ASD at age 10 if they screened positive on the M-CHAT at age 2. At the same time four out of five ELGANs screening positive on the M-CHAT did not have autism. This finding indicates that M-CHAT is an inappropriate screening tool for ASD in this population.

Autism Spectrum Disorder at 10 Years

Prevalence

Ninety-two percent of the 966 10-year-old children who were born at 23–27 weeks were rigorously assessed for autism (Joseph et al. 2017b). First, children meeting ASD screening criteria on the SCQ were evaluated with the ADI-R. Next, those meeting ADI-R criteria were assessed with the ADOS-2; a positive score was the criterion for ASD. Of 889 children in the sample, 26 were excluded from an assessment of ASD; 17 because of severe motor impairment and severe intellectual disability (ID), seven for functional blindness, and two for severe motor impairment, blindness, and ID combined. Six other children who did not return to complete the ASD assessment were excluded, as were 13 children who did not have an IQ assessment.

A total of 61 children met ADOS-2 criteria for ASD, resulting in an overall sample ASD prevalence of 7.1% (95% CI: 5.5–9.0), much higher than the 1.5% prevalence observed in 2014 by the Autism and Developmental Disabilities Monitoring Network (p < 0.001) (Developmental Disabilities Monitoring Network Surveillance 2014). That study, it should be noted, derived its ASD diagnosis from review of medical records, not from direct assessment as in ELGAN.

ASD risk increased with decreasing gestational age at delivery, from 3.4% (95% CI 1.6–6.1) at 27 weeks to 15.0% (95% CI 10.0–21.2) at 23–24 weeks, and 6.5% (95% CI 4.2–9.4) at 25–26 weeks gestational age (Fig. 14.1).

The male-to-female ratio of children with ASD was 2.1:1 (95% CI 51.2:1–3.5:1), lower than the 4:1 ratio observed in 2014 by the Autism and Developmental Disabilities Monitoring Network (Developmental Disabilities Monitoring Network Surveillance 2014). This sex ratio was similar in children with ASD and intellectual impairment (ID) (2.4:1) and in children with ASD with normal intelligence (2.0:1).

Antecedents

Because previous studies provided evidence that risk factors may differ by co-occurrence of ID, we assessed antecedents for combinations of ASD and ID (Joseph et al. 2017a). Of the 840 children assessed for both ASD and intelligence, ASD+/ID- was diagnosed in 27 (3.2%), ASD+/ID+ in 32 (3.8%), and

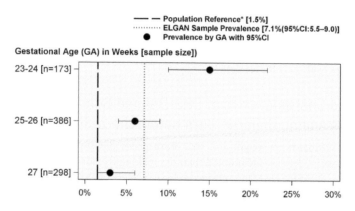

Figure 14.1   Autism Spectrum Disorders Prevalence Rate (%) with 95% Confidence Intervals (CI). [CI that do not cross the general population reference line* are statistically different]. Adapted from Joseph et al. (2017b) with permission from Wiley.

ASD–/ID+ in 71 (8.5%). Time-oriented analysis of risk was performed to identify antecedents for each of these outcomes compared to the absence of both conditions (Table 14.1). First, maternal report of cervical-vaginal infection during pregnancy (mainly bacterial vaginosis or infection with yeast, tricho-monas, or chlamydia) was associated with increased risk of ASD+/ID+ (odds ratio [OR], 2.7; 95% CI, 1.2–6.4). Second, a birth weight Z-score 2 standard deviations or more below the median birth weight for gestational age in a referent sample (Yudkin et al. 1987) that excluded pregnancies delivered for

Table 14.1   Odds ratios and 95% confidence intervals for the associations of ASD+/ID–, ASD+/ID+, ASD–/ID+, and ASD–/ID- with the antecedents listed on the left calculated using a time-oriented multinomial logistic regression model that added variables sequentially as they were identified. Earlier occurring variables that were significantly associated could not be displaced in later models

	ASD+/ID– (n = 27)	ASD+/ID+ (n = 32)	ASD–/ID+ (n = 71)	ASD–/ID– (n = 710)
Pregnancy epoch[a]				
Cervical-vaginal infection	0.9 (0.2, 4.1)	**2.7 (1.2, 6.4)**	0.7 (0.3, 1.6)	1.0
Receipt of antibiotic	**0.1 (0.01, 0.7)**	0.8 (0.4, 1.9)	1.3 (0.9, 2.3)	1.0
Delivery epoch[b]				
Fever at delivery	3.6 (0.98, 13)	0.6 (0.1, 4.4)	**2.9 (1.2, 6.7)**	1.0
Newborn epoch[c]				
Male	2.1 (0.9, 5.0)	**2.9 (1.3, 6.8)**	**2.1 (1.2, 3.6)**	1.0
GA 23–24 weeks	**4.4 (1.7, 11)**	**2.9 (1.3, 6.6)**	**1.8 (1.03, 3.3)**	1.0
BW Z-score < –2	**9.9 (3.3, 30)**	2.1 (0.5, 9.9)	2.0 (0.7, 5.3)	1.0

[a] Both fixed effects (independent variables) were included in the same multinomial logistic regression model. [b] Adjusted for fixed effects that were significantly associated with ASD–/ID+ risk in the pregnancy epoch model. [c] Adjusted for fixed effects that were significantly associated with ASD–/ID+ risk in the pregnancy and delivery epoch models; odds ratios above 1.0 are interpreted as indicating increased risk of the outcome listed at the top of the column for women or children who were exposed to what is described on the left, whereas odds ratios below 1.0 indicate decreased risk, and confidence intervals that do not include 1.0 indicate statistically significant associations (indicated by bold font). Reprinted from Joseph et al. (2017a), Copyright 2017, with permission from Elsevier.

preeclampsia or fetal indications was strongly associated with increased risk of ASD+/ID- (OR, 9.9; 95% CI, 3.3–30). Third, the lowest gestational age category (23–24 weeks) was associated with increased risk of ASD+/ID+ (OR, 2.9; 95% CI, 1.3–6.6) and ASD+/ID- (OR, 4.4; 95% CI, 1.7–11) compared to the highest gestational age category in our data (27 weeks).

Prevalence and Characteristics of SRS-Defined Social Impairment at Age 10 Years among Children Born before the 28th Week of Gestation

Compared to their normal-birth weight and term-born peers, preterm and low-birth-weight children are at higher risk of social deficits, including difficulties making friends, peer problems, and social withdrawal (Ritchie et al. 2015). Sometimes given the label 'preterm behavioral phenotype' (Johnson and Wolke 2013), these deficits seem to be intertwined with emotional and behavior problems, as well as executive and other academic dysfunctions that occur more commonly in children born very preterm than in others (Escovar et al. 2016; Linsell et al. 2016).

Because no validated instrument had been used to characterize the constellation of social deficits considered typical of the 'preterm behavioral phenotype', we evaluated how well the SRS performed. The SRS, a brief, parent-completed questionnaire, assesses a child's social abilities, including social awareness, social cognition, social communication, social motivation, and autistic mannerisms. Sometimes used to screen for ASD (Pine et al. 2006; Azad et al. 2016; Moody et al. 2017) high scores on this instrument that are below the threshold that suggest ASD are often seen as describing 'autism symptoms'. The SRS has thus been used to assess social-communicative limitations that do not meet formal ASD criteria (Hong et al. 2011).

Restricting our attention to the 628 10-year-old children with IQs in the normal range (>85) and who did not meet the rigorous ASD criteria in use in ELGAN, 16% had SRS total scores ≥65, a score at the 96th percentile in 1600 typically developing children (Constantino and Gruber 2005), and used to define social impairment). Among the 148 children who had IQs <85, 27% had SRS-defined social impairment. The prevalence of high SRS sub-component scores ranged from 11% to 32% in the two IQ groups (Fig. 14.2), about three to eight times higher than the 4% prevalence expected based on normative data.

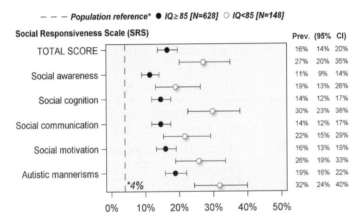

Figure 14.2 Prevalence rate (%) of SRS scores ≥65 with 95% Confidence Intervals (CI). [CI that do not cross the general population reference line* are statistically different]. Reproduced from Korzeniewski (2017b) with permission from Wolters Kluwer.

Among children whose IQ was ≥85, mothers of children with SRS total scores ≥65 were more likely than mothers of children with lower scores to report indicators of social disadvantage (i.e. unmarried; eligible for government-provided medical care insurance). Children born weighing more than 1 standard deviation below the expected mean for gestational age had SRS-defined social impairment more frequently than their expected birth-weight-for-gestational-age peers whose IQ was also ≥85.

Children who had high SRS scores were more likely than their peers to have low scores on the DAS-II, NEPSY-II, and OWLS assessments, with the sole exception of two subtests – DAS-II Nonverbal Reasoning and NEPSY-II Inhibition. Children with high SRS scores were also much more likely than others to have low scores on each of the structural language and pragmatic language subtests of the CCC-2. Consequently, they were also more likely to have low general communication composite scores.

According to parent report, children who had SRS-defined social impairment were more likely than others to be classified as screening positive for attention deficit hyperactivity disorder (ADHD), oppositional defiant or conduct disorder, generalized or separation anxiety, major depression, dysthymic disorder, and/or social phobia. According to teacher report, children who had SRS-defined social impairment were more likely than others to screen positive for ADHD. Teachers preferentially identified the inattentive form of ADHD among children with an SRS-defined social impairment. Children who had high SRS scores were also much more likely than others to be classified by their teachers as having generalized anxiety.

Elevated Protein Concentrations in Newborn Blood and the Risks of Autism Spectrum Disorder, and of Social Impairment, at Age 10 Years among Children Born Extremely Preterm

Because neonatal systemic inflammation (and related-phenomena) (Dammann and Leviton 2014) appear to raise the risk of developing brain alterations (Van Steenwincke et al. 2014), exposure to systemic inflammation during the first postnatal month might also contribute to an increased risk of ASD (Schumann et al. 2010; Movsas et al. 2013; Yang et al. 2016) and of social limitations assessed by the SRS (Grecucci et al. 2016; Hogeveen et al. 2016; Sato et al. 2017). Since growth factors with neurotrophic properties have the potential to minimize this risk (Riikonen 2016; Zheng et al. 2016; Bethlehem et al. 2017), we compared the systemic-inflammation and neurotrophic-protein newborn blood profiles among three groups of children: children diagnosed with ASD, children with high SRS scores but without ASD, and children in neither category.

Because elevated concentrations of inflammation-related proteins on only one day are less likely to convey information about the risk of developmental disabilities than are elevated concentrations on multiple days (Dammann and Leviton 2014), and because elevated concentrations of an inflammation-related protein on multiple days was best evaluated depending on elevated concentrations of neurotrophic proteins (Allred et al. 2017), we examined combinations of top quartile inflammation-related and neurogenic proteins in blood on multiple days in early and late epochs (i.e. postnatal days 1, 7, 14, 21, and 28 respectively).

Table 14.2 summarizes how high concentrations of proteins with anti-inflammatory properties (IL-6R, MMP-9, RANTES, rows 2–4) and proteins with neurotrophic properties (EPO, NT-4, BDNF, bFGF, IGF-1, VEGF, VEGF-R1, VEGF-R2, PIGF, Ang-1, Ang-2, rows 5–15) appear to modulate the risk of ASD and SRS-defined social impairment that was associated with high concentrations of selected pro-inflammatory proteins (e.g. SAA, IL-6, TNF-α, or IL-8) occurring on multiple days of the early or late epoch.

Elevated levels in the first 14 days of life of 11 of the 14 anti-inflammatory or neurotrophic proteins mitigated the association between SAA and ASD. Five of these proteins, when in the upper quartile in the 3rd and 4th week of life, were associated with reduced risk of ASD in the presence of elevated IL-6,

Table 14.2 ▽ indicates increased risk of the entity indicated in the column heading when the protein listed in the first row is *reduced* and the protein listed on the left is *elevated*. ▲ indicates increased risk of the entity indicated in the column heading when the concentrations of the pro-inflammatory protein listed in the first row is *elevated* and the protein listed on the left is *elevated*. In all cases, elevated means in the top quartile, reduced means in the bottom three quartiles

		Early epoch (postnatal days 1, 7, and 14)					Late epoch (postnatal days 21 and 28)				
		ASD (n = 35)			SRS ≥ 65 (n = 127)		ASD (n = 31)			SRS ≥ 65 (n = 84)	
		1	2	3	4	5	6	7	8	9	
1	Protein	SAA	TNF-α	IL-8	TNF-α	IL-8	IL-6	TNF-α	IL-8	TNF-α	IL-8
2	IL-6R	▽									▲
3	MMP-9	▽					▽				▽
4	RANTES	▽	▲		▲	▲	▽				
5	EPO	▽					▽				▽
6	NT-4	▲					▲	▽	▲		▽
7	BDNF	▽					▲	▲		▽	
8	bFGF						▲	▲	▲		
9	IGF-1	▽									▽
10	VEGF	▽									
11	VEGF-R1						▽				
12	VEGF-R2	▽					▽				
13	PlGF	▽									
14	Ang-1	▽									▽
15	Ang-2	▽						▽			▽

Reprinted from Korzeniewsk (2018) under the Creative Commons license: http://creativecommons.org/licenses/by/4.0/.

and six proteins were associated with reduced risk of SRS-defined social impairment in the presence of elevated IL-8. The association between elevated TNF-α and both outcomes was, however, only occasionally mitigated by elevations of the proteins listed on the left, and only in the late epoch.

On the other hand, at times some of these proteins were associated with elevated risks of ASD or high SRS scores in the early or late epochs. The most prominent examples of these were elevations of NT-4, BNDF, and bFGF, which were associated with increased risks in the presence of elevated pro-inflammatory proteins.

MAIN FINDINGS AND INFERENCES TO BE DRAWN

Prevalence

AUTISM SPECTRUM DISORDER

The ELGAN study provided evidence of an extremely high prevalence of ASD at age 10 years among children born prior to the 28th week of gestation, rivaling that found in sibling studies. The overall estimates of risk in ELGAN's are comparable to the general sibling risk of ASD, which in large population-based studies is between 7% and 10% (Gronborg et al. 2013; Risch et al. 2014; Sandin et al. 2014). At the earliest gestational age interval of 23–24 weeks, the 15% prevalence we observed is similar to the prevalence described in the highest risk sibling comparison – boys with an older female sibling with autism (Palmer et al. 2017).

The ASD prevalence overall and with respect to co-occurring intellectual disability is consistent with reports from two other studies. The 7.1% prevalence of ASD in the ELGAN cohort is in agreement with the 7% prevalence estimated by a meta-analysis of 18 studies of children born at a median gestational age of 28 weeks (Agrawal et al. 2018). The prevalence of ASD with or without co-occurring intellectual disability is also consistent with observations reported in the population-based Stockholm Youth Cohort Study (respectively 3.8% and 3.2% in ELGAN and 3.1% and 4.1% in Stockholm) (Xie et al. 2017a). On the other hand, the ASD prevalence in the ELGAN cohort is closer to the prevalence estimated by the French EPICURE study (8%) (Johnson et al. 2010) than to the 16% prevalence reported in a population-based study of Flemish children born prior to the 27th week of gestation (Verhaeghe et al. 2016).

SRS-Defined Social Impairment

The prevalence of non-autistic social impairment is several-fold higher in the ELGAN cohort (Korzeniewski et al. 2017b) than found in the normative data used to develop the SRS (Constantino and Gruber 2005; Korzeniewski et al. 2017b). This is generally consistent with a previous report of increasing SRS scores with decreasing gestational length (Movsas and Paneth 2012). Our finding of a 27% prevalence of social impairment among children with intellectual disability is comparable to the 22% prevalence of SRS total score ≥96 reported among 71 intellectually disabled participants in a recent case-control study (Franck et al. 2018).

The multiplicity of brain functioning deficits we observed among children who suffered social impairment is also generally consistent with a subsequent report from the population-based Generation-R study that found children with SRS-defined social deficits scored lower on all neuropsychological performance domains assessed using the Developmental NEuroPSYchological Assessment-II (Hyseni et al. 2018). A smaller study also found that higher SRS scores tended to be associated with lower Child Behavior Checklist competency scores (Crehan et al. 2018). Our findings additionally agree with evidence that social limitations frequently co-occur with attention and behavior problems in children born very preterm (Hille et al. 2001; Gardner et al. 2004; Reijneveld et al. 2006; Loe et al. 2011; Scott et al. 2012; Rogers et al. 2012; Arpi and Ferrari 2013; Johnson and Wolke 2013; Jones et al. 2013; Peralta-Carcelen et al. 2013; Treyvaud et al. 2013; Joo et al. 2015; Taylor et al. 2015; Montagna and Nosarti 2016; Broring et al. 2018). Together, these results are in keeping with the concept of a 'preterm behavioral phenotype' (Johnson and Wolke 2013).

Antecedents of ASD and Social Impairment

The antecedents of ASD and non-autistic social impairment identified in the ELGAN study cohort can be grouped under the following three themes: (1) maternal infection and inflammation, (2) fetal growth restriction, and (3) physiologic immaturity.

Maternal Infection

Maternal report of cervical-vaginal infection more than doubles the risk of ASD with intellectual disability in the ELGAN cohort, while peripartum fever is associated with about a three-fold increased risk of ASD without intellectual disability, although the latter finding is not statistically significant. These findings are generally consistent with a meta-analysis of 15 studies involving more than 40 000 children with ASD that found maternal infection is associated with moderately increased ASD risk (Jiang et al. 2016). Maternal infection or its correlates may contribute to non-autistic social impairment too, based on evidence from a small exploratory cohort study that found maternal seropositivity for cytomegalovirus is associated with increased social deficits in offspring (Slawinski et al. 2018).

FETAL GROWTH RESTRICTION

Children in the ELGAN cohort who are born with severe fetal growth restriction are 10 times more likely than their appropriately grown peers to meet rigorous criteria for ASD *without intellectual* disability at 10 years (Joseph et al. 2017a), and a three-fold risk of any ASD (Korzeniewski et al. 2017a). Compared to their ELGAN peers who are not growth restricted, they are also more likely to have social awareness impairments and autistic mannerisms identified by the SRS, difficulties with speech coherence, context, non-verbal communication, and interests identified by the Children's Communication Checklist-2, as well as diminished social and psychosocial function and quality of life identified by the Pediatric Quality of Life Inventory™. Children who are less severely growth restricted at birth (≥-2 birth weight Z-score <-1) are also at increased risk of low scores on the Oral Expression subtest of the Oral and Written Language Scales. Together, these findings support the concept of fetal growth restriction as a continuum and not an either/or phenomenon.

While we did not find any other large study of fetal growth restriction and neurocognitive and behavioral outcomes in adolescents born prior to the 28th week of gestation, our findings for ASD parallel cognitive findings in two population-based cohorts of children born before the 32nd week of gestation. In a Dutch cohort of school-aged children born very preterm or very low birth weight (<1500g), prenatally growth restricted children more often developed speech and language deficits and received special education (Kok et al. 1998). Similarly, in the EPIPAGE cohort, 5–8-year-olds born small for gestational age were nearly twice as likely to have minor cognitive difficulties, inattention-hyperactivity symptoms and school difficulties than their appropriately grown peers (Guellec et al. 2011, 2016).

Because many ELGANs with fetal growth restriction are born to women who had severe preeclampsia, our findings are also consistent with a prior study of adults born preterm who weighed <2000g that found increased ASD risk in offspring of mothers who experienced hypertension in pregnancy (Korzeniewski et al. 2013). Additional support comes from recent meta-analyses and systematic reviews whose results are consistent with increased ASD risk with exposure to preeclampsia (Dachew et al. 2018; Maher et al. 2018; Xu et al. 2018).

PHYSIOLOGIC IMMATURITY AND REPEATED OR SUSTAINED POSTNATAL SYSTEMIC INFLAMMATION

The ELGAN study confirmed that irrespective of intellectual disability status, the prevalence of ASD and non-autistic social impairment increases with decreasing gestational age prior to the 28th week of gestation (Joseph et al. 2017a, 2017b; Korzeniewski et al. 2017b). These findings are consistent with the relationship between gestational age and the prevalence of ASD subsequently reported in the Stockholm Youth Cohort Study.

We also found that repeated or sustained systemic inflammation during the first postnatal month is associated with increased risk of ASD in the ELGAN cohort, and high concentrations of neurotrophins appear to modulate this relationship (Korzeniewski et al. 2018). A comparable pattern of association occurred with SRS-defined social impairment, but only during the second half of the first postnatal month. Neurotrophins appear to have not only anti-inflammatory capabilities (Zhang et al. 2016; Skaper 2017) but also the ability to promote survival and repair of nerve cells (Barker et al. 2018; Cacialli et al. 2018). Consequently, we are not sure how neurotrophins modulate the presumed damaging effects of systemic inflammation, or indeed, if the systemic inflammation is a consequence and not a contributor to brain damage (Xing and Lo 2017).

We were unable to find cohort studies of children born very preterm that measured protein concentrations during the first postnatal month in relation to increased risk of ASD or non-autistic social impairment in adolescents. However, our findings are generally consistent with prior studies that found under-expression of VEGF (Masi et al. 2017), TGF-β1 (Masi et al. 2015), NT-3 (Nelson et al. 2006), NT-4 (Abdallah et al. 2013; Segura et al. 2015), HGF (Russo 2013a), EGF (Suzuki et al. 2007; Russo 2013a; Russo 2013b), and IP-10 (Shen et al. 2016) in blood obtained from children with a diagnosis of autism. Affected children are also more likely than others to have high blood concentrations (or mRNA expression) of some neurotrophic proteins (e.g. BDNF [Connolly et al. 2006; Qin et al. 2016; Zheng et al. 2016] and NT [Angelidou et al. 2010]) and such inflammation-related proteins as IL-1b (Ashwood et al. 2011; Inga Jacome et al. 2016; Krakowiak et al. 2017; Masi et al. 2017), IL-1RA (Suzuki et al. 2011), IL-4 (Krakowiak et al. 2017), IL-5 (Suzuki et al. 2011), IL-6 (Ashwood et al. 2011; Inga et al. 2016), IL-8 (Tonhajzerova et al. 2015), IL-12 (p40) (Ashwood et al. 2011), IL-12 (p70) (Suzuki et al. 2011), IL-13 (Suzuki et al. 2011), IL-17 (Inga et al. 2016), GRO-α (Suzuki et al. 2011), TNF-α (Makinodan et al. 2017; Xie et al. 2017b), RANTES (Shen et al. 2016), MIP-1-α (Shen et al. 2016), MCP-1 (Zerbo et al. 2014), MIP-1α (Shen et al. 2016), and MIP-1β (Shen et al. 2016). Some blood protein levels also appear to convey information about risk of social motivation and social communication in children with ASD, including NCAM1 (Yang et al. 2019) and IL-6sR (Napolioni et al. 2013).

Interrelationships among Antecedents and their Correlates

The risk profiles we observed might involve interrelationships among antecedents and their correlates. For example, growth restricted newborns have more intense systemic inflammatory responses during the first postnatal month than their appropriately grown peers (McElrath et al. 2013), and both fetal growth restriction and early systemic inflammation are associated with increased ASD risk in the ELGAN cohort. A combination of fetal growth restriction and repeated or sustained systemic inflammation during the first postnatal month is also associated with increased risk of neurosonographic white matter injury (WMI) (Movsas et al. 2013), which is a correlate of ASD (Pagnozzi et al. 2018) and social dysfunctions (Ritchie et al. 2015; d'Albis et al. 2018). There is some evidence that white matter hypoconnectivity appears to underlie the social communication deficits observed in ASD (Lo et al. 2017; Herringshaw et al. 2018).

Our finding that increased risk of social dysfunctions is associated with both antenatal characteristics (i.e. fetal growth restriction as well as inflammation) and the postnatal characteristic of systemic inflammation (Yanni et al. 2017; Korzeniewski et al. 2018) is consistent with the 'multiple hit' hypothesis that we have applied to preterm lung and brain damage (Dammann et al. 2004). Our preference for time-oriented risk analysis (Joseph et al. 2017a) reflects the inference that multiple exposures can cumulatively raise the risks of ASD and social impairment in children born very preterm.

ASD Screening at 24 Months

The ELGAN study provided evidence that sensorimotor and cognitive impairments, emotional/behavioral dysregulation, and indicators of socioeconomic deprivation appear to contribute significantly to M-CHAT misclassifications at 24 months in children born extremely preterm. While sensitivity was lower in the ELGAN cohort than the pooled estimates from a meta-analysis of 12 studies of high-risk cohorts, specificity was appreciably higher (Yuen et al. 2018). Despite differences in designs and participants that limit direct comparisons, these findings support the inference that clinicians should consider children's age and developmental problems when interpreting M-CHAT scores.

CONCLUSION

Extremely low gestational age babies are especially susceptible to autism and non-autistic social impairment, and this risk increases with the degree of prematurity. Babies in the most premature category, born at 23–24 weeks gestation, have a risk of formally diagnosed ASD of 15%, a figure not dissimilar to the risk reported for siblings of children with ASD. Fetal growth restriction shows a very strong relationship with ASD without ID. Sustained or repeated post-natal systemic inflammation is associated with increased risk of autism and non-autistic social impairment in the ELGAN cohort. The observations described in this chapter prompt us to infer that inflammation and its correlates play key roles in the causal chain in raising the risk of ASD and social impairment by limiting brain maturation and/or disrupting neuroprotective processes before and after birth (Ohja et al. 2018). At the same time, neuroprotective proteins may modulate some of this inflammatory risk, and understanding the antecedents of these proteins may suggest opportunities for ASD prevention.

REFERENCES

Abdallah MW, Mortensen EL, Greaves-Lord K et al. (2013) Neonatal levels of neurotrophic factors and risk of autism spectrum disorders. *Acta Psychiatr Scand* **128**: 61–9.

Agrawal S, Rao SC, Bulsara MK, Patole SK (2018) Prevalence of Autism Spectrum Disorder in Preterm Infants: A Meta-analysis. *Pediatrics* **142**: e20180134.

Allred EN, Dammann O, Fichorova RN et al. (2017) Systemic inflammation during the first postnatal month and the risk of attention deficit hyperactivity disorder characteristics among 10-year-old children born extremely preterm. *J Neuroimmune Pharmacol* **12**: 531–43.

Angelidou A, Francis K, Vasiadi M et al. (2010) Neurotensin is increased in serum of young children with autistic disorder. *J Neuroinflammation* **7**: 48.

Arpi E, Ferrari F (2013) Preterm birth and behaviour problems in infants and preschool-age children: a review of the recent literature. *Dev Med Child Neurol* **55**: 788–96.

Ashwood P, Krakowiak P, Hertz-Picciotto I, Hansen R, Pessah I, Van de Water J (2011) Elevated plasma cytokines in autism spectrum disorders provide evidence of immune dysfunction and are associated with impaired behavioral outcome. *Brain Behav Immun* **25**: 40–5.

Azad G, Reisinger E, Xie M, Mandell DS (2016) Parent and teacher concordance on the social responsiveness scale for children with autism. *School Ment Health* **8**: 368–76.

Barker RA, Gotz M, Parmar M (2018) New approaches for brain repair-from rescue to reprogramming. *Nature* **557**: 329–34.

Bethlehem RAI, Lombardo MV, Lai MC et al. (2017) Intranasal oxytocin enhances intrinsic corticostriatal functional connectivity in women. *Transl Psychiatry* **7**: e1099.

Broring T, Oostrom KJ, van Dijk-Lokkart EM, Lafeber HN, Brugman A, Oosterlaan J (2018) Attention deficit hyperactivity disorder and autism spectrum disorder symptoms in school-age children born very preterm. *Res Dev Disabil* **74**: 103–12.

Cacialli P, Palladino A, Lucini C (2018) Role of brain-derived neurotrophic factor during the regenerative response after traumatic brain injury in adult zebrafish. *Neural Regen Res* **13**: 941–4.

Connolly AM, Chez M, Streif EM et al. (2006) Brain-derived neurotrophic factor and autoantibodies to neural antigens in sera of children with autistic spectrum disorders, Landau-Kleffner syndrome, and epilepsy. *Biol Psychiatry* **59**: 354–63.

Constantino J, Gruber C (2005) *Social Responsive Scale (SRS) Manual*. Los Angeles, CA: Western Psychological Services.

Corradi-Dell'Acqua C, Koban L, Leiberg S, Vuilleumier P (2016) Editorial: What determines social behavior? Investigating the role of emotions, self-centered motives, and social norms. *Front Hum Neurosci* **10**: 342.

Crehan ET, Baer J, Althoff RR, Constantino JN (2018) Tracking the influence of autistic traits on competencies among school aged children with subthreshold autistic traits: a longitudinal study. *Child Psychiatry and Human Development* **49**: 941–55.

d'Albis MA, Guevara P, Guevara M et al. (2018) Local structural connectivity is associated with social cognition in autism spectrum disorder. *Brain* **141**: 3472–81.

Dachew BA, Mamun A, Maravilla JC, Alati R (2018) Pre-eclampsia and the risk of autism-spectrum disorder in offspring: meta-analysis. *Br J Psychiatry* **212**: 142–7.

Dammann O, Leviton A (2014) Intermittent or sustained systemic inflammation and the preterm brain. *Pediatr Res* **75**: 376 80.

Dammann O, Leviton A, Bartels DB, Dammann CE (2004) Lung and brain damage in preterm newborns. Are they related? How? Why? *Biol Neonate* **85**: 305–13.

Developmental Disabilities Monitoring Network, Centers for Disease Control and Prevention (2014) Prevalence of autism spectrum disorder among children aged 8 years – autism and developmental disabilities monitoring network, 11 sites, United States, 2010. *MMWR Surveill Summ* **63**: 1–21.

Escovar E, Rosenberg-Lee M, Uddin LQ, Menon V (2016) The empathizing-systemizing theory, social abilities, and mathematical achievement in children. *Sci Rep* **6**: 23011.

Franck LS, McLemore MR, Cooper N et al. (2018) A novel method for involving women of color at high risk for preterm birth in research priority setting. *J Vis Exp* **131**, 56220. https://doi.org/10.3791/56220.

Gardner F, Johnson A, Yudkin P et al. (2004) Behavioral and emotional adjustment of teenagers in mainstream school who were born before 29 weeks' gestation. *Pediatrics* **114**: 676–82.

Grecucci A, Rubicondo D, Siugzdaite R, Surian L, Job R (2016) Uncovering the social deficits in the autistic brain. A source-based morphometric study. *Front Neurosci* **10**: 388.

Gronborg TK, Schendel DE, Parner ET (2013) Recurrence of autism spectrum disorders in full- and half-siblings and trends over time: a population-based cohort study. *JAMA Pediatr* **167**: 947–53.

Guellec I, Lapillonne A, Marret S et al. (2016) Effect of intra- and extrauterine growth on long-term neurologic outcomes of very preterm infants. *J Pediatr* **175**: 93–9 e1.

Guellec I, Lapillonne A, Renolleau S et al. (2011) Neurologic outcomes at school age in very preterm infants born with severe or mild growth restriction. *Pediatrics* **127**: e883–91.

Happe F, Conway JR (2016) Recent progress in understanding skills and impairments in social cognition. *Curr Opin Pediatr* **28**: 736–42.

Herringshaw AJ, Kumar SL, Rody KN, Kana RK (2018) Neural correlates of social perception in children with autism: local versus global preferences. *Neuroscience* **395**: 49–59.

Hille ETM, den Ouden AL, Wolke DFH et al. (2001) Behavioral problems reported in children who weigh 1000g or less at birth in four countries. *Lancet* **357**: 1641–3.

Hogeveen J, Salvi C, Grafman J (2016) 'Emotional intelligence': lessons from lesions. *Trends Neurosci* **39**: 694–705.

Hong DS, Dunkin B, Reiss AL (2011) Psychosocial functioning and social cognitive processing in girls with Turner syndrome. *J Dev Behav Pediatr* **32**: 512–20.

Hyseni F, Blanken LME, Muetzel R, Verhulst FC, Tiemeier H, White T (2018) Autistic traits and neuropsychological performance in 6- to-10-year-old children: a population-based study. *Child Neuropsychology: A Journal on Normal and Abnormal Development in Childhood and Adolescence* **25**: 352–69.

Inga Jacome MC, Morales Chacon LM, Vera Cuesta H et al. (2016) Peripheral Inflammatory Markers Contributing to Comorbidities in Autism. *Behav Sci (Basel)* **6**: 29.

Johnson S, Hollis C, Kochhar P, Hennessy E, Wolke D, Marlow N (2010) Autism spectrum disorders in extremely preterm children. *J Pediatr* **156**: 525–31 e2.

Johnson S, Wolke D (2013) Behavioural outcomes and psychopathology during adolescence. *Early Hum Dev* **89**: 199–207.

Jones KM, Champion PR, Woodward LJ (2013) Social competence of preschool children born very preterm. *Early Hum Dev* **89**: 795–802.

Joo JW, Choi JY, Rha DW, Kwak EH, Park ES (2015) Neuropsychological outcomes of preterm birth in children with no major neurodevelopmental impairments in early life. *Ann Rehabil Med* **39**: 676–85.

Joseph RM, Korzeniewski SJ, Allred EN et al. (2017a) Extremely low gestational age and very low birthweight for gestational age are risk factors for autism spectrum disorder in a large cohort study of 10-year-old children born at 23–27 weeks' gestation. *Am J Obstet Gynecol* **216**: 304 e1–e16.

Joseph RM, O'Shea TM, Allred EN et al. (2017b) Prevalence and associated features of autism spectrum disorder in extremely low gestational age newborns at age 10 years. *Autism Res* **10**: 224–32.

Kok JH, den Ouden AL, Verloove-Vanhorick SP, Brand R (1998) Outcome of very preterm small for gestational age infants: the first nine years of life. *Br J Obstet Gynaecol* **105**: 162–8.

Korzeniewski SJ, Allred EN, Joseph RM et al. (2017a) Neurodevelopment at age 10 years of children born <28 weeks with fetal growth restriction. *Pediatrics* **140**: e20170697.

Korzeniewski SJ, Allred EN, O'Shea TM, Leviton A, Kuban KCK, ELGAN study investigators (2018) Elevated protein concentrations in newborn blood and the risks of autism spectrum disorder, and of social impairment, at age 10 years among infants born before the 28th week of gestation. *Transl Psychiatry* **8**: 115.

Korzeniewski SJ, Joseph RM, Kim SH et al. (2017b) Social responsiveness scale assessment of the preterm behavioral phenotype in 10-year-olds born extremely preterm. *J Dev Behav Pediatr* **38**: 697–705.

Korzeniewski SJ, Pinto-Martin JA, Whitaker AH et al. (2013) Association between transient hypothyroxinaemia of prematurity and adult autism spectrum disorder in a low-birthweight cohort: an exploratory study. *Paediatr Perinat Epidemiol* **27**: 182–7.

Krakowiak P, Goines PE, Tancredi DJ et al. (2017) Neonatal cytokine profiles associated with autism spectrum disorder. *Biol Psychiatry* **81**: 442–51.

Kuban KC, O'Shea TM, Allred EN, Tager-Flusberg H, Goldstein DJ, Leviton A (2009) Positive screening on the Modified Checklist for Autism in Toddlers (M-CHAT) in extremely low gestational age newborns. *J Pediatr* **154**: 535–40 e1.

Linsell L, Malouf R, Johnson S, Morris J, Kurinczuk JJ, Marlow N (2016) Prognostic Factors for behavioral problems and psychiatric disorders in children born very preterm or very low birth weight: a systematic review. *J Dev Behav Pediatr* **37**: 88–102.

Lo YC, Chen YJ, Hsu YC, Tseng WI, Gau SS (2017) Reduced tract integrity of the model for social communication is a neural substrate of social communication deficits in autism spectrum disorder. *J Child Psychol Psychiatry* **58**: 576–85.

Loe IM, Lee ES, Luna B, Feldman HM (2011) Behavior problems of 9–16 year old preterm children: biological, sociodemographic, and intellectual contributions. *Early Hum Dev* **87**: 247–52.

Lord C, Rutter M, DiLavore PC, Risi S, Gotham K, Bishop S (2012) *Autism Diagnostic Observation Schedule™, Second edition*. Torrance, CA: Western Psychological Services.

Lipscombe B, Boyd RN, Coleman A, Fahey M, Rawicki B, Whittingham K (2016) Does early communication mediate the relationship between motor ability and social function in children with cerebral palsy? *Res Dev Disabil* **53–4**: 279–86.

Luyster RJ, Kuban KC, O'Shea TM et al. (2011) The Modified Checklist for Autism in Toddlers in extremely low gestational age newborns: individual items associated with motor, cognitive, vision and hearing limitations. *Paediatr Perinat Epidemiol* **25**: 366–76.

Maher GM, O'Keeffe GW, Kearney PM et al. (2018) Association of hypertensive disorders of pregnancy with risk of neurodevelopmental disorders in offspring: a systematic review and meta-analysis. *JAMA Psychiatry* **75**: 809–19.

Makinodan M, Iwata K, Ikawa D et al. (2017) Tumor necrosis factor-alpha expression in peripheral blood mononuclear cells correlates with early childhood social interaction in autism spectrum disorder. *Neurochem Int* **104**: 1–5.

Masi A, Breen EJ, Alvares GA et al. (2017) Cytokine levels and associations with symptom severity in male and female children with autism spectrum disorder. *Mol Autism* **8**: 63.

Masi A, Quintana DS, Glozier N, Lloyd AR, Hickie IB, Guastella AJ (2015) Cytokine aberrations in autism spectrum disorder: a systematic review and meta-analysis. *Mol Psychiatry* **20**: 440–6.

McElrath TF, Allred EN, Van Marter L, Fichorova RN, Leviton A, ELGAN study investigators (2013) Perinatal systemic inflammatory responses of growth-restricted preterm newborns. *Acta Paediatr* **102**: e439–42.

Montagna A, Nosarti C (2016) Socio-emotional development following very preterm birth: pathways to psychopathology. *Front Psychol* **7**: 80.

Moody EJ, Reyes N, Ledbetter C et al. (2017) Screening for autism with the SRS and SCQ: variations across demographic, developmental and behavioral factors in preschool children. *J Autism Dev Disord* 47: 3550–61.

Movsas TZ, Paneth N (2012) The effect of gestational age on symptom severity in children with autism spectrum disorder. *J Autism Dev Disord* 42(11): 2431–9.

Movsas TZ, Pinto-Martin JA, Whitaker AH et al. (2013) Autism spectrum disorder is associated with ventricular enlargement in a low birth weight population. *J Pediatr* 163: 73–8.

Napolioni V, Ober-Reynolds B, Szelinger S et al. (2013) Plasma cytokine profiling in sibling pairs discordant for autism spectrum disorder. *J Neuroinflammation* 10: 38.

Nelson PG, Kuddo T, Song EY et al. (2006) Selected neurotrophins, neuropeptides, and cytokines: developmental trajectory and concentrations in neonatal blood of children with autism or Down syndrome. *Int J Dev Neurosci* 24: 73–80.

Ohja K, Gozal E, Fahnestock M et al. (2018) Neuroimmunologic and neurotrophic interactions in autism spectrum disorders: Relationship to neuroinflammation. *Neuromolecular Med* 20: 161–73.

Pagnozzi AM, Conti E, Calderoni S, Fripp J, Rose SE (2018) A systematic review of structural MRI biomarkers in autism spectrum disorder: a machine learning perspective. *Int J Dev Neurosci* 71: 68–82.

Palmer N, Beam A, Agniel D et al. (2017) Association of sex with recurrence of autism spectrum disorder among siblings. *JAMA Pediatr* 171: 1107–12.

Peralta-Carcelen M, Bailey K, Rector R, Gantz M, NICHD Neonatal Research Network (2013) Behavioral and socioemotional competence problems of extremely low birth weight children. *J Perinatol* 33: 887–92.

Pine E, Luby J, Abbacchi A, Constantino JN (2006) Quantitative assessment of autistic symptomatology in preschoolers. *Autism* 10: 344–52.

Qin XY, Feng JC, Cao C, Wu HT, Loh YP, Cheng Y (2016) Association of peripheral blood levels of brain-derived neurotrophic factor with autism spectrum disorder in children: a systematic review and meta-analysis. *JAMA Pediatr* 170: 1079–86.

Reijneveld SA, de Kleine MJ, van Baar AL et al. (2006) Behavioural and emotional problems in very preterm and very low birthweight infants at age 5 years. *Arch Dis Child Fetal Neonatal Ed* 91: F423–8.

Riikonen R (2016) Treatment of autistic spectrum disorder with insulin-like growth factors. *Eur J Paediatr Neurol* 20: 816–23.

Risch N, Hoffmann TJ, Anderson M, Croen LA, Grether JK, Windham GC (2014) Familial recurrence of autism spectrum disorder: evaluating genetic and environmental contributions. *Am J Psychiatry* 171: 1206–13.

Ritchie K, Bora S (2015) Social development of children born very preterm: a systematic review 57: 899–918.

Ritchie K, Bora S, Woodward LJ (2015) Social development of children born very preterm: a systematic review. *Dev Med Child Neurol* 57(10): 899–918.

Robins DL, Fein D, Barton ML, Green JA (2001) The Modified Checklist for Autism in Toddlers: an initial study investigating the early detection of autism and pervasive developmental disorders. *J Autism Dev Disord* 31: 131–44.

Rogers CE, Anderson PJ, Thompson DK et al. (2012) Regional cerebral development at term relates to school-age social-emotional development in very preterm children. *J Am Acad Child Adolesc Psychiatry* 51: 181–91.

Russo AJ (2013a) Correlation between Hepatocyte Growth Factor (HGF) and Gamma-Aminobutyric Acid (GABA) plasma levels in autistic children. *Biomark Insights* 8: 69–75.

Russo AJ (2013b) Decreased Epidermal Growth Factor (EGF) associated with HMGB1 and increased hyperactivity in children with autism. *Biomark Insights* 8: 35–41.

Rutter M, Bailey A, Lord C (2003a) *The Social Communication Questionnaire*. Los Angeles, CA: Western Psychological Services.

Rutter M, Le Couteur A, Lord C (2003b) *Autism Diagnostic Interview – Revised*. Los Angeles, CA: Western Psychological Services.

Sandin S, Lichtenstein P, Kuja-Halkola R, Larsson H, Hultman CM, Reichenberg A (2014) The familial risk of autism. *JAMA* 311: 1770–7.

Sato W, Kochiyama T, Uono S et al. (2017) Reduced gray matter volume in the social brain network in adults with autism spectrum disorder. *Front Hum Neurosci* 11: 395.

Schumann CM, Bloss CS, Barnes CC et al. (2010) Longitudinal magnetic resonance imaging study of cortical development through early childhood in autism. *J Neurosci* 30: 4419–27.

Scott MN, Taylor HG, Fristad MA et al. (2012) Behavior disorders in extremely preterm/extremely low birth weight children in kindergarten. *J Dev Behav Pediatr* **33**: 202–13.

Segura M, Pedreno C, Obiols J et al. (2015) Neurotrophin blood-based gene expression and social cognition analysis in patients with autism spectrum disorder. *Neurogenetics* **16**: 123–31.

Shen Y, Ou J, Liu M et al. (2016) Altered plasma levels of chemokines in autism and their association with social behaviors. *Psychiatry Res* **244**: 300–5.

Skaper SD (2017) Nerve growth factor: a neuroimmune crosstalk mediator for all seasons. *Immunology* **151**: 1–15.

Slawinski BL, Talge N, Ingersoll B et al. (2018) Maternal cytomegalovirus sero-positivity and autism symptoms in children. *Am J Reprod Immunol* **79**: e12840.

Suzuki K, Hashimoto K, Iwata Y et al. (2007) Decreased serum levels of epidermal growth factor in adult subjects with high-functioning autism. *Biol Psychiatry* **62**: 267–9.

Suzuki K, Matsuzaki H, Iwata K et al. (2011) Plasma cytokine profiles in subjects with high-functioning autism spectrum disorders. *PLoS One* **6**: e20470.

Taylor HG, Margevicius S, Schluchter M, Andreias L, Hack M (2015) Persisting behavior problems in extremely low birth weight adolescents. *J Dev Behav Pediatr* **36**: 178–87.

Tonhajzerova I, Ondrejka I, Mestanik M et al. (2015) Inflammatory activity in autism spectrum disorder. *Adv Exp Med Biol* **861**: 93–8.

Treyvaud K, Ure A, Doyle LW et al. (2013) Psychiatric outcomes at age seven for very preterm children: rates and predictors. *J Child Psychol Psychiatry* **54**: 772–9.

Van Steenwinckel J, Schang AL, Sigaut S et al. (2014) Brain damage of the preterm infant: new insights into the role of inflammation. *Biochem Soc Trans* **42**: 557–63.

Verhaeghe L, Dereu M, Warreyn P, De Groote I, Vanhaesebrouck P, Roeyers H (2016) Extremely preterm born children at very high risk for developing autism spectrum disorder. *Child Psychiatry Hum Dev* **47**: 729–39.

Xie S, Heuvelman H, Magnusson C et al. (2017a) Prevalence of autism spectrum disorders with and without intellectual disability by gestational age at birth in the Stockholm youth cohort: a register linkage study. *Paediatr Perinat Epidemiol* **31**: 586–94.

Xie J, Huang L, Li X et al. (2017b) Immunological cytokine profiling identifies TNF-α as a key molecule dysregulated in autistic children. *Oncotarget* **8**: 82390–8.

Xing C, Lo EH (2017) Help-me signaling: non-cell autonomous mechanisms of neuroprotection and neurorecovery. *Prog Neurobiol* **152**: 181–99.

Xu RT, Chang QX, Wang QQ et al. (2018) Association between hypertensive disorders of pregnancy and risk of autism in offspring: a systematic review and meta-analysis of observational studies. *Oncotarget* **9**: 1291–301.

Yang DY, Beam D, Pelphrey KA, Abdullahi S, Jou RJ (2016) Cortical morphological markers in children with autism: a structural magnetic resonance imaging study of thickness, area, volume, and gyrification. *Mol Autism* **7**: 11.

Yang X, Zou M, Pang X et al. (2019) The association between NCAM1 levels and behavioral phenotypes in children with autism spectrum disorder. *Behav Brain Res* **359**: 234–8.

Yanni D, Korzeniewski SJ, Allred EN et al. (2017) Both antenatal and postnatal inflammation contribute information about the risk of brain damage in extremely preterm newborns. *Pediatr Res* **82**: 691–6.

Yudkin PL, Aboualfa M, Eyre JA, Redman CW, Wilkinson AR (1987) New birthweight and head circumference centiles for gestational ages 24 to 42 weeks. *Early Hum Dev* **15**: 45–52.

Yuen T, Penner M, Carter MT, Szatmari P, Ungar WJ (2018) Assessing the accuracy of the Modified Checklist for Autism in Toddlers: a systematic review and meta-analysis. *Dev Med Child Neurol* **60**: 1093–100.

Zerbo O, Yoshida C, Grether JK et al. (2014) Neonatal cytokines and chemokines and risk of autism spectrum disorder: the Early Markers for Autism (EMA) study: a case-control study. *J Neuroinflammation* **11**: 113.

Zhang JC, Yao W, Hashimoto K (2016) Brain-derived Neurotrophic Factor (BDNF)-TrkB signaling in inflammation-related depression and potential therapeutic targets. *Curr Neuropharmacol* **14**: 721–31.

Zheng Z, Zhang L, Zhu T, Huang J, Qu Y, Mu D (2016) Peripheral brain-derived neurotrophic factor in autism spectrum disorder: a systematic review and meta-analysis. *Sci Rep* **6**: 312–41.

Psychiatric and Behavioral Outcomes at Age 2 and 10 Years in Individuals Born Extremely Preterm

Jean A Frazier, Hannah Zamore, and Stephen R Hooper

INTRODUCTION

Changes in perinatal care of extremely low gestational age newborns (ELGANs) over the past four decades have led to increased survival and perhaps also to decreased morbidity rates (Stoll et al. 2015). However, infants born preterm are at risk for a variety of neurodevelopmental concerns, including higher rates of emotional and behavioral disorders across the lifespan (Saigal et al. 2003; Hack et al. 2004; Indredavik et al. 2005; Walshe et al. 2008; Spittle et al. 2009), including the incidence of some some specific outcomes such as attention deficit hyperactivity disorder (ADHD) (Sucksdorff et al. 2015).

The ELGAN study was designed to explore exposure-outcome associations among infants born extremely preterm (EP), <28 weeks gestational age (GA). In keeping with the aims of our study, we explored the prevalence of emotional and behavioral problems and the relationship of antecedent factors with psychiatric outcomes in the ELGAN cohort at age 2 and 10 years. We hypothesized that youth in the ELGAN cohort would have higher rates of psychiatric symptoms compared to normative samples, and that these outcomes would be associated with early life inflammation. Autism spectrum disorders are covered in detail in Chapter 14.

PSYCHIATRIC OUTCOMES IN ELGANS AT AGE 2

Social and Emotional Delays

The evaluation of behavioral competencies in preterm born children is an important line of investigation that has the promise of informing clinical care. We sought to assess the antecedents and correlates of emotional regulation (ER) and orientation/engagement (O/E) at age 2 years in 904 children who were born EP and had a Bayley Scales of Infant Development, second edition (BSID-II) assessment and the associated Bayley Behavior Rating Scale (BRS) (Bayley 1993). We found that 31% of the EP children had difficulties (nonoptimal or questionable scores) with ER and 27% had difficulties with O/E as rated on the BRS. Additionally, children with difficulties were more likely to have BSID-II Mental Development Index (MDI) and Psychomotor Development Index (PDI) scores of <70 than children without difficulties on ER and O/E. The lower the scores on MDI and PDI, the higher the frequency of difficulties with ER and O/E; some 20% of children with MDI scores ≥70 had nonoptimal or questionable scores on both O/E and ER, but more than half with MDI scores of <55 scored as having difficulties on both O/E and ER. About a third of twins and triplets had difficulties with O/E, while male sex and socioeconomic disadvantage were risk factors for ER (Boyd et al. 2013). These data suggest that a significant subset of EP children evaluated at age 2 years had socio-emotional delays (Boyd et al. 2013).

Attention Problems

ADHD affects 5–7% of the general population (Polanczyk et al. 2007; Thomas et al. 2015) and EP children are at even greater risk of having ADHD (Hack et al. 2009; O'Shea et al. 2013; Johnson et al. 2016). Because few studies have evaluated EP toddlers for attention problems (Downey et al. 2015; Johnson et al. 2016), we assessed the correlates and antecedents of attention problems in EP children at the age of 2 years GA-adjusted age. The prevalence of attention problems (empirically based scores) at age 2 years was 11% and for DSM-oriented attention deficit hyperactivity problems (ADHP), as identified by parent report on the Child Behavioral Checklist (CBCL) (Achenbach and Rescorla 2000), was 8% (Downey et al. 2015). EP children were at significantly increased risk of having attention problems or of having ADHP if they were born to a mother with no more than a high school education (adjusted risk ratio (ARR) for attention problems 2.2; ADHP 3.0) or a mother who was exposed to second-hand smoke (ARR for attention problems 1.9; ADHP 2.4). If the placenta had fetal stem vessel thrombosis, the ARRs were 2.5 and 3.1 respectively, while recovery of bacteria from a tracheal aspirate was the only postnatal factor associated with increased risk of having attention problems (ARR for attention problems 1.9). All the above ARRs were statistically significant (Downey et al. 2015).

Emotion and Behavior

EP children are not only at heightened risk of having attention problems, they are also at increased risk for emotional and behavioral dysregulation, which can result in difficulties in school (Frazier et al. 2015). Thus early identification and effective interventions prior to school entry hold the promise of improving outcomes. Unfortunately, few studies have evaluated children during infancy and preschool for emotional and behavioral dysregulation (Delobel-Ayoub et al. 2009). We assessed EP children at age 2 years using the CBCL-Dysregulation Profile (CBCL-DP; a combination of the CBCL attention problems, aggression and anxious/depressed subscales) since it has been defined as a syndrome that portends significant psychopathology and poor outcomes in youth (Ayer et al. 2009). While the CBLC-DP occurs in 1–5% of community samples of slightly older youth (Hudziak et al. 2005, Volk and Todd 2007), we found that 9% of the EP ELGAN children had a CBCL-DP at age 2 years adjusted age. We also found that low maternal education, passive smoking exposure and recovery of Mycoplasma from the placenta were associated with a significantly increased risk of having the CBCL-DP. The multivariable-adjusted odds ratios for these three exposures were 3.2, 1.9, and 2.5 respectively (Frazier et al. 2015). Histologic chorioamnionitis was significantly associated with reduced risk (multivariable-adjusted OR = 0.4), suggesting the possibility of benefit from a pre-conditioning exposure (Hagberg et al. 2004).

Post-natal factors that might mediate the association between extreme preterm birth and psychiatric outcomes have received little attention in the literature. One etiopathologic hypothesis for heighted risk of psychiatric outcomes in preterm born infants involves inflammation, given that children born preterm are more likely than term-born children to have early systemic inflammation (Dammann and Leviton 2014),

The ELGAN Study

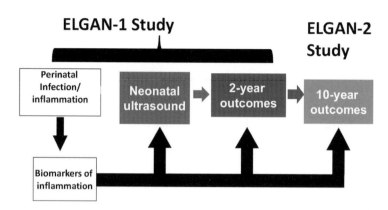

Figure 15.1   The ELGAN study examines the extent to which early life inflammation is predictive of structural brain disorders and of neurodevelopmental impairments in the ELGAN cohort. These relationships have been studied at age 2 and 10 years. A color version of this figure can be found in the color plate section.

and early inflammation has been associated with indicators of brain damage (Hagberg et al. 2015; Allred et al. 2017). During the first postnatal month, we measured concentrations of both inflammatory and neurotrophic proteins in serial blood samples, uniquely poising the ELGAN study to assess the relationship between both early postnatal inflammation and early concentrations of neurotrophic proteins to the risk of psychiatric outcomes assessed at both ages 2 and 10 years of age, and, in the field now, at age 15–16 (Allred et al. 2017).

We have found associations between elevated inflammation-related proteins in neonatal blood of ELGANs with a variety of neurodevelopmental outcomes, such as microcephaly, cerebral white matter injury, developmental delay and cerebral palsy, at age 2 years (Leviton et al. 2011a, 2011b; O'Shea et al. 2012; Kuban et al. 2014). We also evaluated the associations between early inflammation and attention problems in ELGANS assessed at age 2 years adjusted age using the CBCL for ages 1.5–5 (O'Shea et al. 2014). Children were considered to have attention problems if the subscale score was ≥93rd percentile (see Fig. 15.1). Persistent or recurrent inflammatory protein elevation was defined as having a concentration in the highest quartile on at least 2 days, a week apart during the postnatal period. Ten percent of the children who had both a CBCL at age 2 and first-month blood spots for the measurement of early inflammation had an attention problem. Persistent or recurrent elevations of a number of inflammatory proteins (MPO, IL-6, TNF-R1, IL-8, ICAM-3, VEGF-R1, VEGF-R2) were associated with a 2- to 3.9-fold increased risk of having attention problems in EP children.

PSYCHIATRIC OUTCOMES IN ELGANS AT AGE 10

We enrolled 1506 newborns in ELGAN (2002–2004). Of those, 308 died and 232 did not have newborn blood specimens so were unavailable or ineligible to participate in the age 10 year assessment wave. Of the 966 eligibles, 77 either were lost to follow-up or declined to participate. We therefore assessed 889 participant families (92% of eligible children) at age 10 years. We used the parent (n = 871) and teacher report forms (n = 640) of the Child Symptom Inventory-4 (CSI-4) as our primary outcome measure for psychiatric symptoms (Gadow and Sprafkin 2002; Sprafkin et al. 2002). The CSI-4 Checklist screens for Disruptive Behavior Disorders, Anxiety Disorders, Mood Disorders, and other disorders such as autism. We considered CSI-4 disorders as valid indicators of screening positive for a disorder, but not for definitely having the disorder. Thus our CSI-4 classifications are indicators of psychiatric risk for the disorders described.

Attention Deficit Hyperactivity Disorder (ADHD)

At age 10 years, we found that 21% of EP children had ADHD symptoms based on parent report and 23% based on teacher report forms of the CSI-4 (Leviton et al. 2017), with only fair to poor agreement between parent and teachers (Kappa values <0.41). Children identified by parent report as having ADHD symptoms were more likely to have indicators of social dysfunction than children identified by teachers or physicians as having symptoms of ADHD. We also found that ADHD identified by a single observer provided important information about a child's functioning within that particular setting, suggesting that when there is disagreement between reporters, a single reporter's endorsement of ADHD symptoms should be considered as valuable even when a second reporter from another setting does not endorse symptoms of ADHD.

We also found that compared to EP children without ADHD symptoms, EP children with ADHD symptoms were more likely to have neurocognitive impairment and more likely to have low IQ scores (Scott et al. 2017). For example, ADHD symptoms were significantly associated with Z-scores ≤ -1 on all School-Age Differential Ability Scales, Second Edition (DAS-II) (Elliott, 2007), Oral and Written Language Scales (OWLS; Carrow-Woolfolk 1996), and Wechsler Individual Achievement Test-III (WIAT-III) (Wechsler 2009) subtests as well as all but two NEPSY-II (*A Developmental NEuroPSYchological Assessment*, Second Edition; Korkman, Kemp, and Kirk, 1998) subtests and for a Latent Profile Analysis (LPA) based level of executive function, after adjusting for three newborn characteristics (male sex, gestational age 23–24 weeks, and birth weight Z-scores <-2) and for three maternal characteristics (identification as black, age <21 years and eligibility for government provided medical care insurance). Children with ADHD symptoms and a normal intelligence quotient were less likely to have global neurocognitive limitations. However, even children with ADHD symptoms and normal IQ scores were more likely than children without ADHD symptoms to score lower on cognitive tests. For example, when the sample was restricted to children with ADHD and a normal IQ, the adjusted risk of a Z-score ≤ -1 SD below the median remained the same for WIAT-II Word Reading, Pseudoword Decoding and Spelling, NEPSY-II Auditory Response, DAS-II Working Memory, and for the LPA-based measure of executive functioning.

As at age 2, we found that several inflammatory proteins found to be elevated during the first postnatal month were associated with ADHD symptoms (by teacher report on the CSI-4) at age 10 years in individuals with an IQ ≥ 70, and that elevations of various neurotrophic proteins modified that increased risk (Allred et al. 2017). Specifically, we found the top quartile elevations of IL-6R, TNF-$\propto$, IL-8, and VEGF-R2 on 2 days a week apart during the first two postnatal weeks were associated with increased risk of having ADHD symptoms (Odds Ratios ranged from 1.7 to 2.3). In addition, we found top quartile elevations of VEGF, VEFG-R1 and VEGF-R2 on both the 21st and 28th postnatal days were associated with increased risk of having ADHD symptoms (odd ratios ranged from 2.1 to 2.4). At the same time, top quartile elevations of neurotrophic proteins, such as IL-6R, EPO,RANTES, NT-4, bFG-F,BDNF, IGF-1, PIGF, Ang-1, and Ang-2, modulated the increased risk for ADHD symptoms. In other words, children were found to be at increased risk for ADHD symptoms when IL-6R, TNF-$\propto$, IL-8, VEGF, VEFG-R1, and VEGF-R2 were in the top quartile on multiple days only when the neurotrophic proteins listed above were below the top quartile (odds ratios range from 1.7 to 3.6). We are unaware of any other publication describing the relationship between neonatal inflammatory and neurotrophic proteins and ADHD symptoms assessed at school age.

Psychiatric Comorbidity

To date, the impact and burden of psychiatric comorbidity on children born preterm has not been reported in a systematic way. Studies conducted in general child outpatient practices that assess the burden associated with psychiatric disorders highlight the impact of co-occurring psychiatric disorders on daily functioning and underscore the critical need for such assessments in the preterm born population (Staller, 2006; Biederman et al. 2011; Basten et al. 2013). Towards that end, the ELGAN study team identified psychiatric symptoms, co-occurrence of and sex-related differences in these classifications, and the functional outcomes, allowing for the assessment of psychiatric burden at age 10 years. We found that EP children evaluated at age 10 years compared to the CSI-4 normative sample had significantly higher rates of Generalized Anxiety Disorder (5.3% vs 1.6%), Dysthymic Disorder (4% vs 0.7%), Social Phobia (4.8% vs 0.8%), Oppositional Defiant disorder (8.4% vs 5.3%), ADHD inattentive (11.5% vs 3.6%), ADHD Combined (5.5% vs 1.6%), Autism (3% vs 0.5%), and Asperger's disorder (4.5% vs 0%). Additionally, EP boys were more likely to screen positively for ADHD hyperactive/impulsive (5.7% vs 2.3%) and for Autistic Disorder (4.9% vs 0.7%), compared to boys of the CSI-4 normative sample (these differences were not statistically significant in girls). EP girls were more likely compared to the CSI-4 normative sample to have Dysthymic Disorder (4% vs 0%) and this difference was not statistically significant in boys. Boys in ELGAN were more likely than girls to screen positive for an externalizing disorder (30% vs 20%). However, boys and girls had similar screen positive rates for internalizing disorders (Dvir et al. in press). Fifteen percent of ELGAN subjects screened positive for one psychiatric disorder, 7% for two, 3% for three, and 4% for four or more psychiatric disorders, indicating that in total about 30% of ELGAN children were screened positively by their parents for at least one psychiatric disorder. Regarding diagnostic groupings, externalizing and internalizing disorders were the most likely to co-occur (8% of the total ELGAN sample) based on positive screens, followed by externalizing disorders and ASD (3%). Boys were more likely to have one or two psychiatric disorders; however, when three or more disorders were rated as screen positive, there were no sex differences.

ELGAN subjects who screened positively for a higher number of psychiatric disorders were more likely to have low quality of life in the domains of physical, emotional, or social functioning. For example, low physical functioning was characteristic of 15% of children with no psychiatric disorder screen positive, 24% of children with a screen positive for one psychiatric disorder, 33% of children with two screen positives for psychiatric disorders, and 40% of children with screen positives for three or more psychiatric disorders. Similar patterns were observed for emotional, social, and school functioning. In addition, certain maternal characteristics (i.e. older maternal age, higher levels of education, being married, having private health insurance) were protective and predicted lower numbers of psychiatric disorders (Dvir et al. in press).

HOW THE ELGAN STUDY RESULTS COMPARE WITH OTHER RESEARCH FINDINGS

Although still not as common as studies of other health conditions, studies have documented emotional/behavioral outcomes in preterm born children and ELGAN findings are consistent with other studies in terms of the prevalence and typology of emotional and behavioral outcomes in severe prematurity. The literature suggests that children born preterm are at increased risk for ADHD, anxiety, depression, and behavioral problems in early and middle childhood (Hille et al. 2001; Elgen et al. 2002; Delobel-Ayoub et al. 2006, 2009; Hack et al. 2009; Johnson et al. 2010, 2016; Huhtala et al. 2011; Treyvaud et al. 2013; Sucksdorff et al. 2015; Elgen et al. 2017; Ask et al. 2018). The increased frequency of externalizing and internalizing disorders in the ELGAN cohort is consistent with prior studies (Szatmari et al. 1990; Pharoah et al. 1994; Taylor et al. 2000; Miller et al. 2001; Elgen et al. 2002; Hoff et al. 2004; Reijneveld et al. 2006; Samara et al. 2008; Delobel-Ayoub et al. 2009; Hack et al. 2009; Conrad et al. 2010; Johnson et al. 2016). Taken together, this convergence in the literature implicates significant neuropsychiatric risk in preterm born children, particularly in the extremely preterm, as they move into childhood and early adolescence.

ELGAN EMOTIONAL AND BEHAVIORAL OUTCOMES AT AGE 2 COMPARED WITH RESULTS OF OTHER STUDIES FOCUSED ON OUTCOMES DURING INFANCY AND PRESCHOOL (SEE TABLE 15.1)

We have selected 10 representative manuscripts from other studies that have evaluated emotional and behavioral outcomes during infancy and preschool in preterm born individuals. The majority of these studies have relatively small numbers of subjects and three of them enrolled based on birth weight or some combination of birth weight and GA, and thus include the biases introduced by increased presence of children with fetal growth retardation. Six of these manuscripts included a control group. Of the three studies with large numbers of participants that are most comparable to ELGAN, 2 enrolled based on GA and only one enrolled based on GA similar to the ELGAN cohort (Gray et al. 2004; Delobel-Ayoub et al. 2006; Johnson et al. 2016).

Social Emotional Delays

At age 2 years, we found that 31% of children born preterm had difficulties with ER and 27% had difficulties with O/E on the BRS. Children with Mental Development Index and Psychomotor Development Index scores of <70 were more likely to have difficulties with ER and O/E. Multi-fetal pregnancy was associated with difficulties with O/E and male sex and socioeconomic disadvantage were associated with both ER and OE (Boyd et al. 2013). Our findings are consistent with other studies that have reported that preterm born infants have poorer emotional and behavioral regulation compared to term born controls and highlight the importance of assessing social-emotional functioning in addition to cognitive and motor functions in preterm born infants (Delobel-Ayoub et al. 2006; Spittle et al. 2009; Woodward et al. 2017). Finally, a European study in infants born <32 weeks GA found 18% and 13% of the children in their cohort, who did not have severe disabilities, scored non-optimally on the O/E and ER respectively (Janssen et al. 2008). However, this particular study did not report on maternal or child pre- or perinatal antecedents of the BRS.

Attention Problems

We found that the ELGAN participants were at increased risk for attention problems at age 2 years (O'Shea et al. 2014; Downey et al. 2015). Our findings are consistent with the work of others reporting higher rates of inattention and hyperactivity in preterm born individuals assessed during infancy and preschool (Delobel-Ayoub et al. 2006; Johnson et al. 2016; Palumbi et al. 2018). We also reported that several potentially modifiable prenatal and postnatal antecedents were associated with increased risk of attention problems and ADHP at age 2 (e.g. maternal education ≤ high school, maternal second-hand

Table 15.1 Summary of selected studies of psychiatric outcomes during infancy and preschool in individuals born preterm

Author	Study participants	Assessment	Findings	Comment
Weisglas-Kuperus et al. (1998)	114 VLBW (<1500g or GA < 36 weeks) born between 1985 and 1986 and reassessed at age 3.5 years	Used CBCL (2/3)	VLBW youth had more depressed behavior (11 vs 2.1%) and more internalizing problems (34.2 vs 12.5%) by parent report and had greater total problem scores (21.9 vs 9.9%) than the comparison group. Cognition influenced behavior problems per clinician report and home environment affected behavior per parent report	Dutch
Gray et al. (2004)	<2500 grams bwt born 1985 (n = 869)	CBCL, General Health Questionnaire at 3, 5, and 8 years of age	Prevalence of behavior problems was about 20% at each age; moderate stability over time; correlates of behavior problems were lower maternal age, maternal smoking	Data about predictive validity over time
Delobel-Ayoub et al. (2006)	22–32 weeks and full term controls born 1997 at 3 years of age (n = 1228)	Strength and Difficulties Questionnaire (SDQ)	Total difficulties, hyperactivity, conduct problems, emotional problems, peer problem, and prosocial behavior all were more prevalent among preterm, as compared to controls; in multivariate analysis, risk factors for high total difficulties score were low maternal age, low maternal education, major cerebral ultrasound lesions, developmental delay; re-hospitalization in first year, poor health as judged by parents	Most comparable to ELGAN with regard to sample size; includes analysis of risk factors; relied solely on parent report
Janssens et al. (2009)	25–35 weeks born 2003–2005 and controls, assessed at 12 months (n = 69)	Diagnostic Classification Zero to Three	Preterms more likely than controls to have multi-system developmental disorders and regulatory disorders	
Spittle et al. (2009)	188 very preterm (GA < 30 weeks or BW < 1250g) and 70 full-term children assessed at 2 years corrected age	Infant Toddler Social and Emotional Assessment	Very preterm children had higher internalizing and dysregulation scores and lower competence scores than peers. Lower social competence scores were associated with female sex, Lower BW Z-scores, WM abnormalities and postnatal corticosteroids	
Huhtala et al. (2011)	VLBW at 3 years (n = 14)	CBCL for child at 3 years and for parents, when child was 2 years old: Beck Depression Inventory, Parenting Stress Index, Sense of Coherence Scale	BDI, PSI, and SOC were correlated with internalizing, externalizing, and total problems scores on CBCL	

(Continued)

Table 15.1   Summary of selected studies of psychiatric outcomes during infancy and preschool in individuals born preterm (Continued)

Author	Study participants	Assessment	Findings	Comment
Johnson et al. (2015)	638 LMPT (32–36 weeks) 765 Controls at age 2 (corrected age)	- BITSEA for behavioral problems and social competence - Parent Report of Children's Abilities-R for cognitive development	LMPT infants were at significantly increased risk of delay in social competence compared with controls. No significant group difference for the prevalence of behavior problems	- Significantly later term than ELGAN - Only evaluates social competence - Large sample size
Johnson et al. (2016)	EPT (<26 weeks) born Mar–Dec 1995 at 2.5 (n = 283), 6 (n = 160), and 11 (n = 219) years 160 Controls	2.5: - MDI - PDI - BSID-II 6: - NEPSY - K-ABC - SDQ 11: - Du Paul Scale-IV (ADHD)	- EP rated with greater symptoms of inattention than controls - No breast feeding associated with higher inattention and hyperactivity/impulsivity - higher inattention and externalizing symptoms at age 2.5 associated with inattention at 11 years - cognitive impairment, lower MDI and PDI scores, functional disability and smaller head circumference associated with symptoms of inattention and hyperactivity/impulsivity (effect size greater for inattention) - pervasive conduct problems at 6 associated with higher inattention and hyperactivity/impulsivity at 11	- similar GA to ELGAN - evaluates antecedents not prevalence, expands on prevalence work
Woodward et al. (2017)	110 VPT (<32 weeks) 113 Controls at 2 and 4 (corrected age) and 9 years (born 1998–2000)	2 and 4: - Modified Emotion Regulation Checklist - BSID-III - SDQ - Elley-Irving Socioeconomic Index - Hospital Anxiety and Depression Scale (maternal) 9: - Development and Well-being Assessment Interview (DSM-IV) - Woodcock Johnson-III Tests of Achievement	- VPT had poorer emotional and behavioral regulation - VPT had higher rates of DSM-IV mental health disorder and educational delay at 9 years - Poorer self-regulation at 2 and 4 associated with increased risk of ADHD, CD, anxiety disorders at 9	- self-regulation as an antecedent to mental health issues

(Continued)

Table 15.1 Summary of selected studies of psychiatric outcomes during infancy and preschool in individuals born preterm (Continued)

Author	Study participants	Assessment	Findings	Comment
Palumbi et al. (2018)	n = 68 (45M, and 23F) ages 2–16.3; late preterm infants admitted to the C/A Neuropsychiatric unit – University of Bari Jan 2014–March 2016	Leiter-R, WPPSI-III, WISC-IV, MT group reading Tests for Primary School; MT group Advanced Reading for Mathematics Tests for the first biennium of Secondary School; Battery for the Evaluation of Developmental Dyslexia and Dysorthograpgy for Primary and Middle school; Evaluation Tests of Calculation Ability for Primary School and Evaluation Tests of Calculation Ability and Problem Solving for Middle School, CBCL	Language disorder: 32.4%, ADHD: 23.5%, Specific Learning Disorder: 22.1%, Developmental Coordination Disorder: 19.1%, Intellectual Disability 17.6%, Autism Spectrum Disorder: 13.2% 30.8% had internalizing problems Co-morbidities 28%; LD and DCD: 13.23%, ASD and ID: 8.8%, ADHD and ASD: 5.9%	

• Studies include if they have the first wave of assessments starting in infancy or preschool age even if they included subsequent waves in school age, adolescence or adulthood.

Key: ADHD, attention deficit hyperactivity; BDI, Beck depression inventory; BITSEA, Brief Infant Toddler Social and Emotional Assessment; BPD, bronchopulmonary dysplasia; BSID-II, Bayley Scale of Infant Development-second edition; BSID-III, Bayley Scale of Infant Development-third edition; BW, birth weight; BWT, birth weight; CBCL, child behavior checklist; DCD, developmental coordination disorder; ELGAN, extremely low gestational age newborn; FSIQ, full scale Intelligence quotient; GA, gestational age; ID, intellectual disability; ITSEA, Infant Toddler Social Emotional Assessment; K-ABC, Kaufman Assessment Battery for Children; LD, learning disorder; LMPT, late and moderately preterm; MDI, mental developmental index; NEPSYA, Developmental Neuropsychological Assessment; PDI, psychomotor developmental index; PSI, parenting stress index; SDQ, strengths and difficulties questionnaire; SOC, Sense of coherence scale; VLBW, very low birth weight; VPT, very preterm; WISC-IV, Wechsler Intelligence Scale for Children, fourth edition; WM, white matter; WPPSI-III, Wechsler Preschool and Primary Scale of Intelligence.

smoke exposure, placenta with fetal stem vessel thrombosis, bacteria recovered from tracheal aspirates) (Downey et al. 2015). This information could help in the development of preventative strategies such as educating pregnant women about avoiding secondhand smoke, reducing days on ventilators to reduce tracheal colonization, and trying to identify placental infection earlier.

Emotion and Behavior

The CBCL-DP (a combination of the CBCL attention problems, aggression, and anxious/depressed subscales) has been defined as a syndrome that portends significant psychopathology and poor outcomes in youth (Ayer et al. 2009). We are unaware of any other publication that has assessed the CBCL-DP in a preterm born cohort. We found that 9% of the EP ELGAN children had a CBCL-DP at age 2 years, adjusted age (Hudziak et al. 2005; Volk and Todd 2007). Preterm youth with emotional and behavioral dysregulation differed in multiple ways from their preterm peers who did not have emotional and behavioral dysregulation (Frazier et al. 2015). We also identified several potentially modifiable risk factors (low maternal education, passive smoking exposure and recovery of Mycoplasma from the placenta) for the CBCL-DP that could be the target of future educational and intervention strategies.

ELGAN PSYCHIATRIC OUTCOMES AT AGE 10 COMPARED WITH THE RESULTS OF OTHER STUDIES FOCUSED ON OUTCOMES DURING SCHOOL AGE (SEE TABLE 15.2)

We have selected 30 representative manuscripts from other studies that have evaluated mental health outcomes during school-age in preterm born individuals. The majority of these studies have relatively small numbers of subjects and 19 of them enrolled based on birth weight or some combination of birth weight and GA so they include the biases introduced by the correlates of fetal growth retardation. Twenty-six of these manuscripts included a control group. Of the six studies with large numbers of participants that are most comparable to ELGAN, two were birth cohorts with all GAs included, two enrolled based on GA and or birthweight, and two enrolled based on GA (only one enrolled based on GA similar to the ELGAN cohort).

Attention Deficit Hyperactivity Disorder (ADHD)

We found that 21% of EP children had ADHD symptoms based on parent report and 23% based on teacher report forms of the CSI-4 (Leviton et al. 2017). Having higher rates of ADHD is consistent with reports of other investigators who enrolled EP children based on GA (or in birth cohorts assembled on the basis of GA) and assessed the children during school-age (Stjernqvist and Svenningsen 1999; Farooqi et al. 2007; Samara et al. 2008; Delobel-Ayoub et al. 2009; Johnson et al. 2010, 2016; Loe et al. 2011; Treyvaud et al. 2013; Sucksdorff et al. 2015; Ask et al. 2018; Linsell et al. 2018). At age 10, we found that EP children with ADHD symptoms were more likely to have neurocognitive impairment; and in those with a normal intelligence quotient, ADHD symptoms were associated with executive function deficits (Scott et al. 2017). Our findings are similar to recent efforts exploring these relationships that have shown high infant activity levels being related to later ADHD symptoms at age 7 (Meeuwsen et al. 2018), with one study showing slower motor processing speed as being uniquely related to inattentive symptoms in very preterm children (Retzler et al. 2018). Finally, we found poor agreement between parent and teacher identified symptoms of ADHD on

Table 15.2 Summary of selected studies of psychiatric outcomes during school age in individuals born preterm

Author	Study participants	Assessment	Findings	Comment
Szatmari et al. (1990)	<1000 gm bwt born 1980–1982 and controls at 5 years of age (n = 82)	CBCL to identify ADHD, conduct disorder, and emotional disorder (a combination of anxiety, obsessive-compulsive, and depressive symptoms)	7.3% ADHD (OR = 5.4); 15.9% either classified hyperactive by parent or teacher (OR = 2.6); no difference between ELBW and controls for conduct and emotional disorders	
Sommerfelt et al. (1993)	29 LBW infants compared to 29 matched term controls at 8 years	Personality Inventory for Children-scales describe child behavior, psychopathology, and social and cognitive function	VLBW children had more learning and school related problems, more conduct and emotional problems in the VLBW boys. VLBW boys had higher scores on the somatic concern scale and on the development scale	Norway
Pharoah et al. (1994)	233 8–9 years with BW <2000g compared with 233 matched controls and 46 unmatched children attending special schools	Rutter Behavior Scale (parent and teacher)	LBW infants had more behavioral problems (36 vs 22% on parent and 27 vs 12 on teacher). LBW boys had more hyperactivity (21 vs 5). More emotional and conduct problems (40 vs 30 on parent –35 vs 7 on teacher and 29 vs 11 on parent, and 22 vs 16 on teacher respectively)	UK
Stjernqvist and Svenningsen (1999)	<29 weeks born 1985–1986 and full-term controls evaluated at 10 years (n = 52)	CBCL	Preterm children had higher total problems score, internalizing, externalizing, social competence problems, and attention problems; 20% of preterms (RR = 2.5) had ADHD	
Taylor et al. (2000)	Bwt < 750 g (n = 60), 750–1499 (n = 55), and term born 1982–1986 and evaluated at 7 and 11 years	CBCL and Teacher Report Form and Children's Depression Inventory	Those with bwt <750 grams were 4.8 times more likely to meet criteria for ADHD and 5 times more likely to have total problem score >63	
Miller et al. (2001)	500–999 grams bwt born 1985–1988 assessed at 5 and 8 years (n = 46)	CBCL parent and teacher; T score >63 and Conners Rating Scales parent and teacher T ≥ 65	15.6% had total behavior problems score in clinical range at 5 years and 27.7% at 8 years; on Conners, conduct problems increased from 7.9% to 17%; impulsive/hyperactive increased from 10.5 to 14.9%, and anxiety increased from 7.9 to 10.6% between 5 and 8 years	

(Continued)

Table 15.2 Summary of selected studies of psychiatric outcomes during school age in individuals born preterm (Continued)

Author	Study participants	Assessment	Findings	Comment
Nadeau et al. (2001)	<29 week and <1500 grams born 1987–1990 and normal BW controls assessed at 7 years (n = 61)	CBCL and Teacher Report Form and assessment by school peers	Perceived by peers to be more sensitive/isolated, by teacher as more inattentive, and by parents as hyperactive	
Elgen (2002)	<2000 grams bwt without major handicaps and controls born 1986–1988 at 11 years of age (n = 130)	CBCL (parents and teachers); psychometric scales of the Yale children's inventory; children assessment schedule; psychometric scale of Asperger syndrome diagnostic interview	ADHD in 10% (OR = 9.6); depression in 2% and oppositional defiant in 1%	
Weindrich et al. (2003)	VLBW born 1986–1988 and normal bwt controls assessed at 11 years of age (n = 29)	CBCL	VLBW had higher scores on all CBCL syndrome scales other than aggressive behavior	
Hoff et al. (2004)	244 Extremely Pre-mature (GA < 28 weeks or BW < 1000g) and 76 matched term controls assessed at age 5 years	Conners Abbreviated Symptom Questionnaire for Parents and questions on social skills and anxious/ withdrawn and outward reacting behavior	Index children had more hyperactive behavior (17.5 vs 4.2%) and poorer social skills (30.9 vs 16.7%). Lower FSIQ associated with outward reacting, hyperactive behavior and poorer social skills. Sensitive parenting was associated with less outward reacting and less hyperactive behavior. Controlling for FSIQ and parenting, index children continued to have increase hyperactivity but not poorer social skill	Denmark
Reijneveld et al. (2006)	<32 weeks or <1500 grams at 5 years (n = 431)	CBCL	Compared to population controls, very preterm or very low BW scored higher on all scales of CBCL except sex problems and anxious/depressed; higher internalizing, externalizing, and total problem scores	
Farooqi et al. (2007)	<26 weeks, born 1990–1992 and controls; assessed at 11 years of age (n = 86)	CBCL (parents and teachers); children completed depression self-rating scale	Depression self-rating not different; by parent report, ELGANs more likely to have score >90th percentile for anxious/depressed, withdrawn, attention problems, internalizing, and total problems. All of these were confirmed by teacher report, plus more likely to score high on somatic complaints, social problems, and thought problems	CBCL competence scales were also analyzed Sweden

(Continued)

Table 15.2 Summary of selected studies of psychiatric outcomes during school age in individuals born preterm (Continued)

Author	Study participants	Assessment	Findings	Comment
Greenley et al. (2007)	Bwt < 750 gms (n = 48), bwt 750–1499 (n = 46), and term controls evaluated at 11 and 17 years	CBCL and Teacher Report Form	Among those <750 grams, increasing adolescent-perceived conflict in family was associated with increase in total behavior problems and externalizing problems	
Gray et al. (2008)	26–33 weeks with (n = 78) or without (n = 60) BPD at school age	CBCL and Teacher Report Form	Syndrome scales: BPD higher scores for withdrawn, somatic complaints but not anxious/depressed or attention problems	Analysis of risk factors
Samara et al. (2008)	EpiCure cohort (<26 weeks born 1995) and controls at 6 years of age (n = 200)	Strengths and Difficulties Questionnaire (SDQ)	Extremely preterm children scored higher on overall behavioral difficulties, emotional problems (boys only), conduct problems, hyperactivity problems, peer problems, and prosocial behavior	
Delobel-Ayoub et al. (2009)	22–32 weeks and full-term controls born 1997 at 5 years of age (n = 1095)	SDQ	Preterms had two-fold higher prevalence of hyperactivity/inattention, emotional symptoms, and peer problems; correlates of behavioral problems were low cognitive performance, developmental delay, hospitalizations of the child, young maternal age, and poor maternal mental well-being	Most comparable to ELGAN with regard to sample size; includes analysis of risk factors; relied solely on parent report
Hack et al. (2009)	BWT <1000 gm born 1992–1995 and normal bwt controls at 8 years of age (n = 219)	Child Symptom Inventory-4 (CSI-4)	ELBW had higher scores for inattentive, hyperactive, and combined types of ADHD: higher scores for generalized anxiety and autistic and Asperger's Disorders; differences in both boys and girls except for generalized anxiety (present only in girls); higher rates of any ADHD, inattentive ADHD, combined ADHD, social phobia; correlates of ADHD were lower SES, male sex (hyperactive type), but no neonatal risk factors; autistic and Asperger's were correlated with BPD, days on postnatal steroids, and duration of hospital stay	Pertinent to the analyses of CSI-4 problems in ELGAN-2

(Continued)

Table 15.2   Summary of selected studies of psychiatric outcomes during school age in individuals born preterm (Continued)

Author	Study participants	Assessment	Findings	Comment
Rautava et al. (2010)	588 VLBW (GA < 32 weeks or BW<1,500 g) and 176 controls at 5 years of age	Five to Fifteen questionnaire	VLBW had lower developmental and behavioral scores in all FTF domains. The scores were lower the lower the GA	Finland
Johnson et al. (2010)	<26 weeks born 1995 and controls assessed at 11 years (n = 219)	Development and Well Being Assessment, a structured psychiatric assessment, via telephone interview (92%) or online (8%) from which DSM-IV diagnoses assigned	Extremely preterm more likely to have any ADHD disorder 11.5% (OR = 4.3); inattentive ADHD 7.1% (OR = 10.5); any emotional disorder 9% (OR = 4.6); any autism spectrum disorder 8% (versus none in controls)	This is the study that is most comparable to ELGAN study UK
Conrad et al. (2010)	31 ELBW and 18 VLBW and controls born 1992–1997 at age 7–16 years (n = 49)	Pediatric Behavior Scale-30	Preterm group had higher scores on depression/anxiety and hyperactivity/inattention	
Loe et al. (2011)	<36 weeks and controls at 9–16 years (n = 63)	CBCL	Preterm more likely to have syndrome scale T score >60 for anxious/depressed −34% (OR 10) and attention problems −39% (OR 10); preterm had higher internalizing and total problem scores	
Treyvaud et al. (2013)	177 VPT and 65 term controls At 7 years	DAWBA	VPT children 3x odds for meeting any psychiatric diagnosis at age 7. Most common were anxiety disorders (11 vs 8%), ADHD (10 vs 3%) and ASD (4.5 vs 0%)	Neonatal brain abnormalities, social-emotional problems at age 5 and those with higher social risk at age 7 were more likely to meet criteria for a psychiatric disorder at age 7

(Continued)

Table 15.2 Summary of selected studies of psychiatric outcomes during school age in individuals born preterm (Continued)

Author	Study participants	Assessment	Findings	Comment
Scott et al. (2012)	Bwt < 1000 gm born 2001–2003 and controls at 5 years of age (n = 148)	CBCL and Teacher Report Form, Behavior Rating Inventory of Executive Function and School Social Behavior Scales	ELBW had higher prevalence of ADHD combined – 33% (OR – 2.5); ADHD inattentive – 21% (OR 2.6); ADHD hyperactive –28% (OR – 2.5); social phobia (p = 0.056); ADHD DSM-oriented syndrome –15% (OR 2.9); social competence composite in at-risk or high-risk range –19% (OR 5.99); peer relations in at-risk or high-risk range –22% (OR 6.88)	
Elgen et al. (2015)	213 EP/ELBW (22–27 weeks or <1000 g) at age 5	- Yale Children's Inventory	- minor NDIs (Neurodevelopmental impairments) associated with higher mean YCI scores - decreased hearing, IQ, and male gender associated with higher scores on the attention scale	- compares EP with NDI to those without - no control group
Sucksdorff et al. (2015)	10 321 patients with ADHD 38 355 Controls matched for gender, date and place of birth (all Finnish, born between 1991 and 2005, all singletons)	- ADHD diagnosis according to the ICD-9/10 (depending on year of birth)	- Risk of ADHD increased by each declining week of gestation - elevated risk also seen among late preterm and early term infants - increased risk for ADHD when BW was 1 SD below or 2 SD above mean for GA	- huge sample size - risk assessed for each week of GA - risk assessed in relationship with BW and GA - expands previous findings about ADHD risk and prevalence in this population

(*Continued*)

Table 15.2   Summary of selected studies of psychiatric outcomes during school age in individuals born preterm (Continued)

Author	Study participants	Assessment	Findings	Comment
Breeman et al. (2016)	260 VP/VLBW (<32 weeks or <1500 g) 229 Controls at ages 6, 8, and 26	- CBCL at 6 and 8 years - YACBL at 26 years - TRCB at 6 and 8 years for attention span - TRAB at 26 for attention span - Mannheim Parent Interview for ADHD dx at 6 and 8 - DSM-IV based ADHD adult rating scale for dx at 26	VP/VLBW had higher attention problem scores than controls in both childhood and adulthood. VP/VLBW were more often diagnosed with ADHD in childhood and adulthood than controls. VP/VLBW more often had ADHD-inattentive or combined types in childhood. For both groups attention span increased over time. Parent-rated attention problems in VP/VLBW decreased from ages 6 to 8, but increased from 8 to 26. VP/VLBW had more stable ADHD diagnoses over time than controls	- results consistent with previous studies regarding rates of ADHD - evaluates prevalence, as well as long term diagnostic stability
Elgen Fevang et al. (2017)	216 EP/ELBW (<28 weeks, or <1000 g) 1882 Controls at 11 years	- Strengths and Difficulties Questionnaire (SDQ) (Parent and Teacher)	EP/ELBW children had significantly higher scores and/or increased risk of parent, teacher, combined rated hyperactivity/inattention, emotional, and peer problems. Parents reported the EP/ELBW children to be at increased risk for conduct problems. For both populations low maternal education at birth was significantly associated with mental health problems at age 11	Similar cohort to ELGAN (born 1999–2000, <28 weeks GA, evaluated age 11)
Linsell et al. (2018)	infants <26 weeks, born in the UK or Republic of Ireland from March 1st to December 31st 1995 – 315 surviving infants were assessed at age 6, 9, 11, 16, and 19; term based controls were matched based on age, race, and sex	Child behavioral checklist, Strength and Difficulties Questionnaire, Bayley's scale of infant development, Kaufamman Assessment Battery for Children, Weschler Abbreviated Scale of Intelligence	SDQ total difficulties score of the EPT higher than their term born peers at age 6 and with similar longitudinal trajectories in both groups. EPT had increased risk of having overall difficulties in the clinically significant range on the SDQ compared to term controls. There was a significant difference in every subscale of the SDQ at age 6; greatest differences were in the hyperactivity/inattention scale and peer relationship problems. Emotional symptoms were shown to increase overtime in both groups but to a greater extent in the EPT group relative to controls. CBCL classification of clinical behavioral problems at age 2.5 years old was strongly associated with high SDQ total difficulties score from 6 years forward. Moderate/severe cognitive impairment at the last assessment was associated with higher SDQ total difficulties in the EPT subjects	

(Continued)

Table 15.2   Summary of selected studies of psychiatric outcomes during school age in individuals born preterm (Continued)

Author	Study participants	Assessment	Findings	Comment
Jaekel et al. (2018)	200 VPT/VLBW children from South Bavaria, Germany that were born during a 15 month period between 1985 and 1986 and 196 healthy term infants that were born in the same obstetric hospital, at age 6, were recruited and matched for variables. Participants were assessed at age 6, 8, and 26	Structured Mannheimer Parent Interview (MEI), Munich Composite International Interview Diagnostic Interviews, Life Course Interview and the Young Adult Self-Report	Study did not show persistently increased risk of anxiety or mood disorder over time. Study did show increased risk of anxiety disorder at age 8 and mood disorder at age 26 in VP/VLBW however these findings did not survive correction for multiple testing	
Ask et al. (2018)	n = 113 227 total children born at various GAs were included (55, 187 were born at 40 weeks GA, including 33, 081-siblings). children were assessed at age 5 and 8 years of age for symptoms of ADHD	Conner's Parent Rating Scale-Revised; Parent/Teacher Rating Scale for Disruptive Behavior Disorders	After accounting for unmeasured factors (genetic/environmental), early preterm birth was associated with a higher levels of ADHD symptoms in At age 5 and was associated with inattentive but not hyperactive symptoms at age 8-year-old	

Studies included if they have the first wave of assessments starting at school age even if they include waves of older individuals during adolescence or adulthood.

Key: ADHD, attention deficit hyperactivity; BPD, bronchopulmonary dysplasia; BWT, birth weight; CBCL, child behavior checklist; CSI-4, Child Symptom Inventory; DAWBA, developmental and well-being assessment; ELBW, extremely low birth weight; ELGAN, extremely low gestational age newborn; EP, extremely preterm; EPT, extremely preterm; FSIQ, full scale intelligence quotient; FTF, Five to Fifteen questionnaire; GA, gestational age; ICD, International Classification of Disease; LBW, low birth weight; MEI, Mannheimer Parent Interview; NDI, Neurodevelopmental Disorder Impairment; OR, odds ratio; RR, relative risk; SDQ, strengths and difficulties questionnaire; SES, Socioeconomic status; TRAB, Tester's Rating of Adult Behavior; TRCB, Teacher's Rating of Child Behavior; VLBW, very low birth weight; VPT, very preterm; YACBL, The Young Adult Behavior Checklist; YCI, Yale Children's Inventory.

the CSI-4 at age 10, and we have suggested that ADHD symptoms, even when identified by only a single observer, may provide valuable information about a child's functioning informing intervention efforts to help improve school performance (Leviton et al. 2017; O'Shea et al. 2013).

Psychiatric Comorbidity

We know of no other study that has assessed the burden of psychiatric comorbidity in EP children. We have found higher rates of internalizing and externalizing disorders as well as a significant number of psychiatric co-occurences in the ELGAN study that predicted school functioning, psychotropic medication exposure, and overall functioning (i.e. physical, emotional, social) (Dvir et al. in press). The greater the co-occurence of positive screens for psychiatric disorders, the more impairment in school, physical, emotional, and social functioning. Certain maternal characteristics were protective and predicted lower numbers of positive screens for psychiatric disorders (Dvir et al. in press). An enhanced understanding of the functional correlates of EP children screening positive on the CSI-4 for individual psychiatric disorders will provide information that has the potential to improve identification, treatment, and prevention efforts. In addition, the frequency of psychiatric co-occurence in EP children and its impact on day-to-day functioning are of central importance to the field as it will help guide clinicians in their diagnostic and treatment decisions.

POTENTIAL MECHANISM FOR PSYCHIATRIC OUTCOMES

There is increasing evidence in the psychiatric literature of an association between inflammation and psychiatric diagnoses. Unfortunately, the bulk of the literature assesses inflammatory markers at the time of the diagnosis and the literature provides little information about cause and effect or timing of the inflammation activation relative to the onset of the psychiatric disorder. A recent study found an association between elevated childhood interleukin 6 and hypomania in young adulthood (Hayes et al. 2017). Other evidence that inflammation precedes psychiatric symptom onset exists in the clinical domain in patients with pediatric acute-onset neuropsychiatric syndrome. In this disorder, infection always precedes the onset of neuropsychiatric disorders by definition (Swedo et al. 1998; Murphy et al. 2014), which is consistent with the possibility that inflammation contributes to the pathogenesis of these disorders. Just one experimental study directly addresses the temporal relationship between inflammation and psychiatric symptoms, in this case anxiety. Healthy male volunteers (19–30 years) were intravenously injected with endotoxin or saline in two experimental sessions. They then completed psychological questionnaires. Endotoxin induced a significant increase in several inflammatory markers and cortisol, and also an increase in anxiety levels. Increased anxiety appeared to be related to cytokine elevations, rather than hypothalamic pituitary axis system activation (Reichenberg et al. 2001).

Consistent with our original hypothesis that inflammation activation is associated with adverse neurodevelopmental outcomes, we found that persistent/recurrent elevations of seven inflammatory proteins during the first 2 weeks, were associated with a two- to 3.9-fold increased risk of having an attention problem (O'Shea et al. 2014). Similar to the findings at age 2, we found that a number of elevated inflammatory proteins during the first postnatal month were associated with ADHD symptoms at age 10 years as identified by the teacher, and that elevations of various neurotrophic proteins modified that increased risk (Allred et al. 2017). These findings have implications for possible early identification of those at highest risk for ADHD symptoms and for early intervention strategies that could target inflammation and decrease the risk of symptoms of ADHD.

The ELGAN study design affords us the opportunity to assess the temporal relationship between inflammation and mental health outcomes in EP born children as we found in our inflammatory protein and ADHD outcome papers. These relationships may inform future research work on psychiatric diagnosis onset and inflammation in both preterm and term born individuals. Towards that end, data analyses are currently underway exploring the associations between inflammatory and neurotrophic protein elevations and other psychiatric outcomes (e.g. CBCL-DP at age 2 and anxiety and depression at age 10). In addition, we will be adding new data points at age 15 that will further inform this work.

STRENGTHS AND WEAKNESSES OF THE ELGAN STUDY

The overall strengths of the ELGAN cohort are numerous including our large sample size, the representation of children born in three different regions of the United States, the selection of subjects based on gestational age and not birth weight, and the prospective longitudinal design with very little loss to follow-up (assessments at birth, age 2, age 10, now at age 15, and hopefully at age 18). A large number of subjects have returned for follow-up assessment at each time point allowing us to provide reliable estimates of psychiatric outcome prevalence rates. Limitations of the ELGAN study include our lack of a control group, and no direct evaluation of maternal psychiatric health at birth, age 2, and at age 10. In addition, the observational nature of the study design relied on parent and teacher reports both at age 2 and 10 years, using the CBCL and then the CSI-4, both of which are screening tools and not diagnostic instruments (Achenbach and Rescorla 2000; Gadow and Sprafkin 2002; Sprafkin et al. 2002); thus, not allowing us to draw strong conclusions regarding psychiatric disorders per se in ELGANs.

FUTURE DIRECTIONS

Given these limitations, the next important step will be to obtain maternal mental health information and to conduct comprehensive, standardized psychiatric diagnostic interviews, both of which we are doing in our next two waves of planned assessments (at age 15 years and 18 years). In addition, we will be looking at the placenta as a modulator of the inflammatory process (see Fig. 15.2) and the

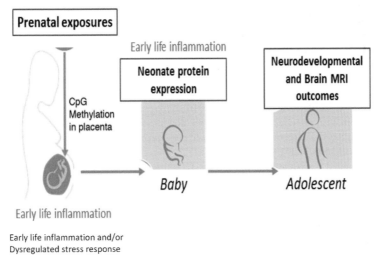

Figure 15.2   The ELGAN study focuses on the placenta, as a sensor and transducer of prenatal exposures such as inflammation and response to stress in the fetus. The relationships that have been studied (age 2 and 10 years) and will be studied (age 15 and 18 years) within ELGAN include: prenatal exposures, early life inflammation indicators, and later life health outcomes, including mental health outcomes. A color version of this figure can be found in the color plate section.

association of placental differences with various later life health outcomes including mental health outcomes.

Our prior findings and future directions should continue to advance our understanding of the associations of early inflammatory processes in children born extremely premature and later neuropsychiatric outcomes, and perhaps provide a neurobiological basis for early and aggressive intervention with this population of children.

REFERENCES

Achenbach TM, Rescorla LA (2000) *Manual for the ASEBA Preschool Forms and Profiles.* Burlington, VT: University of Vermont, Research Center for Children, Youth, & Families.

Allred EN, Dammann O, Fichorova RN et al. (2017) Systemic inflammation during the first postnatal month and the risk of attention deficit hyperactivity disorder characteristics among 10-year-old children born extremely preterm. *Journal of Neuroimmune Pharmacology* **12**: 531–43. doi: 10.1007/s11481-017-9742-9.

Ask H, Gustavson K, Ystrom E et al. (2018) Association of gestational age at birth with symptoms of attention-deficit/hyperactivity disorder in children. *JAMA Pediatrics* **172**: 749–56. doi: 10.1001/jamapediatrics.

Ayer L, Althoff R, Ivanova M et al. (2009) Child Behavior Checklist Juvenile Bipolar Disorder (CBCL-JBD) and CBCL Posttraumatic Stress Problems (CBCL-PTSP) scales are measures of a single dysregulatory syndrome. *Journal of Child Psychology and Psychiatry, and Allied Disciplines* **50**: 1291–300. doi: 10.1111/j.1469-7610.2009.02089.

Basten M, Althoff R, Tiemeier H et al. (2013) The dysregulation profile in young children: empirically defined classes in the Generation R study. *Journal of the American Academy of Child and Adolescent Psychiatry* **52**: 850.e2. doi: 10.1016/j.jaac.2013.05.007.

Bayley N (1993) *Bayley Scales of Infant Development: Manual.* New York: Psychological Corporation.

Biederman J, Petty CR, Clarke A, Lomedico A, Faraone SV (2011) Predictors of persistent ADHD: an 11-year follow-up study. *Journal of Psychiatric Research* **45**: 150–5. doi: 10.1016.

Boyd LA, Msall ME, O'Shea TM, Allred EN, Hounshell G, Leviton A (2013) Social–emotional delays at 2 years in extremely low gestational age survivors: correlates of impaired orientation/engagement and emotional regulation. *Early Human Development* **89**: 925–30. doi: 10.1016.

Breeman LD, Jaekel J, Baumann N, Bartmann P, Wolke D (2016) Attention problems in very preterm children from childhood to adulthood: the Bavarian Longitudinal Study. *Journal of Child Psychology and Psychiatry* **57**: 132–40. doi: 10.1111/jcpp.12456.

Carrow-Woolfolk E (1996) *Oral and Written Language Scales: Written Expression Scale Manual.* Circle Pines, MN: American Guidance Service.

Conrad AL, Richman L, Lindgren S, Nopoulos P (2010) Biological and environmental predictors of behavioral sequelae in children born preterm. *Pediatrics* **125**: 83. doi: 10.1542/peds.2009-0634 [doi].

Dammann O, Leviton A (2014) Intermittent or sustained systemic inflammation and the preterm brain. *Pediatr Res* **75**: 376–80. doi: 10.1038/pr.2013.238.

Delobel-Ayoub M, Arnaud C, White-Koning M et al. (2009) Behavioral problems and cognitive performance at 5 years of age after very preterm birth: the EPIPAGE study. *Pediatrics* **123**: 1485–92. doi: 10.1542/peds.2008-1216.

Delobel-Ayoub M, Kaminski M, Marret S et al. (2006) Behavioral outcome at 3 years of age in very preterm infants: the EPIPAGE study. *Pediatrics* **117**: 1996–2005. doi: 10.1542/peds.2005-2310.

Downey LC, O'Shea TM, Allred EN et al. (2015) Antenatal and early postnatal antecedents of parent-reported attention problems at 2 years of age. *The Journal of pediatrics* **166**: 25 e1. doi: 10.1016/j.jpeds.2014.08.004.

Dvir Y, Frazier J, Joseph R, Moore P et al. (in press) Psychiatric symptoms: prevalence and co-occurrence among extremely low gestational age newborns at age ten years. *Journal of Developmental and Behavioral Pediatrics.*

Elgen Fevang S, Hysing M, Sommerfelt K (2017) Mental health assessed by the Strengths and Difficulties Questionnaire for children born extremely preterm without severe disabilities at 11 years of age: a Norwegian, national population-based study. *European Child & Adolescent Psychiatry* **26**: 1523–31. doi: 10.1007/s00787-017-1007-x.

Elgen I, Sommerfelt K, Markestad T (2002) Population based, controlled study of behavioural problems and psychiatric disorders in low birthweight children at 11 years of age. *Archives of Disease in Childhood. Fetal and Neonatal Edition* **87**: 128. doi: 10.1136/fn.87.2.F128.

Elgen SK, Sommerfelt K, Leversen KT, Markestad T (2015) Minor neurodevelopmental impairments are associated with increased occurrence of ADHD symptoms in children born extremely preterm. *European Child & Adolescent Psychiatry* **24**: 463–70. doi: 10.1007/s00787-014-0597-9.

Elliott CD (2007) *Differential Ability Scales–Second edition (DAS-II).* San Antonio, TX: Harcourt Assessment.

Farooqi A, Hägglöf B, Sedin G, Gothefors L, Serenius F (2007) Mental health and social competencies of 10- to 12-year-old children born at 23 to 25 weeks of gestation in the 1990s: a Swedish national prospective follow-up study. *Pediatrics* **120**: 118–33. doi: 10.1542/peds.2006-2988.

Frazier JA, Wood ME, Ware J et al. (2015) Antecedents of the child behavior checklist-dysregulation profile in children born extremely preterm. *Journal of the American Academy of Child and Adolescent Psychiatry* **54**: 816–23. doi: 10.1016/j.jaac.2015.07.008.

Gadow KD, Sprafkin JN (2002) *Child Symptom Inventory 4: Screening and Norms Manual.* Stony Brook, NY: Checkmate Plus.

Gray PH, O'Callaghan MJ, Poulsen L (2008) Behaviour and quality of life at school age of children who had bronchopulmonary dysplasia. *Early Human Development* **84**: 1–8. doi: 10.1016/j.earlhumdev.2007.01.009.

Gray R, Indurkhya A, McCormick M (2004) Prevalence, stability, and predictors of clinically significant behavior problems in low birth weight children at 3, 5, and 8 years of age. *Pediatrics* **114**: 736–43. doi: 10.1542/peds.2003-1150-L.

Greenley RN, Taylor HG, Drotar D, Minich NM (2007) Longitudinal relationships between early adolescent family functioning and youth adjustment: an examination of the moderating role of very low birth weight. *Journal of Pediatric Psychology* **32**: 453–62. doi: 10.1093/jpepsy/jsl027.

Hack M, Taylor HG, Schluchter M, Andreias L, Drotar D, Klein N (2009) Behavioral outcomes of extremely low birth weight children at age 8 years. *Journal of developmental and behavioral pediatrics: JDBP* **30**: 122, doi: 10.1097/DBP.0b013e31819e6a16.

Hack M, Youngstrom EA, Cartar L et al. (2004) Behavioral outcomes and evidence of psychopathology among very low birth weight infants at age 20 years. *Pediatrics* **114**: 932–40. doi: 10.1542/peds.2003-1017-L.

Hagberg H, Dammann O, Mallard C, Leviton A (2004) Preconditioning and the developing brain. *Semin Perinatol* **28**: 389–95. [PubMed: 15693395].

Hagberg H, Mallard C, Ferriero DM et al. (2015) The role of inflammation in perinatal brain injury. *Nature Reviews Neurology* **11**: 192. doi: 10.1038/nrneurol.2015.13.

Hayes JF, Khandaker GM, Anderson J et al. (2017) Childhood interleukin-6, C-reactive protein and atopic disorders as risk factors for hypomanic symptoms in young adulthood: a longitudinal birth cohort study. *Psychological Medicine* **471**: 23–33. doi: 10.1017/S0033291716001574.

Hille ET, den Ouden AL, Saigal S et al. (2001) Behavioral problems in children who weigh 1000 g or less at birth in four countries. *Lancet* **357**: 1641–3. doi: 10.1016/S0140-6736(00)04818-2.

Hoff B, Hansen BM, Munck H, Mortensen EL (2004) Behavioral and social development of children born extremely premature: 5-year follow-up. *Scandinavian Journal of Psychology* **45**: 285–92. doi: 10.1111/j.1467-9450.2004.00407.x.

Hudziak JJ, Althoff RR, Derks EM, Faraone SV, Boomsma DI (2005) Prevalence and genetic architecture of Child Behavior Checklist-juvenile bipolar disorder. *Biological Psychiatry* **58**: 562–8. doi: 10.1016/j.biopsych.2005.03.024.

Huhtala M, Korja R, Lehtonen L et al. (2011) Parental psychological well-being and cognitive development of very low birth weight infants at 2 years. *Acta Paediatrica* **100**: 1555–60. doi: 10.1111/j.1651-2227.2011.02428.x.

Indredavik MS, Skranes JS, Vik T et al. (2005) Low-birth-weight adolescents: psychiatric symptoms and cerebral MRI abnormalities. *Pediatric Neurology* **33**: 259–66. doi: 10.1016/j.pediatrneurol.2005.05.002.

Jaekel J, Baumann N, Bartmann P, Wolke D (2018) Mood and anxiety disorders in very preterm/very low-birth weight individuals from 6 to 26 years. *Journal of Child Psychology and Psychiatry* **59**: 88–95. doi: 10.1111/jcpp.12787.

Janssen A, Nijhuis-van der Sanden M, Akkermans R, Oostendorp R, Kollée L (2008) Influence of behaviour and risk factors on motor performance in preterm infants at age 2 to 3 years. *Developmental Medicine and Child Neurology* **50**: 926–31. doi: 10.1111/j.1469-8749.2008.03108.x.

Janssens A, Uvin K, Van Impe H, Laroche S, Van Reempts P, Deboutte D (2009) Psychopathology among preterm infants using the diagnostic classification zero to three. *Acta Paediatrica* **98**: 1988–93. doi: 10.1111/j.1651-2227.2009.01488.x.

Johnson S, Hollis C, Kochhar P, Hennessy E, Wolke D, Marlow N (2010) Autism spectrum disorders in extremely preterm children. *The Journal of Pediatrics* **156**: 531 e2. doi: 10.1016/j.jpeds.2009.10.041.

Johnson S, Kochhar P, Hennessy E, Marlow N, Wolke D, Hollis C (2016) Antecedents of attention-deficit/hyperactivity disorder symptoms in children born extremely preterm. *Journal of Developmental and Behavioral Pediatrics: JDBP* **37**: 285. doi: 10.1097/DBP.0000000000000298.

Johnson S, Matthews R, Draper ES et al. (2015) Early emergence of delayed social competence in infants born late and moderately preterm. *Journal of Developmental & Behavioral Pediatrics* **36**: 690–9. doi: 10.1097/DBP.0000000000000222.

Korkman M, Kemp SL, Kirk U (1998) *NEPSY – A Developmental Neuropsychological Assessment.* San Antonio, TX: Psychological Corporation.

Kuban KC, O'Shea TM, Allred EN et al. 2014, Systemic inflammation and cerebral palsy risk in extremely preterm infants. *Journal of Child Neurology* **29**: 1692–8. doi: 10.1177/0883073813513335 [doi].

Leviton A, Hunter SJ, Scott MN et al. (2017) Observer variability identifying attention deficit/hyperactivity disorder in 10-year-old children born extremely preterm. *Acta Paediatrica* **106**: 1317–22. doi: 10.1111.

Leviton A, Kuban KC, Allred EN et al. 2011a, Early postnatal blood concentrations of inflammation-related proteins and microcephaly two years later in infants born before the 28th post-menstrual week. *Early Human Development* **87**: 325–30. doi: 10.1016/j.earlhumdev.2011.01.043 [doi].

Leviton A, Kuban K, O'Shea TM et al. (2011b) The relationship between early concentrations of 25 blood proteins and cerebral white matter injury in preterm newborns: the ELGAN study. *The Journal of Pediatrics* **158**: 5. doi: 10.1016/j.jpeds.2010.11.059 [doi].

Linsell L, Johnson S, Wolke D, Morris J, Kurinczuk JJ, Marlow N (2018) Trajectories of behavior, attention, social and emotional problems from childhood to early adulthood following extremely preterm birth: a prospective cohort study. *European Child & Adolescent Psychiatry* **28**: 531–42. doi: 10.1007/s00787-018-1219-8.

Loe IM, Lee ES, Luna B, Feldman HM (2011) Behavior problems of 9–16 year old preterm children: biological, sociodemographic, and intellectual contributions. *Early Human Development* **87**: 247–52. doi: 10.1016/j.earlhumdev.2011.01.023.

Meeuwsen M, Perra O, van Goozen SH, Hay DF (2018) Informants' ratings of activity level in infancy predict ADHD symptoms and diagnoses in childhood. *Development and Psychopathology* 1–15. doi: 10.1017/S0954579418000597.

Miller M, Bowen JR, Gibson FL, Hand PJ, Ungerer JA (2001) Behaviour problems in extremely low birthweight children at 5 and 8 years of age. *Child: Care, Health and Development* **27**: 569–81. doi: 10.1046/j.1365-2214.2001.00223.x.

Murphy T, Gerardi D, Leckman J (2014) Pediatric acute-onset neuropsychiatric syndrome. *Psychiatr Clin North Am* **37**: 353–74. doi: 10.1016/j.psc.2014.06.001.

Nadeau L, Boivin M, Tessier R, Lefebvre F, Robaey P (2001) Mediators of behavioral problems in 7-year-old children born after 24 to 28 weeks of gestation. *Journal of Developmental & Behavioral Pediatrics* **22**: 1–10. doi: 0196-206X/00/2201-0001.

O'Shea T, Joseph, R, Kuban, K et al. (2014) Elevated blood levels of inflammation-related proteins are associated with an attention problem at age 24 mo in extremely preterm infants. *Pediatric Research* **75**: 781. doi: 10.1038/pr.2014.41.

O'Shea T, Allred E, Kuban K et al. (2012) Elevated concentrations of inflammation-related proteins in postnatal blood predict severe developmental delay at 2 years of age in extremely preterm infants. *The Journal of Pediatrics* **160**: 401.e4. doi: 10.1016/j.jpeds.2011.08.069 [doi].

O'Shea T, Downey L, Kuban K (2013) Extreme prematurity and attention deficit: epidemiology and prevention. *Frontiers in Human Neuroscience* **7**: 578. doi: 10.3389/fnhum.2013.00578.

Palumbi R, Peschechera A, Margari M et al. (2018) Neurodevelopmental and emotional-behavioral outcomes in late-preterm infants: an observational descriptive case study. *BMC Pediatrics* **18**: 318. doi: 10.1186/s12887-018-1293-6.

Pharoah PO, Stevenson CJ, Cooke RW, Stevenson RC (1994) Prevalence of behaviour disorders in low birthweight infants. *Archives of Disease in Childhood* **70**: 271–4. doi: 10.1136/adc.71.4.386.

Polanczyk G, de Lima MS, Horta BL et al. (2007) The worldwide prevalence of ADHD: a systematic review and metaregression analysis. *Am J Psychiatry* **164**: 942–8.

Rautava L, Andersson S, Gissler M et al. (2010) Development and behaviour of 5-year-old very low birthweight infants. *European Child & Adolescent Psychiatry* **19**: 669–77. doi: 10.1007/s00787-010-0104-x.

Reichenberg, A, Yirmiya, R, Schuld, A et al. (2001) Cytokine-associated emotional and cognitive disturbances in humans. *Archives of General Psychiatry* **58**: 445–52. doi: 10.1001/archpsyc.58.5.445.

Reijneveld SA, De Kleine M, van Baar AL et al. (2006) Behavioural and emotional problems in very preterm and very low birthweight infants at age 5 years. *Archives of Disease in Childhood-fetal and Neonatal Edition* **91**: F428. doi: 10.1136/adc.2006.093674.

Retzler J, Johnson S, Groom M, Hollis C, Budge H, Cragg, L (2018) Cognitive predictors of parent-rated inattention in very preterm children: the role of working memory and processing speed. *Child Neuropsychology* **25**: 617–35. doi: 10.1080/09297049.2018.1510908.

Saigal S, Pinelli J, Hoult L, Kim MM, Boyle M (2003) Psychopathology and social competencies of adolescents who were extremely low birth weight. *Pediatrics* **111**: 969–75. doi: 10.1542/peds.111.5.969.

Samara M, Marlow N, Wolke D (2008) Pervasive behavior problems at 6 years of age in a total-population sample of children born at ≤ 25 weeks of gestation. *Pediatrics* **122**: 562–73. doi: 10.1542/peds.2007-3231.

Scott MN, Hunter SJ, Joseph RM et al. (2017) Neurocognitive correlates of ADHD symptoms in children born at extremely low gestational age. *Journal of Developmental and Behavioral Pediatrics: JDBP* **38**: 249. doi: 10.1097/DBP.0000000000000436.

Scott MN, Taylor HG, Fristad MA et al. (2012) Behavior disorders in extremely preterm/extremely low birth weight children in kindergarten. *Journal of Developmental and Behavioral Pediatrics* **33**: 202. doi: 10.1097/DBP.0b013e3182475287.

Sommerfelt K, Ellertsen B, Markestad T (1993) Personality and behaviour in eight-year-old, non-handicapped children with birth weight under 1500 g. *Acta Paediatrica* **82**: 723–8. doi: 10.1111/j.1651-2227.1993.tb12546.x.

Spittle AJ, Treyvaud K, Doyle LW et al. (2009) Early emergence of behavior and social-emotional problems in very preterm infants. *Journal of the American Academy of Child and Adolescent Psychiatry* **48**: 909–18. doi: 10.1097/CHI.0b013e3181af8235.

Sprafkin J, Gadow KD, Salisbury H, Schneider J, Loney J (2002) Further evidence of reliability and validity of the Child Symptom Inventory-4: parent checklist in clinically referred boys. *Journal of Clinical Child and Adolescent Psychology* **31**: 513–24. doi: 10.1207/S15374424JCCP3104_10.

Staller JA (2006) Diagnostic profiles in outpatient child psychiatry. *American Journal of Orthopsychiatry* **76**: 98–102. doi: 10.1037/0002-9432.76.1.98.

Stjernqvist K, Svenningsen NW (1999) Ten-year follow-up of children born before 29 gestational weeks: health, cognitive development, behaviour and school achievement. *Acta Paediatrica (Oslo, Norway: 1992)* **88**: 557–62. doi: 10.1111/j.1651-2227.1999.tb00175.x.

Stoll BJ, Hansen NI, Bell EF et al. (2015) Trends in care practices, morbidity, and mortality of extremely preterm neonates, 1993–2012. *Jama* **314**: 1039–51. doi: 10.1001/jama.2015.10244.

Sucksdorff M, Lehtonen L, Chudal R et al. (2015) Preterm birth and poor fetal growth as risk factors of attention-deficit/hyperactivity disorder. *Pediatrics* **136**: e599–608. doi: 10.1542/peds.2015-1043.

Swedo SE, Leonard HL, Garvey M et al. (1998) Pediatric autoimmune neuropsychiatric disorders associated with streptococcal infections: clinical description of the first 50 cases. *Focus* **155**: 264–71. doi: 10.1176/ajp.155.2.264.

Szatmari P, Saigal S, Rosenbaum P, Campbell D, King S (1990) Psychiatric disorders at five years among children with birthweights less than 1000g: a regional perspective. *Developmental Medicine and Child Neurology* **32**: 954–62. doi: 10.1111/j.1469-8749.1990.tb08117.x.

Taylor HG, Klein N, Minich NM, Hack M (2000) Middle-school-age outcomes in children with very low birth-weight. *Child Development* **71**: 1495–511. doi: 10.1111/1467-8624.00242.

Thomas R, Sanders S, Doust J et al. (2015) Prevalence of attention-deficit/hyperactivity disorder: a systematic review and meta-analysis. *Pediatrics* **135**: e994–1001.

Treyvaud K, Ure A, Doyle LW et al. (2013) Psychiatric outcomes at age seven for very preterm children: rates and predictors. *Journal of Child Psychology and Psychiatry* **54**: 772–9. doi: 10.1111/jcpp.12040.

Volk HE, Todd RD (2007) Does the Child Behavior Checklist juvenile bipolar disorder phenotype identify bipolar disorder?. *Biological Psychiatry* **62**: 115–20. doi: 10.1016/j.biopsych.2006.05.036.

Walshe M, Rifkin L, Rooney M et al. (2008) Psychiatric disorder in young adults born very preterm: role of family history. *European Psychiatry* **23**: 527–31. doi: 10.1016/j.eurpsy.2008.06.004.

Wechsler D (2009) *The Wechsler Individual Achievement Test-III*. Oxford, UK: Pearson Assessment.

Weindrich D, Jennen-Steinmetz C, Laucht M, Schmidt MH (2003) Late sequelae of low birthweight: mediators of poor school performance at 11 years. *Developmental Medicine and Child Neurology* **45**: 463–9. doi: 10.1017/S0012162203000860.

Weisglas-Kuperus N, Koot HM, Baerts W, Feeter WPF, Sauer PJJ (1998) Behaviour Problems of Very Low-Birthweight Children. *Developmental Medicine and Child Neurology* **35**: 406–16. doi: 10.1111/j.1469-8749.1993.tb11662.x.

Woodward LJ, Lu Z, Morris AR, Healey DM (2017) Preschool self regulation predicts later mental health and educational achievement in very preterm and typically developing children. *The Clinical Neuropsychologist* **31**: 404–22. doi: 10.1080/13854046.2016.1251614.

Concluding Chapter
Please Draw Your Own Conclusions

Alan Leviton, Olaf Dammann, T Michael O'Shea, and Nigel Paneth

This concluding chapter, like the introductory chapter, is about ideas, but in the introductory chapter the ideas are those that influenced the ELGAN study. In this chapter, the ideas are those we think the ELGAN study influenced. After you read this chapter, try to answer the question, 'What if the ELGAN study never happened?'

Before we proceed to the ideas/themes/concepts that are the essence of the ELGAN study, we address the issue of data quality. We begin at the beginning.

DATA QUALITY

In keeping with the axiom that the higher the data quality, the more accurate the inferences based on the data, we emphasized data quality early and throughout. We standardized data collection by creating manuals and data collection forms that minimized ambiguity. We then assessed how our colleagues used them, and subsequently made modifications until we felt we had minimized observer variability. We did this for data collected by the research nurses/assistants, sonologists, ophthalmologists, pathologists, developmentalists, and neurologists (Kuban et al. 2005, 2007, 2008; O'Shea et al. 2009).

Some of our 'exposure' variables posed a challenge. For example, we collected information about mothers' education and Medicaid (government-provided medical care insurance) eligibility at the time of birth and Medicaid eligibility at 24 months. Each is a valid indicator/correlate of socio-economic disadvantage. For reports based on follow-up assessments, we used Medicaid eligibility at 24 months as our indicator of socio-economic disadvantage because the 'missing rate' was lowest. We recognized that states varied in their eligibility criteria for Medicaid (more stringent in Michigan and North Carolina than in Massachusetts), but enrollment rates were invariably high for pregnant women in all states.

Because little was known about the quality of the data generated by our protein-concentration-measurement capability, we felt a strong need to go beyond the coefficient of variation and provide whatever evidence we could that our assessments were biologically valid (content validity). We showed that the recovery of organisms from the placenta was what would be expected based on placenta histology (Hecht et al. 2008) and newborn blood protein concentrations (Fichorova et al. 2011). Similarly, the placenta histology findings were consistent with the protein-measurement data (Hecht et al. 2011; Leviton et al. 2011c). In addition, the placenta bacteriology, the placenta histology, and the protein-measurement findings supported our dichotomy of indications for extremely preterm delivery (McElrath et al. 2008, 2011).

Neurocognition includes the abilities to concentrate, remember things, process information, learn, speak, and understand (National Cancer Institute). These are among the most important functions we wanted to assess at 10 years, and, cognizant of age-related limitations, at age 2 years. We wanted to identify limitations/impairments of attention, executive functions, language, reading, quantitative abilities, and social sensitivity/awareness.

We chose 'outcome' assessments that are standardized and well-accepted. While we still regard the Bayley Scales of Infant Development-Second Edition (BSID-II) as a reasonable choice for our assessment of cognitive and motor function at age 2 years, almost two-thirds of children who had a low BSID-II Mental Development Index (MDI) at age 2 years had a normal IQ ($\geq$70) at age 10 years (O'Shea et al. 2018).

Similarly, our screening instrument for autism spectrum disorders (ASD), the Modified Checklist for Autism in Toddlers (M-CHAT), identified high rates of screening positive among children who had a low BSID-II MDI, motor (Psychomotor Development Index; PDI), and vision or hearing impairments (Kuban et al. 2009). To maximize the validity of our ASD assessment at age 10 years, cases were identified based on a positive score on the Autism Diagnostic Observation Schedule-2 (ADOS-2) (Joseph et al. 2017). Among children in our cohort who satisfied this rigorous criterion for ASD at 10 years, almost half were not correctly screened by the M-CHAT at age 2 years (Kim et al. 2016b). In addition to a sensitivity of 52%, the M-CHAT had a specificity of 84%, a positive predictive value of 20%, and a negative predictive value of 96%. False-positive and false-negative rates were high among children with hearing and vision impairments. High false-positive rates also were associated with lower socioeconomic status (SES), motor and cognitive impairments and emotional/behavioral dysregulation at age 2 years.

Less easily handled were other disorders. Several authoritative groups recommend that when attention deficit disorders (ADD) are assessed with subjective criteria, information should be collected from multiple sources (e.g. parents and teachers) (Cao et al. 2014; Laplante et al. 2015). However, we found that parents and teachers often disagreed about whether or not a child had symptoms of ADD. On the other hand, when both teachers and parents agreed, the rate of identifying children who had an individual education plan, repeated a grade, or was assigned to a remedial class was minimally higher than when only the teacher identified the child as likely ADD or when only a parent identified the child as likely ADD (Leviton et al. 2017c). This prompted us to accept these single observer reports separating children identified by teachers and those identified by parents (Allred et al. 2017; Leviton et al. 2018c).

Executive dysfunctions represented another challenge. Executive functions have been divided into three separable but interacting components: working memory, inhibitory control, and mental shifting/cognitive flexibility (Diamond 2013). This trichotomy led us to assess children's performance on three corresponding measures individually: DAS-II Working Memory composite, NEPSY-II Inhibition Inhibition, and NEPSY-II Inhibition Switching, and a composite of these three (Leviton et al. 2018e, 2018f). Children who had a Z-score $\leq$−1 were considered to have that dysfunction.

At least 24 studies have reported that children and adults born very preterm have poorer social competence than others (Ritchie et al. 2015). We did not find any consensus about how best to define social awareness, social cognition, social information processing, social communication, and social motivation. The Social Responsiveness Scale (SRS) is a brief, parent-completed questionnaire designed to evaluate these social abilities (Constantino and Gruber 2012). We dichotomized scores at 65 (i.e. the 96th percentile in the general population) in order to maximize our identifying children who have clinically significant social limitations (Korzeniewski et al. 2017b, 2018; Babata et al. 2018).

To assess 'laterality preference', we used a modified version of the Dean Laterality Preference Schedule (Dean 1978). We found that 'mixed-handed' children were more likely than right-handed children to have limitations in verbal and nonverbal intellectual skills, attention, working memory, set-shifting, academic progress, and fine and gross motor function (Burnett et al. 2018). They were also more likely to satisfy criteria for ASD. Left-handed children did not differ appreciably from right-handed children.

THEMES

Gestational Age/Maturity

We view gestational age as the best available single measure of maturation. However, we also recognize how limited it is in summarizing maturity, and how much other information it also conveys (Leviton et al. 2005). Not all infants born at 25 weeks are similarly mature. Among the many variables that we collected that provide supplemental information about maturation are the Score for Neonatal Acute Physiology (SNAP-II) and its 'Perinatal Extension' (SNAP-PE-II), illness-severity scores that measure physiologic instability and provide information about the risk of death (Richardson et al. 2001).

One of the components of the SNAPs is lowest mean blood pressure. Some feel that ELGANs with their limited cerebral blood flow autoregulation are particularly susceptible to brain damage that might result from low blood pressure (du Plessis 2009).

Another component of the SNAPs is the lowest ratio of PaO_2/FiO_2, which can be viewed as an indicator of respiratory function, as well as an indicator of hypoxemia. Hypoxemia has also been viewed as a risk factor for brain damage in ELGANs. As recently as 2014, the author of a textbook on neonatal neurology wrote that the premyelinating oligodendrocyte (pre-OL) 'was demonstrated in experimental models to be vulnerable to injury by hypoxia ischemia and inflammation, the two key insults leading to human PVL' (Volpe 2014: 756). However, we have been unable to find documentation that hypoxia ischemia leads to human periventricular leukomalcia (PVL) (Gilles et al. 2018).

What the ELGAN Study Found

SNAPs

ELGANs who had high SNAP-II and SNAP-PE-II scores, indicative of physiologic instability, tended to receive relatively fewer kcal/kg/day than their peers (Bartholomew et al. 2013). They were also more likely than others to have morphologic abnormalities seen on cranial ultrasound scans obtained in the intensive care nursery (Dammann et al. 2010; Sisman et al. 2014) strabismus at age 2 years (VanderVeen et al. 2016), and at age 10 years have cognitive impairment (IQ, executive function, language ability), adverse neurological outcomes (epilepsy, impaired gross motor function), behavioral abnormalities (attention deficit disorder and hyperactivity), social dysfunction (autistic spectrum disorder), and education-related adversities (low school achievement and need for educational supports) (Logan et al. 2017, 2018d).

While physiologic instability may be in the causal chain between immaturity and brain injury (e.g. via hypoxemia and hypotension), it might also function as a correlate of postnatal events and characteristics associated with brain damage (e.g. bacteremia, necrotizing enterocolitis [NEC], BPD/CLD, systemic inflammation). We also invoke the high probability that physiologic instability conveys information about immaturity/vulnerability characteristics associated with brain damage (paucity of proteins with brain-protecting and brain-damage-repair capabilities).

HYPOXEMIA AND OTHER BLOOD GAS ABNORMALITIES

Every blood gas derangement (hypoxemia, hyperoxemia, hypocapnia, hypercapnia, and acidosis) during the first 72 postnatal hours (defined as a top quartile measurement on 1 day, and separately on 2 days) was associated with multiple indicators of brain damage (an echolucent/hypoechoic lesion or ventriculomegaly on a scan in the intensive care nursery, quadriparetic, diparetic, and hemiparetic cerebral palsy, microcephaly, and low BSID MDI and PDI at age 2 years) (Leviton et al. 2010b) and at age 10 years with a multiple different indicators, including low scores on components of the NEPSY-II (A Developmental NEuroPSYchological Assessment-II), WIAT-III (Wechsler Individual Achievement Test–Third Edition), and parent report of an individual education plan, repeating a grade or special remedial class placement (Leviton et al. 2017a).

Children who had a blood gas derangement were also more likely to have a high illness severity score during the first 12 postnatal hours (SNAP-II™) (Richardson et al. 2001). This supports the possibility that the blood gas derangements are indicators of physiologic instability/vulnerability/immaturity rather than contributors to brain damage. Because physiologically unstable newborns are at increased risk of all sorts of disorders and complications, it should come as no surprise that children with a blood gas derangement were more likely than their peers to have systemic inflammation during the first two postnatal weeks (Leviton et al. 2011a).

HYPOTENSION

Blood pressure in extremely premature infants increased directly with both increasing gestational age and postnatal age (Laughon et al. 2007). The decision to treat hypotension varied widely among the 14 medical centers of the ELGAN study. Indeed, treatment was associated more strongly with the center where care was provided than with gestational age and postnatal age. Systemic hypotension, however, was not associated with cerebral white matter lesions (Logan et al. 2011b), cerebral palsy (Logan et al. 2011b), or Bayley Scales Mental and Psychomotor indices of <70 (Logan et al. 2011a).

DEVELOPMENTAL REGULATION/MATURATION-DEPENDENT VULNERABILITY

We have applied the term 'developmental regulation' to all the developmental processes that change with increasing gestational age.

Oligodendrocyte precursors are much more vulnerable to adversities than are mature oligodendrocytes (Butts et al. 2008). In humans, this vulnerability is presumed to be maximum near gestational age 24 weeks. Growth factors that enhance oligodendrocyte development and survival are known as oligotrophins (Dammann and Leviton 1999).

Similarly, growth factors that that promote the development, survival, and function of neurons are considered to have neurotrophic properties and are identified as neurotrophins. Those that also influence the formation and maintenance of blood vessels are known as angioneurins (Zacchigna et al. 2008). The relationship between blood vessels and surrounding brain tissue has prompted recognition of the neurovascular unit (NVU) and its ability to regulate regional cerebral blood flow (CBF) and nutrient delivery (Iadecola 2017).

Our interest in neurotrophins began in the 1990s with two publications. The first had the following quote, 'massive cell death' that is part of the development of the vertebrate nervous system 'is thought to reflect the failure of … neurons to obtain adequate amounts of specific neurotrophic factors that are produced by the target cells and that are required for the neurons to survive. … These survival signals seem to act by suppressing an intrinsic cell suicide program' (Raff et al. 1993: 695). The second, just a year later, had this quote, 'Some of the developmental problems experienced by preterm newborns reflect a deprivation of placenta-provided hormones and growth factors during crucial stages of neurodevelopment' (Reuss et al. 1994: 743). This was the origin of what we have called the 'paucity of protectors' hypothesis mentioned in the introductory chapter. Most likely a consequence of developmental regulation (Dammann and Leviton 2004), this paucity reflects the ELGAN's inability to synthesize adequate amounts of growth factors capable of protecting the developing brain and other organs against adversities (Reuss et al. 1996; Dammann and Leviton 1999; Leviton et al. 1999). In utero, the mother and/or placenta provide what is needed. Ex utero, however, the very preterm newborn is deprived.

The 'paucity of protectors' hypothesis provides a potential explanation for why ELGANs are at such heightened risk of brain-related dysfunctions and limitations. If ELGANS were not yet able to provide the brain with sufficient neurotrophins to allow normal development, let alone protect against adversity, might exogenous neurotrophins allow normal brain development and protection? We found support within just a few years. 'In vitro studies have identified a class of biologic response modifiers loosely referred to as growth factors, which stimulate the cellular events of tissue regeneration' (Graves 1997). That same year, others wrote, 'Because of its potent neuroprotective actions in the developing brain, brain-derived neurotrophic factor (BDNF) may be a potential treatment for … forms of acute injury in the perinatal period' (Cheng et al. 1997). Additional support for BDNF as a protector, followed soon after (Tong and Perez-Polo 1998) as did support for neuregulin-1 as a protector (Dammann et al. 2008), and basic fibroblast growth factor (bFGF) as a protector/enhancer of repair (Ay et al. 1999).

These reports prompted us to include in our ELGAN study grant proposal the concept that some biologic response modifiers could function as protectors (damage minimizers, whether by reducing the extent of damage, or by enhancing repair) (Dammann and Leviton 2000). Because we were beginning to recognize that white matter damage included damage to axons (and neurons) as well as oligodendrocytes, we included in our wish list of proteins to measure those with oligotrophic and/or neurotrophic properties (Dammann et al. 2001).

What the ELGAN Study Found

Top-quartile concentrations of angioneurins (the collective name for all the proteins with angiogenic, neurotrophic, and oligotrophic properties) were associated with modestly reduced risks of ventriculomegaly (Leviton et al. 2018a), ADHD (Allred et al. 2017), learning limitations (Leviton et al. 2018b), social impairment (Korzeniewski et al. 2018), and more prominently reduced risks of executive dysfunctions (Leviton et al. 2018f).

'PLACENTAL INSUFFICIENCY' AND 'PLACENTAL DYSFUNCTION'

The terms 'placental insufficiency' and 'placental dysfunction', most commonly used for poor placental function, are often imprecisely defined or not defined at all (Hunt et al. 2016). Usually associated with preeclampsia and fetal growth restriction (FGR) (Fleiss et al. 2019), we use the term for the broad concept of the placenta's limited ability to transfer nutrients from the gravida to her fetus.

Placental insufficiency/dysfunction has been associated with altered expression of BDNF in the brain of the offspring (at least in sheep) (Reiss et al. 2004) and guinea pigs (Dieni and Rees 2005), and low placenta expression of bFGF (Seidmann et al. 2013). In addition, insulin-like growth factors (IGFs) in the placenta appear to control placental resource allocation needed for optimal fetal growth (Sferruzzi-Perri et al. 2017). Nevertheless, growth factor deficiency has only recently been added to the list of placenta dysfunctions (Abd Ellah et al. 2015).

What the ELGAN Study Found

ELGANs delivered for severe FGR and/or disorders associated with impaired placenta implantation were more likely than others to have low postnatal day-1 concentrations of insulin-like growth factor 1 (IGF) (Leviton et al. 2019), vascular endothelial growth factor (VEGF) (Leviton et al. 2017d), VEGF receptor 2 (VEGF-R2) (Leviton et al. 2017d), angiopoietin 1 (Ang-1) (Leviton et al. 2017d), placenta growth factor (PIGF) (Leviton et al. 2017d), neurotrophin 4 (NT-4) (Leviton et al. 2017b), and brain-derived neurotrophic factor (BDNF) (Leviton et al. 2017b).

FETAL GROWTH RESTRICTION (FGR)

At about the time the ELGAN study began, fetal growth restriction (FGR) in term-born children was associated with low placenta weight (Molteni et al. 1978), and with increased risk of low IQ and low academic achievements (Geva et al. 2006), while FGR preterm children (mean gestational age 32.5 weeks (Tolsa et al. 2004), <32 weeks (Regev et al. 2003) were known to have difficulties with attention (Tolsa et al. 2004), and to be at increased risk of bronchopulmonary dysplasia (BPD) (also known as chronic lung disease (CLD) of prematurity), and retinopathy of prematurity (ROP) (Regev et al. 2003).

What the ELGAN Study Found

The ELGAN study confirmed that FGR infants (defined as having a birth weight Z-score <−2) are at heightened risk of a small placenta (Hecht et al. 2007), BPD/CLD (Bose et al. 2009; Laughon et al. 2011b), and prethreshold ROP (Lee et al. 2015). FGR infants were also at increased risk of microcephaly at birth (McElrath et al. 2010). At age 2 years, former FGR ELGANs were at elevated risk of strabismus (VanderVeen et al. 2016). and a low BSID-II MDI (Helderman et al. 2012), while FGR girls, but not FGR boys, were at an increased risk of a low Psychomotor Development Index of the BSID-II (Streimish et al. 2012).

At age 10 years, compared to their peers whose birthweight was appropriate for gestational age, former FGR ELGANs were more likely to have lower scores on assessments of cognition and academic achievement, and also more likely to have phobias, obsessions, compulsions, social awareness impairments, autistic mannerisms, difficulty with semantics and speech coherence, and diminished social and psychosocial functioning (Korzeniewski et al. 2017a). Severe fetal growth restriction was also strongly associated with ASD among children who did not have cognitive limitations (Joseph et al. 2017). In addition, former FGR ELGANs were at increased risk of learning limitations (Leviton et al. 2018d) and an executive dysfunction (defined by low scores on an assessment that measures inhibition in the context of set shifting) (Korkman et al. 1998). The presumed increased risk of ADHD associated with FGR appears to have been masked by associations in our sample between ADHD and magnesium for seizure prophylaxis (Leviton et al. 2018c) (a surrogate for preeclampsia) (van Dijk and Oudejans 2011) and ROP (Lee et al. 2015) (another correlate of FGR).

The profile of elevated concentrations of cytokines, cytokine receptors, chemokines, adhesion molecules, and metalloproteinases seen in day-1 specimens from ELGANs delivered for spontaneous indications (i.e. preterm labor, membrane rupture, abruption, and cervical insufficiency) was rarely seen among ELGANs delivered for fetal indications (almost invariably severe FGR) and maternal indications (almost invariably preeclampsia) (McElrath et al. 2011). Although severely growth-restricted ELGANs were not at increased risk of systemic inflammation shortly after birth, by post-natal day 14 they were significantly more likely than their peers to have elevated concentrations of cytokines, chemokines, adhesion molecules, and a metalloproteinase (McElrath et al. 2013). This propensity continued to some extent to the end of the first postnatal month when FGR ELGANs were more likely than others to have top quartile concentrations of two cytokines, interleukin (IL) 1-beta and tumor necrosis factor (TNF-alpha), a chemokine (IL-8), and an adhesion molecule (intercellular adhesion molecule 1) (ICAM-1) (Leviton et al. 2016b).

As might be expected in light of their tendency to have a small placenta (Hecht et al. 2007) associated with placental insufficiency (Gaccioli and Lager 2016; Audette and Kingdom 2017), FGR ELGANs were also more likely than their peers to have low day-1 concentrations of IGF-1 (Leviton et al. 2019), NT-4 (Leviton et al. 2017b), BDNF (Leviton et al. 2017b), VEGF (Leviton et al. 2017d), VEGF-R2 (Leviton et al. 2017d), Ang-1 (Leviton et al. 2017d), and PlGF (Leviton et al. 2017d).

THE 'STERILE WOMB' HYPOTHESIS

According to the 'sterile womb' hypothesis, the uterus is normally sterile and the newborn first acquires microbes during and after birth (Funkhouser and Bordenstein 2013). This does appear to apply to deliveries at term (Theis et al. 2019). On the other hand, evidence continues to mount that microbial communities are present in the placenta and amniotic fluid of deliveries before term (Willyard 2018).

What the ELGAN Study Found

Even though approximately half of the placentas harbored organisms within the chorionic plate, bacterial deoxyribonucleic acid could not be identified by polymerase chain reaction methods (Onderdonk et al. 2008a). Of all Cesarean deliveries during the 27th week of gestation, a microorganism was cultured from the placenta parenchyma of 43% of infants delivered following labor, 60% of deliveries following membrane rupture, and 23% of deliveries prompted by severe preeclampsia (Onderdonk et al. 2008b). The ELGAN study findings support the existence of a prenatal microbiome among an appreciable percentage of women who deliver months before term.

We consider the recovered microorganisms to be biologically important and not merely contaminants because organism recovery at birth was associated with echolucent brain lesions (Olomu et al. 2009) and ROP (Chen et al. 2011), first evident when the infant was in the intensive care nursery, and at 2 years of age with attention deficit symptoms (Downey et al. 2015), and microcephaly, as well as less extreme reduction in head circumference (Leviton et al. 2010d).

POLYMICROBIAL PLACENTA CULTURES

Polymicrobial infections can be clinically very important and continue to be the focus of exciting research (Stacy et al. 2016; Whiteley et al. 2017; Bowen et al. 2018; Brown et al. 2018; Frost et al. 2018). They are not necessarily indicative of 'contamination.'

What the ELGAN Study Found

More than 30% of the placentas delivered for preterm labor, preterm premature rupture of membrane (pPROM), placental abruption, and cervical insufficiency harbored more than one microorganism, while only 4% of placentas delivered for preeclampsia and 11% of of placentas delivered for fetal indications harbored multiple microorganisms (Onderdonk et al. 2008b).

Polymicrobial placenta cultures predicted both cranial ultrasound-defined echolucent/hypoechoic lesions, as well as diparetic cerebral palsy (Leviton et al. 2010a). Consequently, we are reluctant to consider these organisms contaminants. By documenting the clinical significance of polymicrobial infections of the placenta, we add to the recent literature emphasizing the importance of polymicrobial infections to preterm birth (Payne and Bayatibojakhi 2014).

INFLAMMATION

When compared to adults and infants born at term, ELGANs appear less able to respond effectively to an inflammatory/infectious stimulus (Schuller et al. 2018). In part, this reflects the ELGAN's immune system orientation to maintaining tolerance to maternal antigens and avoiding inflammation-triggered preterm delivery (van Well et al. 2017). On the other hand, newborns can display enhanced (Schultz et al. 2002), excessive (Nanthakumar et al. 2011), and 'robust if not enhanced' (Kollmann et al. 2009) inflammatory responses.

Systemic inflammation can contribute to brain damage in ELGANs (Strunk et al. 2014; Hagberg et al. 2015), as well as be a consequence of brain damage (Morganti-Kossmann et al. 2018).

What the ELGAN Study Found

Our additions to this literature include the fairly consistent observations of decreasing concentrations of inflammation-related proteins with increasing gestational age (Leviton et al. 2011b). We found this inverse pattern both in children whose placenta was inflamed and whose placenta was not inflamed, documenting that our observations were not confounded by the association of low gestational with intra-amniotic inflammation.

Each of the following disorders and limitations has a newborn systemic inflammation signature: early and persistent pulmonary dysfunction (Laughon et al. 2011a; Bose et al. 2013), normal early pulmonary function followed by pulmonary deterioration (Laughon et al. 2011a), prolonged ventilation assistance (Bose et al. 2013), BPD/CLD (Bose et al. 2011), ROP (Holm et al. 2017b), bacteremia (Leviton et al. 2012), ventriculomegaly (Leviton et al. 2016a, 2018a), an echolucent/hypoechoic ultrasound image (Leviton et al. 2018a), neuro-ophthalmologic dysfunctions (Holm et al. 2017a), low intelligence (Leviton et al. 2013, 2016a; O'Shea et al. 2012, 2013; Kuban et al. 2017), microcephaly (Leviton et al. 2016a), overweight and obesity at 2 years (Perrin et al. 2018), cerebral palsy (Kuban et al. 2014), executive dysfunctions (Leviton et al. 2018f), learning disorders (Leviton et al. 2018b), attention-deficit disorder (ADD) (O'Shea et al. 2014; Allred et al. 2017), ASD (Korzeniewski et al. 2018), and social limitations (Korzeniewski et al. 2018).

SUSTAINED INFLAMMATION

The effects of prolonged exposure to inflammatory stimuli have only recently been studied in vivo (Wickens et al. 2018). Even a relatively brief inflammation-provoking exposure can be followed by an inflammatory response lasting weeks (Singer et al. 2016), and even months (Osborne et al. 2017).

What the ELGAN Study Found

When we had measurements for only the first two postnatal weeks, we hedged our bets and identified elevated concentrations of inflammation-related proteins on two or more days a week apart as 'intermittent or sustained' inflammation (Dammann and Leviton 2014). Only with our measuring the concentrations of proteins in specimens collected during the second half of the first postnatal month could we show that the so-called intermittent or sustained inflammation can be sustained for much of the first postnatal month (Dammann et al. 2016).

ELGANs who had elevated concentrations of inflammation-related proteins on two or more days during the first two postnatal weeks were more likely than all others to be at increased risk of a brain dysfunction evident at age 2 years (O'Shea et al. 2012, 2013; Dammann and Leviton 2014). At age 10 years, we also found increased risk of ADD (Allred et al. 2017), executive dysfunctions (Leviton et al. 2018f), low scores on measures of reading and mathematics achievement (Leviton et al. 2018b), ASD (Korzeniewski et al. 2018), and social impairment (Korzeniewski et al. 2018).

Our findings are in keeping with advances in neurobiology. During development, microglia, play a role assisting with neuronal survival and proliferation, synapse pruning, and synapse formation and function (Mosser et al. 2017). Exposure to inflammatory stimuli transform microglia from their physiological surveillant state to a primed state (Mosser et al. 2017). Some of these primed microglia can persist throughout the lifespan of mice (Hammond et al. 2019), and promote damaging processes, apparently via epigenetic regulators such as microRNAs (miRNAs) (Karthikeyan et al. 2016). Because miRNAs play a role in normal brain development (Radhakrishnan and Alwin Prem Anand 2016), altering the miRNA environment has the potential to alter/distort brain development (Srivastav et al. 2018), as well as promote on-going inflammation (Gaudet et al. 2018).

TWO-HITS

The first publication to have two 'hit' and multiple 'hit' in the title was published in 1969 (Ashley 1969). It summarized the evidence that the occurrence of cancer in large populations was best modeled in light of the cumulative exposure to malignancy-provocations.

We first invoked a multi-hit view of organ damage in preterm newborns 35 years later (Dammann et al. 2004), just about the time when basic science data (Eklind et al. 2001; Yang et al. 2004) documented that lipopolysaccharide 'primes the (immature) brain to become more sensitive to later events' (Eklind et al. 2006: 161). Since then, meager evidence has come from the study of preterm humans (Glass et al. 2008).

What the ELGAN Study Found

In the ELGAN study population, virtually all of the indicators of brain damage and dysfunction have both antenatal and postnatal antecedents. On the other hand, we have shown that the two-hit model of brain damage applies at age 2 years to low BSID MDIs (with severe FGR as the first hit and postnatal systemic inflammation as the second hit) (Leviton et al. 2013). Similarly, the combination of placental inflammation (as the first hit) and postnatal systemic inflammation (as the second hit), was associated with increased risk of spastic cerebral palsy (Yanni et al. 2017), and microcephaly (Yanni et al. 2017). We are sensitive to the possibility that the first hit could also diminish the adverse consequences of the second hit (Hagberg et al. 2004).

INFLAMMATION AND GROWTH FACTORS

Our interest in the modulation of risk was enhanced by reports that LPS (a powerful inflammation stimulant) can increase the expression of neurotrophin-3 (NT-3) (Elkabes et al. 1998), nerve growth factor (NGF) (Heese et al. 1998), and BDNF (Miwa et al. 1997) in rodent microglia, and of NGF, BDNF, and NT-3 in mouse splenocytes (Barouch et al. 2000). These findings further increased our interest in communication between immune and central nervous systems (da Silva Meirelles et al. 2017).

What the ELGAN Study Found

Elevated blood concentrations of inflammation-related proteins were at times accompanied by same-day elevated blood concentrations of NT4, BDNF, and bFGF (Leviton et al. 2017b), VEGF, VEGFR-1, VEGFR-2, PIGF, and Ang-1, Ang-2 (Leviton et al. 2017d), as well as IGF-1 and its binding protein, IGFBP-1 (Leviton et al. 2019).

Elevated blood concentrations of angio-neurotrophic proteins appeared to modulate the increased risks of ROP associated with elevated blood concentrations of inflammation-related proteins (Holm et al. 2017b), while elevated blood concentrations of angio-neurotrophic proteins appeared to modulate the increased risks of the following at age 10 years: cognitive impairment (Kuban et al. 2018), low scores on measures of reading and mathematics achievement (Leviton et al. 2018b), ADD (Allred et al. 2017), executive dysfunctions (Leviton et al. 2018f), as well as ASD and high scores on assessments of social impairment (Korzeniewski et al. 2018).

Our findings support the possibility that exogenous neurotrophins can diminish brain damage and dysfunction in ELGANs (Wang et al. 2018). On the other hand, we recognize the potential danger of providing ELGANs with exogenous neurotrophins. Because they play a critical role in regulating neuronal survival and pruning/sculpting synapses (Zagrebelsky and Korte 2014), exogenous neurotrophins pose the danger of altering normal brain development.

INFLAMMATION HAS EPIGENETIC EFFECTS

Bacteria, whether in the gut, or the placenta, can promote epigenetic phenomena (Lu and Claud 2018). So which comes first, epigenetic phenomena or systemic inflammation and does it matter? Although it is highly likely to matter (Fitzgerald et al. 2018), we cannot answer the question based on ELGAN study data. On the other hand, cross-talk does occur between inflammation and epigenetic factors (Shen et al. 2017).

What the ELGAN Study Found

Just as we found that bacteria in the placenta (Fichorova et al. 2011), and inflammation in the bowel (Martin et al. 2013), promote systemic inflammation, we also found that bacteria-dependent epigenetic patterning occurs in the placenta (Tomlinson et al. 2017), and predicts cognitive function at age 10 years (Meakin et al. 2018; Tilley et al. 2018).

SOCIO-ECONOMIC DISADVANTAGES

Children born preterm into families with socioeconomic disadvantages tend to have lower cognition, language, reading, and math achievement scores than their peers born into families with socioeconomic advantages (ElHassan et al. 2018). One of the major explanations for this disparity invokes allostatic load, the term applied to the stress that accompanies/follows from the need for constant adaptation

(McEwen and Wingfield 2010). As they struggle to earn a living, pay bills, and make decisions about what is absolutely essential (Duncan et al. 2017), stressed parents appear less able than others to nurture, stimulate, and respond to their children's needs (Kim et al. 2016a), which is also reflected in the child's academic limitations (Clark and Woodward 2015).

Other explanations invoke the effects of genetics (Plomin and Deary 2015), epigenetic phenomena (Kundakovic and Jaric 2017), pro-inflammatory tendencies (Gilman et al. 2017), and high levels of stress on cortisol synthesis and metabolism (Ursache et al. 2017). One 'biological-embedding' model postulates that early adversity is 'embedded' in immune cells, resulting in a 'pro-inflammatory pheno-type' that persists for years and perhaps decades (Ehrlich et al. 2016).

Evaluations of the relationship between socioeconomic disadvantage and inflammation in children have studied the gravida's blood (Gilman et al. 2017), the placenta (Miller et al. 2017), cord blood (Miller et al. 2017), infant's saliva (David et al. 2017), and the blood of school-age children (Mansur et al. 2016), but had not measured the concentrations of inflammation-related proteins in the blood of ELGANs during the weeks following birth.

What the ELGAN Study Found

The ELGAN study filled in this knowledge gap showing that the risks of top quartile concentrations of multiple inflammation-related proteins on multiple days during the first 2 weeks were increased for each of three indicators/correlates of socioeconomic disadvantage (i.e. mother's eligibility for govern-ment-provided medical care insurance (Medicaid), mother's formal education level, and mother's IQ approximated with the Kaufman Brief Intelligence Test – 2), while the risks of top quartile concentra-tions of selected neurotrophic proteins were reduced (Leviton et al. 2019). Separately, we found that adjustment for socioeconomic disadvantage did not alter the relationships between protein concentra-tions and both low IQ and low working memory 10 years later.

At age 10 years, socioeconomic disadvantage (whether classified by maternal education at birth or 10 years later) was associated in our cohort with significantly poorer neurocognitive and academic outcomes (Joseph et al. 2018). However, adjusting for socioeconomic disadvantage did not reduce the magnitude of the relationships between protein concentrations and both low IQ and low working memory 10 years later. This suggests that our reports of the increased risk of neurocognitive and other limitations at age 10 years associated with high concentrations of inflammatory proteins and low concentrations of proteins with neu-rotropic properties are not confounded by socioeconomic status, but that links between maternal/family socioeconomic disadvantage and the child's neurocognitive function include inflammatory propensities, and diminished abilities to modulate the adverse effects of inflammation.

ELEVATED BODY MASS INDEX

The idea that maternal over-nutrition (pre-pregnancy overweight and obesity) might have adverse effects on fetal brain development is a relatively new idea (Rodriguez et al. 2008). During the early years of ELGAN study data analysis, a flurry of papers added support for what some have called the 'over-nutrition hypoth-esis' (Lawlor et al. 2007) applied to the child's cognition and behavior (Van Lieshout et al. 2011).

What the ELGAN Study Found

In a series of papers exploring the relationship between mother's pre-pregnancy overweight and obesity and her offspring's wellbeing, we found that during the first postnatal month, among ELGANs deliv-ered for maternal or fetal indications (but not for spontaneous indications), those whose mother was overweight or obese were more likely than others to have elevated concentrations of inflammation proteins (van der Burg et al. 2013). At age 2 years, infants born to overweight and obese women were not at increased risk of cerebral palsy (van der Burg et al. 2018), while children born to obese mothers (but not to overweight mothers) were more likely than others to have BSIDs more than 3 standard deviations below the reference mean (van der Burg et al. 2015). Some of this impaired development does not appear to be due to confounding associated with immaturity, socio-economic correlates or neonatal systemic inflammation (van der Burg et al. 2015).

Both maternal pre-pregnancy overweight and obesity were associated with increased risk at 10 years of parent-identified ADD characteristics (van der Burg et al. 2017), and low scores on assessments of verbal IQ, processing speed, visual fine motor control, and spelling (Jensen et al. 2017). Children born to mothers who gained a relatively high or a relatively low amount of weight during the pregnancy were at increased risk of a low score on an oral expression assessment. The children whose mother was in the low weight-gain group were also at increased risk of a low score on a reading assessment.

We remain unsure to what extent inflammation contributes to the cognitive and behavioral limitations of former ELGANs born to overweight and obese mothers. Nevertheless, the ELGAN study's major addition to the literature is probably our exploration of the possibility that inflammation might be involved (van der Burg et al. 2016).

TWINS AND TRIPLETS

When our highly valued coordinator was informed she was carrying twins, we felt the need to explore what was in the ELGAN study relevant to multiple births. We were aware that in decades past, full-term twins tended to have lower IQs than singletons (Voracek and Haubner 2008). In recent years, however, the differences between twins and singletons have diminished (Deary 2012). Explanations for this include improvements in obstetric and neonatal care, and the association of twinning with assisted reproductive technologies, which are more often utilized by women from higher socioeconomic categories, which, in turn, is associated with neurocognitve advantages (Datta et al. 2016).

What the ELGAN Study Found

After adjusting for confounders, the 306 products of multiple birth pregnancies (245 twins, 55 triplets, and six septuplets) performed significantly better on one of six subtests of executive function than their 568 singleton peers (Logan et al. 2019). Otherwise, performance was similar on all other assessments of neurocognitive function. Our findings should provide some reassurance that multi-fetal pregnancy, even among infants born extremely preterm, is not associated with limitations of neurocognitive function.

COMORBIDITIES

Low intelligence, executive dysfunctions, learning disorders, ADD, ASD, social limitations, communication difficulties, and psychiatric disorders tend to occur together in children born extremely preterm (Ding et al. 2018). Indeed, the term 'preterm behavioral phenotype' has been applied to the constellation of 'symptoms and disorders associated with anxiety, inattention, and social and communication problems, and manifest in a significantly higher prevalence of emotional disorders, ADHD and autism' (Johnson and Wolke, 2013: 199) Others have added the word 'complex' to a single entity that tends to co-occur with other entities (e.g. 'complex' attention-deficit hyperactivity disorder) (Koolwijk et al. 2014).

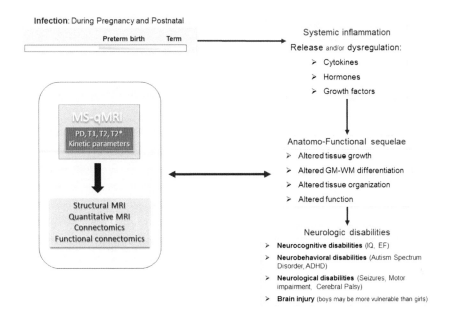

Figure 11.1 The ELGAN hypotheses and the MS-qMRI channels of information.

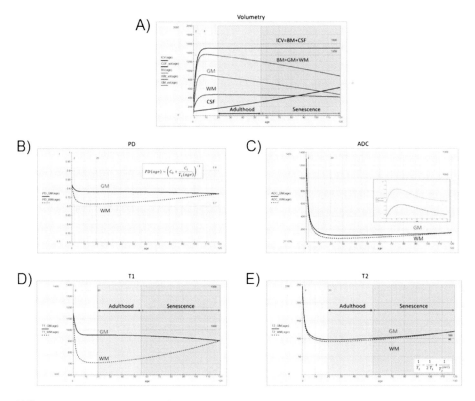

Figure 11.2 Brain qMRI parameters as functions of advancing age.

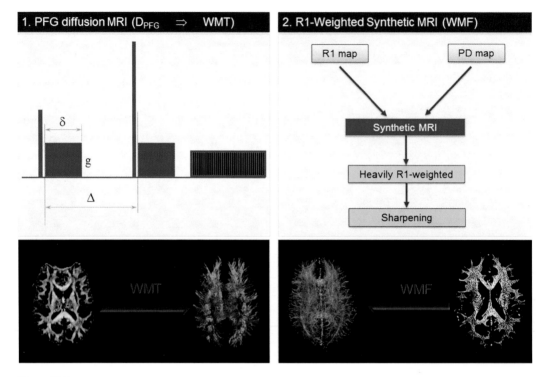

Figure 11.3 dMRI-WMT and WMF.

Theoretical Context: Longitudinal Relaxation in White Matter

$$(R1)_{total} = (R1)_{kin} + (R1)_{MT} + (R1)_{para}$$

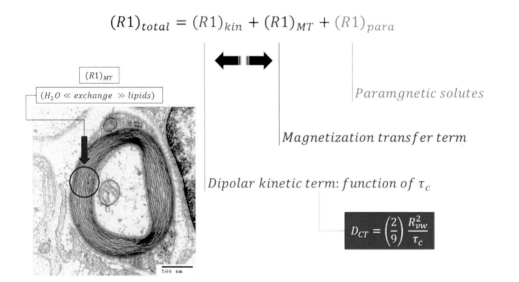

Figure 11.4 The structure of myelin: Implications for qMRI.

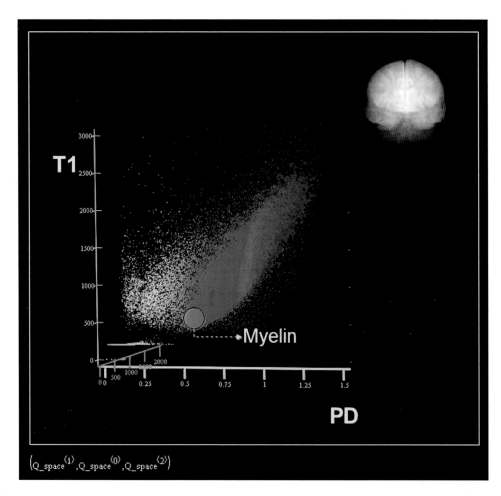

Figure 11.5 qMRI space of normal brain.

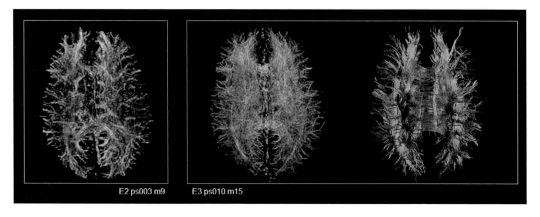

Figure 11.6 WMF: From E2 to E3 and MS-qMRI reports.

The ELGAN Study

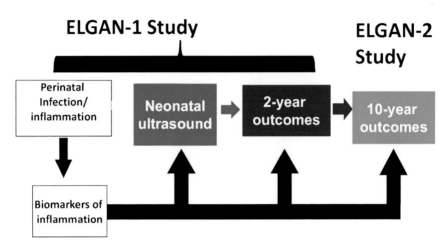

Figure 15.1 The ELGAN study examines the extent to which early life inflammation is predictive of structural brain disorders and of neurodevelopmental impairments in the ELGAN cohort. These relationships have been studied at age 2 and 10 years.

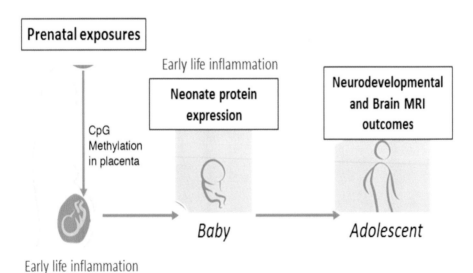

Figure 15.2 The ELGAN study focuses on the placenta, as a sensor and transducer of prenatal exposures such as inflammation and response to stress in the fetus. The relationships that have been studied (age 2 and 10 years) and will be studied (age 15 and 18 years) within ELGAN include: prenatal exposures, early life inflammation indicators, and later life health outcomes, including mental health outcomes.

Comorbidities have been attributed to socioeconomic influences (Deary and Johnson 2010), higher rates of stress and parental psychopathology (Deault 2010), epigenetics (Kiser et al. 2015), limited levels of 'cognitive reserve' (Koenen et al. 2009), common alterations to the connectome (Smyser et al. 2019), and network dynamics and control (Leviton et al. 2015).

What the ELGAN Study Found

Among the disorders identified when the ELGAN was in the intensive care nursery, NEC (Bell stage IIIb) was the only one that clustered with ROP, BPD/CLD, and cerebral white matter damage (defined as an echolucent/hypoechoic lesion, or moderate or severe ventriculomegaly on a protocol cranial ultrasound scan) (Leviton et al. 2010c). The most parsimonious explanation is that the systemic inflammation resulting from NEC (Martin et al. 2013) contributes to the damage of other organs, each of which is associated with systemic inflammation (Bose et al. 2011; Leviton et al. 2011d, 2018a; Holm et al. 2017b). Children who had stage 3+ (severe) ROP were also more likely than others at age 2 years to have low BSID MDIs and PDIs, and a head circumference more than 2 standard deviations below the expected mean (Allred et al. 2014).

When our subjects were 10 years old, we looked for the co-occurrence of four major neurologic impairments, cognitive impairment (defined as IQ and executive function scores more than 1.5 SD below the norm), cerebral palsy (CP), ASD, and epilepsy (Hirschberger et al. 2018). A total of 19% had one diagnosis, 10% had two diagnoses, 3% had three diagnoses, and none had all four diagnoses. Compared to children who were not cognitively impaired, those who had cognitive impairment had more than five times the risk of CP and/or epilepsy, and seven times the risk for having an ASD.

In a separate search for the clustering of other dysfunctions at age 10 years, we separated IQ from executive dysfunctions (impairments of working memory, inhibition, and ability to switch tasks). To see how much co-occurrence of the disorders assessed at age 10 years exceeded what would be expected if the occurrence of each disorder was independent of each other, we calculated observed to expected ratios for each set of disorders. The bottom line of Table 16.1 provides the observed frequency of each dysfunction/disorder. An IQ of less than 70 occurred in 15% of children, while an IQ in the 70–84 range occurred in 18%.

Examples of comorbidity have also been identified in ELGAN study publications about ADD (Scott et al. 2017), learning limitations (Akshoomoff et al. 2017), social sensitivity (Korzeniewski et al. 2017b), BPD (Sriram et al. 2018), SNAP (Logan et al. 2017), latent profile analyses (Heeren et al. 2017), strabismus (VanderVeen et al. 2016), bacteremia (Bright et al. 2017), maternal education (Joseph et al. 2018), visual field defects (Holm et al. 2015), and impaired visual fixation (Phadke et al. 2014).

The expected co-occurrence of two disorders is the product of the observed occurrence of each. A reading learning limitation (defined as a WIAT Word Read Z-score ≤-1) and a math learning limitation (defined as a WIAT Numerical Operations Z-score ≤-1) co-occurred in 23% of children. The expected co-occurrence if each learning limitation was independent of the other is 12%. The probability that the resulting observed/expected ratio of 1.9 occurred by chance is <0.001. Consequently, we draw the inference that these two dysfunctions co-occur more commonly than expected if they were independent. We draw the same inference for all the other statistically significant associations in the table. The ELGAN study is probably unique in having looked at all of them together.

We are not able to explain why co-morbidity is such an important characteristic of the cognitive and behavioral profile. Possible explanations include common antecedents (contributing to enhanced inflammation and epigenetic phenomena), and shared consequences of alterations to the connectome (Smyser et al. 2019).

Table 16.1 The ratio of observed/expected occurrences of two disorders together. **Bolded ratios** are statistically significantly different from 1 at a p-value <0.001. Ratios ≥2 are <u>underlined</u>

		2	3	4	5	6	7	8	9	10	11	12	13
Disorders		WM	II	IS	ED	Read	Math	ADp	ADt	AXp	AXt	SRS	ASD
1a	IQ < 70	2.7	1.6	1.7	3.5	2.9	2.3	1.7	1.8	1.2	1.5	2.2	4.4
1b	IQ 70–84	1.9	1.3	1.6	1.9	1.6	1.6	1.0	1.8	1.0	1.3	1.1	0.9
2	Work Mem		1.4	1.5	2.9	2.1	1.8	1.4	1.7	1.2	1.5	1.6	2.1
3	Inhib-Inhib			1.3	1.8	1.4	1.3	1.2	1.2	0.9	1.2	1.1	1.3
4	Inhib-Switch				1.8	1.5	1.5	1.2	1.3	1.1	1.3	1.3	1.5
5	Exec dysf					2.4	2.0	1.5	1.8	1.0	1.4	4.6	2.5
6	Read						1.9	1.4	1.7	1.0	1.2	1.6	1.9
7	Math							1.4	1.4	1.2	1.3	1.5	1.9
8	ADHD-P								1.8	2.7	1.9	2.4	2.2
9	ADHD-T									1.1	2.0	1.4	1.0
10	Anxiety-P										2.0	1.5	2.3
11	Anxiety-T											1.6	1.4
12	SRS total												3.8
Percent		36%	57%	56%	26%	30%	39%	21%	23%	11%	8%	24%	7%

IQ: Mean of DAS-II Verbal and Nonverbal Reasoning standard scores; **Work Mem**: DAS-II Working Memory Z-score ≤–1; **Ini-Ini**: NEPSY-II Inhibition-Inhibition combined scaled score Z-score ≤–1; **Ini-Switch**: NEPSY-II Inhibition-Switching combined scaled score Z-score ≤–1; **Exec dysf.**: Executive dysfunction surrogate (Work Mem and Ini-Ini and Ini-Switch); Read: WIAT-III Word reading Z-score ≤–1; **Math**: WIAT-III Numerical Operations Z-score ≤–1; **ADHD-P**: Parent CSI-4 screen in on ADHD; **ADHD-T**: Teacher CSI-4 screen in on ADHD; **Anxiety-P**: Parent CSI-4 screen in on Generalized anxiety, or Social phobia, or Separation anxiety; **Anxiety-T**: Teacher CSI-4 screen in on Generalized anxiety or Social phobia; **SRS total**: Social Responsiveness Scale total T score ≥65; **ASD**: Autism Spectrum Disorder diagnosis.

SUMMARY

The achievements of the ELGAN study are broad and not easily summarized. In addition, our own investments in this project limit our ability to take an objective, distant, and dispassionate view of the significance of what the ELGAN study found.

We merely point out that our main goal was to see if inflammatory phenomena outside the brain influenced the risk of brain damage in ELGANs. We have done that by reporting that systemic inflammation during the first postnatal month is associated with histologic placenta inflammation (Hecht et al. 2011; Leviton et al. 2011c), recovery of bacteria from the placenta parenchyma (Fichorova et al. 2011), the pregnancy disorders that initiate spontaneous preterm delivery (i.e. preterm labor, pre-labor rupture of membranes, and cervical 'insufficiency') (McElrath et al. 2008, 2011), fetal growth restriction (McElrath et al. 2013), indicators/correlates of socioeconomic disadvantage (Leviton et al. 2019), assisted ventilation for 14 or more than days (Bose et al. 2013), BPD/CLD (Bose et al. 2011), ROP (Holm et al. 2017b), NEC (Martin et al. 2013), low intelligence (O'Shea et al. 2012, 2013; Leviton et al. 2013; Kuban et al. 2017), cerebral palsy (Kuban et al. 2014), executive dysfunctions (Leviton et al. 2018f), reading and mathematics limitations (Leviton et al. 2018b), ADD (O'Shea et al. 2014; Allred et al. 2017), ASD (Korzeniewski et al.

2018), and social limitations among children who did not satisfy criteria for an ASD (Korzeniewski et al. 2018).

Let history answer the counterfactual question, 'What if the ELGAN study never occurred?'

THE FUTURE

The ELGAN study team continues to study both early life inflammation as well as structural and functional brain disorders. In its third phase of follow-up, ELGAN is broadening its efforts to include new exposures, new outcomes, and new collaborators. In keeping with guidance of the NIH Office of the Director's Environmental Influences on Child Health Outcomes (ECHO), ELGAN study researchers are collecting data about our participants' exposures to environmental chemicals, such as air and water pollutants, and, at age 15 years, updating information collected about psychosocial, family, and community factors, psychiatric disorders, the brain connectome, asthma, obesity, sleep, and quality of life. The ECHO Program components include experienced scientists with expertise in a wide range of research fields, including environmental epidemiology, developmental origins of health and disease, placental biology, genetics, epigenetics, epidemiology of childhood asthma, epidemiology of childhood obesity, developmental psychology, and quality of life. ECHO consists of over 30 cohorts that comprise tens of thousands of children. Thus the ELGAN study is positioned to increase further our understanding of how pre-, peri-, and post-natal factors contribute to risk and resiliency among individuals born extremely preterm. By addressing research questions that, when answered, have implications for practice, policy, and/or programs, the ELGAN study investigators aim to improve the lives of children.

REFERENCES

Abd Ellah, N, Taylor, L, Troja, W et al. (2015) Development of non-viral, trophoblast-specific gene delivery for placental therapy. *PLoS ONE* **10**: e0140879.

Akshoomoff N, Joseph RM, Taylor HG et al. (2017) Academic achievement deficits and their neuropsychological correlates in children born extremely preterm. *J Dev Behav Pediatr* **38**: 627–37.

Allred EN, Capone A, Jr, Fraioli A et al. (2014) Retinopathy of prematurity and brain damage in the very preterm newborn. *J Aapos* **18**: 241–7.

Allred EN, Dammann O, Fichorova RN et al. (2017) Systemic inflammation during the first postnatal month and the risk of attention deficit hyperactivity disorder characteristics among 10 year-old children born extremely preterm. *J Neuroimmune Pharmacol* **12**: 531–43.

Ashley DJ (1969) The two 'hit' and multiple 'hit' theories of carcinogenesis. *Br J Cancer* **23**: 313–28.

Audette MC, Kingdom JC (2017) Screening for fetal growth restriction and placental insufficiency. *Semin Fetal Neonatal Med* **23**: 119–25.

Ay H, Ay I, Koroshetz WJ, Finklestein SP (1999) Potential usefulness of basic fibroblast growth factor as a treatment for stroke. *Cerebrovasc Dis* **9**: 131–5.

Babata K, Bright HR, Allred EN et al. (2018) Socioemotional dysfunctions at age 10 years in extremely preterm newborns with late-onset bacteremia. *Early Hum Dev* **121**: 1–7.

Barouch R, Appel E, Kazimirsky G, Braun A, Renz H, Brodie C (2000) Differential regulation of neurotrophin expression by mitogens and neurotransmitters in mouse lymphocytes. *J Neuroimmunol* **103**: 112–21.

Bartholomew J, Martin CR, Allred E et al. (2013) Risk factors and correlates of neonatal growth velocity in extremely low gestational age newborns: the ELGAN study. *Neonatology* **104**: 298–304.

Bose C, Laughon M, Allred EN et al. (2011) Blood protein concentrations in the first two postnatal weeks that predict bronchopulmonary dysplasia among infants born before the 28th week of gestation. *Pediatr Res* **69**: 347–53.

Bose C, Van Marter LJ, Laughon M et al. (2009) Fetal growth restriction and chronic lung disease among infants born before the 28th week of gestation. *Pediatrics* **124**: e450–6.

Bose CL, Laughon MM, Allred EN et al. (2013) Systemic inflammation associated with mechanical ventilation among extremely preterm infants. *Cytokine* **61**: 315–22.

Bowen WH, Burne RA, Wu H, Koo H (2018) Oral biofilms: pathogens, matrix, and polymicrobial interactions in microenvironments. *Trends Microbiol* **26**: 229–42.

Bright HR, Babata K, Allred EN et al. (2017) Neurocognitive outcomes at 10 years of age in extremely preterm newborns with late-onset bacteremia. *J Pediatr* **187**: 43–9.e1.

Brown SP, Blackwell HE, Hammer BK (2018) The state of the union is strong: a review of ASM's 6th conference on cell-cell communication in bacteria. *J Bacteriol* **200**: e00291–18.

Burnett AC, Anderson PJ, Joseph RM et al. (2018) Hand preference and cognitive, motor, and behavioral functioning in 10-year-old extremely preterm children. *J Pediatr* **195**: 279–82.e3.

Butts BD, Houde C, Mehmet H (2008) Maturation-dependent sensitivity of oligodendrocyte lineage cells to apoptosis: implications for normal development and disease. *Cell Death Differ* **15**: 1178–86.

Cao X, Laplante DP, Brunet A, Ciampi A, King S (2014) Prenatal maternal stress affects motor function in 5(1/2)-year-old children: project ice storm. *Dev Psychobiol* **56**: 117–25.

Chen ML, Allred EN, Hecht JL et al. (2011) Placenta microbiology and histology, and the risk for severe retinopathy of prematurity. *Invest Ophthalmol Vis Sci* **52**: 7052–8.

Cheng Y, Gidday JM, Yan Q, Shah AR, Holtzman DM (1997) Marked age-dependent neuroprotection by brain-derived neurotrophic factor against neonatal hypoxic-ischemic brain injury. *Ann Neurol* **41**: 521–9.

Clark CA, Woodward LJ (2015) Relation of perinatal risk and early parenting to executive control at the transition to school. *Dev Sci* **18**: 525–42.

Constantino JN, Gruber CP (2012) *Social Responsiveness Scale Second Edition (SRS-2)*. Los Angeles: Western Psychological Services.

Da Silva Meirelles L, Simon D, Regner A (2017) Neurotrauma: the crosstalk between neurotrophins and inflammation in the acutely injured brain. *Int J Mol Sci* **18**: 1082.

Dammann O, Allred EN, Fichorova RN, Kuban K, O'Shea TM, Leviton A (2016) Duration of systemic inflammation in the first postnatal month among infants born before the 28th week of gestation. *Inflammation* **39**: 672–7.

Dammann O, Bueter W, Leviton A, Gressens P, Dammann CE (2008) Neuregulin-1: a potential endogenous protector in perinatal brain white matter damage. *Neonatology* **93**: 182–7.

Dammann O, Hagberg H, Leviton A (2001) Is periventricular leukomalacia an axonopathy as well as an oligopathy? *Pediatr Res* **49**: 453–7.

Dammann O, Leviton A (1999) Brain damage in preterm newborns: might enhancement of developmentally-regulated endogenous protection open a door for prevention? *Pediatrics* **104**: 541–50.

Dammann O, Leviton A (2000) Brain damage in preterm newborns: biologic response modification as a strategy to reduce disabilities. *J Pediatr* **136**: 433–8.

Dammann O, Leviton A (2004) Biomarker epidemiology of cerebral palsy. *Ann Neurol* **55**: 158–61.

Dammann O, Leviton A (2014) Intermittent or sustained systemic inflammation and the preterm brain. *Pediatr Res* **75**: 376–80.

Dammann O, Leviton A, Bartels DB, Dammann CE (2004) Lung and brain damage in preterm newborns. Are they related? How? Why? *Biol Neonate* **85**: 305–13.

Dammann O, Naples M, Bednarek F et al. (2010) SNAP-II and SNAPPE-II and the risk of structural and functional brain disorders in extremely low gestational age newborns: the ELGAN study. *Neonatology* **97**: 71–82.

Datta J, Palmer MJ, Tanton C et al. (2016) Prevalence of infertility and help seeking among 15 000 women and men. *Hum Reprod* **31**: 2108–18.

David J, Measelle J, Ostlund B, Ablow J (2017) Association between early life adversity and inflammation during infancy. *Dev Psychobiol* **59**: 696–702.

Dean RS (1978) Reliability and predictive validity of the Dean Laterality Preference Schedule with preadolescents. *Percept Mot Skills* **47**: 1345–6.

Deary IJ (2012) Intelligence. *Annu Rev Psychol* **63**: 453–82.

Deary IJ, Johnson W (2010) Intelligence and education: causal perceptions drive analytic processes and therefore conclusions. *Int J Epidemiol* **39**: 1362–9.

Deault LC (2010) A systematic review of parenting in relation to the development of comorbidities and functional impairments in children with attention-deficit/hyperactivity disorder (ADHD). *Child Psychiatry Hum Dev* **41**: 168–92.

Diamond A (2013) Executive functions. *Annu Rev Psychol* **64**: 135–68.

Dieni S, Rees S (2005) BDNF and TrkB protein expression is altered in the fetal hippocampus but not cerebellum after chronic prenatal compromise. *Exp Neurol* **192**: 265–73.

Ding S, Lemyre B, Daboval T, Barrowman N, Moore GP (2018) A meta-analysis of neurodevelopmental outcomes at 4–10 years in children born at 22–25 weeks gestation. *Acta Paediatr* **108**: 1237–44.

Director NOOT *Environmental Influences on Child Health Outcomes (ECHO) Program* [Online]. Available: https://www.nih.gov/research-training/environmental-influences-child-health-outcomes-echo-program [Accessed February 25, 2019].

Downey LC, O'Shea TM, Allred EN et al. (2015) Antenatal and early postnatal antecedents of parent-reported attention problems at 2 years of age. *J Pediatr* **166**: 20–5.

Du Plessis AJ (2009) The role of systemic hemodynamic disturbances in prematurity-related brain injury. *J Child Neurol* **24**: 1127–40.

Duncan GJ, Magnuson K, Votruba-Drzal E (2017) Moving beyond correlations in assessing the consequences of poverty. *Annu Rev Psychol* **68**: 413–34.

Ehrlich KB, Ross KM, Chen E, Miller GE (2016) Testing the biological embedding hypothesis: is early life adversity associated with a later proinflammatory phenotype? *Dev Psychopathol* **28**: 1273–83.

Eklind S, Mallard C, Arvidsson P, Hagberg H (2006) Effect of lipopolysaccharide on global gene expression in the immature rat brain. *Pediatr Res* **60**: 161–8.

Eklind S, Mallard C, Leverin AL et al. (2001) Bacterial endotoxin sensitizes the immature brain to hypoxic-ischaemic injury. *Eur J Neurosci* **13**: 1101–6.

Elhassan No, Bai S, Gibson N, Holland G, Robbins JM, Kaiser JR (2018) The impact of prematurity and maternal socioeconomic status and education level on achievement-test scores up to 8th grade. *PLoS One* **13**: e0198083.

Elkabes S, Peng L, Black IB (1998) Lipopolysaccharide differentially regulates microglial trk receptor and neurotrophin expression. *J Neurosci Res* **54**: 117–22.

Fichorova RN, Onderdonk AB, Yamamoto H et al. (2011) Maternal microbe-specific modulation of inflammatory response in extremely low gestational age newborns. *mBio* **2**: e00280–10.

Fitzgerald E, Boardman JP, Drake AJ (2018) Preterm birth and the risk of neurodevelopmental disorders – is there a role for epigenetic dysregulation? *Curr Genomics* **19**: 507–21.

Fleiss B, Wong F, Brownfoot F et al. (2019) Knowledge gaps and emerging research areas in intrauterine growth restriction-associated brain injury. *Front Endocrinol* **10**: 188.

Frost I, Smith WPJ, Mitri S et al. (2018) Cooperation, competition and antibiotic resistance in bacterial colonies. *ISME J* **12**: 1582–93.

Funkhouser LJ, Bordenstein SR (2013) Mom knows best: the universality of maternal microbial transmission. *PLoS Biol* **11**: e1001631.

Gaccioli F, Lager S (2016) Placental nutrient transport and intrauterine growth restriction. *Front Physiol* **7**: 40.

Gaudet AD, Fonken LK, Watkins LR, Nelson RJ, Popovich PG (2018) MicroRNAs: roles in regulating neuroinflammation. *Neuroscientist* **24**: 221–45.

Geva R, Eshel R, Leitner Y, Valevski AF, Harel S (2006) Neuropsychological outcome of children with intrauterine growth restriction: a 9-year prospective study. *Pediatrics* **118**: 91–100.

Gilles F, Gressens P, Dammann O, Leviton A (2018) Hypoxia-ischemia is not an antecedent of most preterm brain damage: the illusion of validity. *Dev Med Child Neurol* **60**: 120–5.

Gilman SE, Hornig M, Ghassabian A et al. (2017) Socioeconomic disadvantage, gestational immune activity, and neurodevelopment in early childhood. *Proc Natl Acad Sci USA* **114**: 6728–33.

Glass HC, Bonifacio SL, Chau V et al. (2008) Recurrent postnatal infections are associated with progressive white matter injury in premature infants. *Pediatrics* **122**: 299–305.

Graves DT (1997) The use of biologic response modifiers in human clinical trials. *Ann Periodontol* **2**: 259–67.

Hagberg H, Dammann O, Mallard C, Leviton A (2004) Preconditioning and the developing brain. *Semin Perinatol* **28**: 389–95.

Hagberg H, Mallard C, Ferriero DM et al. (2015) The role of inflammation in perinatal brain injury. *Nat Rev Neurol* **11**: 192–208.

Hammond TR, Dufort C, Dissing–Olesen L et al. (2019) Single-cell RNA sequencing of microglia throughout the mouse lifespan and in the injured brain reveals complex cell-state changes. *Immunity* **50**: 253–71 e6.

Hecht JL, Fichorova RN, Tang VF, Allred EN, McElrath TF, Leviton A (2011) Relationship between neonatal blood protein profiles and placenta histologic characteristics in ELGANs. *Pediatr Research* **69**: 68–73.

Hecht JL, Kliman HJ, Allred EN et al. (2007) Reference weights for placentas delivered before the 28th week of gestation. *Placenta* **28**: 987–90.

Hecht JL, Onderdonk A, Delaney M et al. (2008) Characterization of chorioamnionitis in 2nd-trimester C-section placentas and correlation with microorganism recovery from subamniotic tissues. *Pediatr Dev Pathol* **11**: 15–22.

Heeren T, Joseph RM, Allred EN, O'Shea TM, Leviton A, Kuban KCK (2017) Cognitive functioning at the age of 10 years among children born extremely preterm: a latent profile approach. *Pediatr Res* **82**: 614–9.

Heese K, Fiebich Bl, Bauer J, Otten U (1998) NF-kappaB modulates lipopolysaccharide-induced microglial nerve growth factor expression. *Glia* **22**: 401–7.

Helderman JB, O'Shea TM, Goldstein DJ et al. (2012) Antenatal antecedents of low scores on the Bayley Scales of Infant Development at 24 months among children born before the 28th post-menstrual week. The ELGAN study. *Pediatrics* **129**: 494–502.

Hirschberger RG, Kuban KCK, O'Shea TM et al. (2018) Co-occurrence and severity of neurodevelopmental burden (cognitive impairment, cerebral palsy, autism spectrum disorder, and epilepsy) at age ten years in children born extremely preterm. *Pediatr Neurol* **79**: 45–52.

Holm M, Austeng D, Fichorova RN et al. (2017a) Postnatal systemic inflammation and neuro-ophthalmologic dysfunctions in extremely low gestational age children. *Acta Paediatr* **106**: 454–7.

Holm M, Morken TS, Fichorova RN et al. (2017b) Systemic inflammation-associated proteins and retinopathy of prematurity in infants born before the 28th week of gestation. *Invest Ophthalmol Vis Sci* **58**: 6419–28.

Holm M, Msall ME, Skranes J, Dammann O, Allred E, Leviton A (2015) Antecedents and correlates of visual field deficits in children born extremely preterm. *Eur J Paediatr Neurol* **19**: 56–63.

Hunt K, Kennedy SH, Vatish M (2016) Definitions and reporting of placental insufficiency in biomedical journals: a review of the literature. *Eur J Obstet Gynecol Reprod Biol* **205**: 146–9.

Iadecola C (2017) The neurovascular unit coming of age: a journey through neurovascular coupling in health and disease. *Neuron* **96**: 17–42.

Jensen ET, Van Der Burg JW, O'Shea TM et al. (2017) The relationship of maternal prepregnancy body mass index and pregnancy weight gain to neurocognitive function at age 10 years among children born extremely preterm. *J Pediatr* **187**: 50–7 e3.

Johnson S, Wolke D (2013) Behavioural outcomes and psychopathology during adolescence. *Early Hum Dev* **89**: 199–207.

Joseph RM, Korzeniewski SJ, Allred EN et al. (2017) Extremely low gestational age and very low birthweight for gestational age are risk factors for autism spectrum disorder in a large cohort study of 10-year-old children born at 23–27 weeks' gestation. *Am J Obstet Gynecol* **216**: 304 e1–304 e16.

Joseph RM, O'Shea TM, Allred EN, Heeren T, Kuban KK (2018) Maternal educational status at birth, maternal educational advancement, and neurocognitive outcomes at age 10 years among children born extremely preterm. *Pediatr Res* **83**: 767–77.

Karthikeyan A, Patnala R, Jadhav SP, Eng-Ang L, Dheen ST (2016) MicroRNAs: key players in microglia and astrocyte mediated inflammation in CNS pathologies. *Curr Med Chem* **23**: 3528–46.

Kim P, Capistrano C, Congleton C (2016a) Socioeconomic disadvantages and neural sensitivity to infant cry: role of maternal distress. *Soc Cogn Affect Neurosci* **11**: 1597–607.

Kim SH, Joseph RM, Frazier J et al. (2016b) Predictive validity of the Modified Checklist for Autism in Toddlers (M-CHAT) born very preterm. *J Pediatr* **178**: 101–7.e2.

Kiser DP, Rivero O, Lesch KP (2015) Annual research review: The (epi)genetics of neurodevelopmental disorders in the era of whole-genome sequencing – unveiling the dark matter. *J Child Psychol Psychiatry* **56**: 278–95.

Koenen KC, Moffitt TE, Roberts AL et al. (2009) Childhood IQ and adult mental disorders: a test of the cognitive reserve hypothesis. *Am J Psychiatry* **166**: 50–7.

Kollmann TR, Crabtree J, Rein-Weston A et al. (2009) Neonatal innate TLR-mediated responses are distinct from those of adults. *J Immunol* **183**: 7150–60.

Koolwijk I, Stein DS, Chan E, Powell C, Driscoll K, Barbaresi WJ (2014) 'Complex' attention-deficit hyperactivity disorder, more norm than exception? Diagnoses and comorbidities in a developmental clinic. *J Dev Behav Pediatr* **35**: 591–7.

Korkman M, Kirk U, Kemp S (1998) *NEPSY: A Developmental Neuropsychological Assessment.* New York: The Psychological Corporation.

Korzenicwski SJ, Allred EN, Joseph RM et al. (2017a) Neurodevelopment at age 10 years of children born <28 weeks with fetal growth restriction. *Pediatrics* **140**: e20170697.

Korzeniewski SJ, Allred EN, O'Shea TM, Leviton A, Kuban KCK (2018) Elevated protein concentrations in newborn blood and the risks of autism spectrum disorder, and of social impairment, at age 10 years among infants born before the 28th week of gestation. *Transl Psychiatry* **8**: 115.

Korzeniewski SJ, Joseph RM, Kim SH et al. (2017b) Social responsiveness scale assessment of the preterm behavioral phenotype in 10-year-olds born extremely preterm. *J Dev Behav Pediatr* **38**: 697–705.

Kuban K, Adler I, Allred EN et al. (2007) Observer variability assessing US scans of the preterm brain: the ELGAN study. *Pediatr Radiol* **37**: 1201–8.

Kuban KC, Joseph RM, O'Shea TM et al. (2017) Circulating inflammatory-associated proteins in the first month of life and cognitive impairment at age 10 years in children born extremely preterm. *J Pediatr* **180**: 116–23 e1.

Kuban KC, O'Shea M, Allred E et al. (2005) Video and CD-ROM as a training tool for performing neurologic examinations of 1-year-old children in a multicenter epidemiologic study. *J Child Neurol* **20**: 829–31.

Kuban KC, O'Shea TM, Allred EN et al. (2014) Systemic inflammation and cerebral palsy risk in extremely preterm infants. *J Child Neurol* **29**: 1692–8.

Kuban KC, O'Shea TM, Allred EN, Tager-Flusberg H, Goldstein DJ, Leviton A (2009) Positive screening on the Modified Checklist for Autism in Toddlers (M-CHAT) in extremely low gestational age newborns. *J Pediatr* **154**: 535–40 e1.

Kuban KCK, Allred EN, O'Shea TM et al. (2008) An algorithm for diagnosing and classifying cerebral palsy in young children *J Pediat* **153**: 466–72.e1.

Kuban KCK, Heeren T, O'Shea TM et al. (2018) Among children born extremely preterm a higher level of circulating neurotrophins is associated with lower risk of cognitive impairment at school age. *J Pediatr* **201**: 40–8 e4.

Kundakovic M, Jaric I (2017) The epigenetic link between prenatal adverse environments and neurodevelopmental disorders. *Genes (Basel)* **8**: 104.

Laplante DP, Brunet A, King S (2015) The effects of maternal stress and illness during pregnancy on infant temperament: Project Ice Storm. *Pediatr Res* **79**: 107–13.

Laughon M, Bose C, Allred E et al. (2007) Factors associated with treatment for hypotension in extremely low gestational age newborns during the first postnatal week. *Pediatrics* **119**: 273–80.

Laughon M, Bose C, Allred EN et al. (2011a) Patterns of blood protein concentrations of ELGANs classified by three patterns of respiratory disease in the first 2 postnatal weeks. *Pediatr Res* **70**: 292–6.

Laughon M, Bose C, Allred EN et al. (2011b) Antecedents of chronic lung disease following three patterns of early respiratory disease in preterm infants. *Arch Dis Child Fetal Neonatal Ed* **96**: F114–20.

Lawlor DA, Smith GD, O'Callaghan M et al. (2007) Epidemiologic evidence for the fetal overnutrition hypothesis: findings from the mater-university study of pregnancy and its outcomes. *Am J Epidemiol* **165**: 418–24.

Lee JW, Vanderveen D, Allred EN, Leviton A, Dammann O (2015) Pre-threshold retinopathy in premature infants with intra-uterine growth restriction. *Acta Paediatr* **104**: 27–31.

Leviton A, Allred EN, Dammann O et al. (2019) Socioeconomic status and early blood concentrations of inflammation-related and neurotrophic proteins among extremely preterm newborns. *PLoS One* **14**: e0214154.

Leviton A, Allred EN, Fichorova RN et al. (2016a) Systemic inflammation on postnatal days 21 and 28 and indicators of brain dysfunction 2 years later among children born before the 28th week of gestation. *Early Hum Dev* **93**: 25–32.

Leviton A, Allred EN, Fichorova RN, Kuban KC, O'Shea TM, Dammann O (2016b) Antecedents of inflammation biomarkers in preterm newborns on days 21 and 28. *Acta Paediatr* **105**: 274–80.

Leviton A, Allred, EN, Fichorova RN (2018a) Circulating biomarkers in extremely preterm infants associated with ultrasound indicators of brain damage. *Eur J Paediatr Neurol* **22**: 440–50.

Leviton A, Allred EN, Fichorova RN et al. (2019) Early post-natal IGF-1 and IGFBP-1 blood levels in extremely preterm infants. Relationships with indicators of placental insufficiency and with systemic inflammation. *American Journal of Perinatology* **36**:1442–52.

Leviton A, Allred EN, Joseph RM, O'Shea TM, Kuban KCK (2017a) Newborn blood gas derangements of children born extremely preterm and neurocognitive dysfunctions at age 10 years. *Respir Physiol Neurobiol* **242**: 66–72.

Leviton A, Allred EN, Kuban K (2011a) Blood protein concentrations in the first two postnatal weeks associated with early postnatal blood gas derangements among infants born before the 28th week of gestation. The ELGAN study. *Cytokine* **56**: 392–8.

Leviton A, Allred EN, Kuban KC et al. (2010a) Microbiologic and histologic characteristics of the extremely preterm infant's placenta predict white matter damage and later cerebral palsy. the ELGAN study. *Pediatr Res* **67**: 95–101.

Leviton A, Allred EN, Paneth N et al. (2010b) Early blood gas abnormalities and the preterm brain. *Am J Epidemiology* **172**: 907–16.

Leviton A, Allred EN, Yamamoto H et al. (2017b) Antecedents and correlates of blood concentrations of neurotrophic growth factors in very preterm newborns. *Cytokine* **94**: 21–8.

Leviton A, Blair E, Dammann O, Allred E (2005) The wealth of information conveyed by gestational age. *J Pediatr* **146**: 123–7.

Leviton A, Dammann O, Allred EN (2018b) Neonatal systemic inflammation and the risk of low scores on measures of reading and mathematics achievement at age 10 years among children born extremely preterm. *Int J Dev Neurosci* **66**: 45–53.

Leviton A, Dammann O, Engelke S et al. (2010c) The clustering of disorders in infants born before the 28th week of gestation. *Acta Paediatr* **99**: 1795–800.

Leviton A, Fichorova R, Yamamoto Y et al. (2011b) Inflammation-related proteins in the blood of extremely low gestational age newborns. The contribution of inflammation to the appearance of developmental regulation. *Cytokine* **53**: 66–73.

Leviton A, Fichorova RN, O'Shea TM et al. (2013) Two-hit model of brain damage in the very preterm newborn: small for gestational age and postnatal systemic inflammation. *Pediatr Res* **73**: 362–70.

Leviton A, Gressens P, Wolkenhauer O, Dammann O (2015) Systems approach to the study of brain damage in the very preterm newborn *Front Syst Neurosci* **9**: 58.

Leviton A, Hecht JL, Allred EN, Yamamoto H, Fichorova RN, Dammann O (2011c) Persistence after birth of systemic inflammation associated with umbilical cord inflammation. *J Reprod Immunol* **90**: 235–43.

Leviton A, Hooper SR, Hunter SJ et al. (2018c) Antecedents of screening positive for attention deficit hyperactivity disorder in ten-year-old children born extremely preterm. *Pediatr Neurol* **81**: 25–30.

Leviton A, Hunter SJ, Scott MN et al. (2017c) Observer variability identifying attention deficit/hyperactivity disorder in 10-year-old children born extremely preterm. *Acta Paediatr* **106**: 1317–22.

Leviton A, Joseph RM, Allred EN, O'Shea TM, Kuban KKC (2018d) Antenatal and neonatal antecedents of learning limitations in 10-year old children born extremely preterm. *Early Hum Dev* **118**: 8–14.

Leviton A, Joseph RM, Allred EN, O'SHEA TM, Taylor HG, Kuban KKC (2018e) Antenatal and neonatal antecedents of executive dysfunctions in extremely preterm children. *J Child Neurol* **33**: 198–208.

Leviton A, Joseph RM, Fichorova RN, Allred EN, Taylor HG, O'Shea TM, Dammann O (2018f) Executive dysfunction early postnatal biomarkers among children born extremely preterm. *J Neuroimmune Pharmacol* **14**: 188–99.

Leviton A, Kuban K, Allred EN et al. (2010d) Antenatal antecedents of a small head circumference at age 24-months post-term equivalent in a sample of infants born before the 28th post-menstrual week. *Early Hum Dev* **86**: 515–21.

Leviton A, Kuban K, O'Shea TM et al. (2011d) The relationship between early concentrations of 25 blood proteins and cerebral white matter injury in preterm newborns: The ELGAN study. *J Pediatr* **158**: 897–903.e5.

Leviton A, O'Shea TM, Bednarek FJ, Allred EN, Fichorova RN, Dammann O (2012) Systemic responses of preterm newborns with presumed or documented bacteraemia. *Acta Paediatr* **101**: 355–9.

Leviton A, Paneth N, Reuss ML et al. (1999) Hypothyroxinemia of prematurity and the risk of cerebral white matter damage. *J Pediatr* **134**: 706–11.

Leviton A, Ryan S, Allred EN et al. (2017d) Antecedents and early correlates of low concentrations of angiogenic proteins in very preterm newborns. *Clin Chim Acta* **471**: 1–5.

Logan JW, Allred EN, Msall ME et al. (2019) Neurocognitive function of 10-year-old multiples born less than 28 weeks of gestational age. *J Perinatol* **39**: 237–47.

Logan JW, Dammann O, Allred EN et al. (2017) Early postnatal illness severity scores predict neurodevelopmental impairments at 10 years of age in children born extremely preterm. *J Perinatol* **37**: 606–14.

Logan JW, O'Shea TM, Allred EN et al. (2011a) Early postnatal hypotension and developmental delay at 24 months of age among extremely low gestational age newborns. *Archives of Disease in Childhood* **95**: F321–8.

Logan JW, O'Shea TM, Allred EN et al. (2011b) Early postnatal hypotension, brain ultrasound lesions, and cerebral palsy among extremely low gestational age newborns. *J Perinatol* **96**: F316–7.

Lu L, Claud EC (2018) Intrauterine inflammation, epigenetics, and microbiome influences on preterm infant health. *Curr Pathobiol Rep* **6**: 15–21.

Mansur RB, Cunha GR, Asevedo E et al. (2016) Socioeconomic disadvantage moderates the association between peripheral biomarkers and childhood psychopathology. *PLoS ONE* **11**: e0160455.

Martin CR, Bellomy M, Allred EN, Fichorova RN, Leviton A. (2013) Systemic inflammation associated with severe intestinal injury in extremely low gestational age newborns. *Fetal Pediatr Pathol* **32**: 222–34.

McElrath TF, Allred EN, Kuban KCK et al. (2010) Factors associated with small head circumference at birth among infants born before the 28th week. *Am J Obstet Gynecol* **203**: 138.e1–138.e8.

McElrath TF, Allred EN, Van Marter L, Fichorova RN, Leviton A (2013) Perinatal systemic inflammatory responses of growth-restricted preterm newborns. *Acta Paediatr* **102**: e439–42.

McElrath TF, Fichorova RN, Allred EN et al. (2011) Blood protein profiles of infants born before 28 weeks differ by pregnancy complication. *Am J Obstet Gynecol* **204**: 418.e1–418.e12.

McElrath TF, Hecht JL, Dammann O et al. (2008) Pregnancy disorders that lead to delivery before the 28th week of gestation: an epidemiologic approach to classification. *Am J Epidemiol* **168**: 980–9.

McEwen BS, Wingfield JC (2010) What is in a name? Integrating homeostasis, allostasis and stress. *Horm Behav* **57**: 105–11.

Meakin CJ, Martin EM, Santos HP (2018) Placental CpG methylation of HPA-axis genes is associated with cognitive impairment at age 10 among children born extremely preterm. *Horm Behav* **101**: 29–35.

Miller GE, Borders AE, Crockett AH et al. (2017) Maternal socioeconomic disadvantage is associated with transcriptional indications of greater immune activation and slower tissue maturation in placental biopsies and newborn cord blood. *Brain Behav Immun* **64**: 276–84.

Miwa T, Furukawa S, Nakajima K, Furukawa Y, Kohsaka S (1997) Lipopolysaccharide enhances synthesis of brain-derived neurotrophic factor in cultured rat microglia. *J Neurosci Res* **50**: 1023–9.

Molteni RA, Stys SJ, Battaglia FC (1978) Relationship of fetal and placental weight in human beings: fetal/placental weight ratios at various gestational ages and birth weight distributions. *J Reprod Med* **21**: 327–34.

Morganti-Kossmann MC, Semple BD, Hellewell SC, Bye N, Ziebell JM (2018) The complexity of neuroinflammation consequent to traumatic brain injury: from research evidence to potential treatments. *Acta Neuropathol* **137**: 731–55

Mosser CA, Baptista S, Arnoux I, Audinat E (2017) Microglia in CNS development: shaping the brain for the future. *Prog Neurobiol* **149–50**: 1–20.

Nanthakumar N, Meng D, Goldstein AM et al. (2011) The mechanism of excessive intestinal inflammation in necrotizing enterocolitis: an immature innate immune response. *PLoS One* **6**: e17776.

National Cancer Institute, Dictionary of Cancer Terms (n.d.) https://www.cancer.gov/publications/dictionaries/cancer-terms/def/neurocognitive [Accessed July 3, 2019].

Nourollahpour Shiadeh M, Behboodi Moghadam Z, Adam I, Saber V, Bagheri M, Rostami A (2017) Human infectious diseases and risk of preeclampsia: an updated review of the literature. *Infection* **45**: 589–600.

O'Shea TM, Allred EN, Dammann O et al. (2009) The ELGAN study of the brain and related disorders in extremely low gestational age newborns. *Early Hum Dev* **85**: 719–25.

O'Shea TM, Allred EN, Kuban KC (2012) Elevated concentrations of inflammation-related proteins in postnatal blood predict severe developmental delay at 2 years of age in extremely preterm infants. *J Pediatr* **160**: 395–401 e4.

O'Shea TM, Joseph RM, Allred EN et al. (2018) Accuracy of the Bayley-II mental development index at 2 years as a predictor of cognitive impairment at school age among children born extremely preterm. *J Perinatol* **38**: 908–16.

O'Shea TM, Joseph RM, Kuban KC et al. (2014) Elevated blood levels of inflammation-related proteins are associated with an attention problem at age 24 mo in extremely preterm infants. *Pediatr Res* **75**: 781–7.

O'Shea TM, Shah B, Allred EN et al. (2013) Inflammation-initiating illnesses, inflammation-related proteins, and cognitive impairment in extremely preterm infants. *Brain Behav Immun* **29**: 104–12.

Olomu IN, Hecht JL, Onderdonk AO, Allred EN, Leviton A (2009) Perinatal correlates of *Ureaplasma urealyticum* in placenta parenchyma of singleton pregnancies that end before 28 weeks of gestation. *Pediatrics* **123**: 1329–36.

Onderdonk AB, Delaney ML, Dubois AM, Allred EN, Leviton A (2008a) Detection of bacteria in placental tissues obtained from extremely low gestational age neonates. *Am J Obstet Gynecol* **198**: 110 e1–7.

Onderdonk AB, Hecht JL, McElrath TF M et al. (2008b) Colonization of second-trimester placenta parenchyma. *Am J Obstet Gynecol* **199**: 52.e1–52.e10.

Osborne BF, Caulfield JI, Solomotis SA, Schwarz JM (2017) Neonatal infection produces significant changes in immune function with no associated learning deficits in juvenile rats. *Dev Neurobiol* **77**: 1221–36.

Payne MS, Bayatibojakhi S (2014) Exploring preterm birth as a polymicrobial disease: an overview of the uterine microbiome. *Front Immunol* **5**: 595.

Perrin EM, O'Shea TM, Skinner AC et al. (2018) Elevations of inflammatory proteins in neonatal blood are associated with obesity and overweight among 2-year-old children born extremely premature. *Pediatr Res* **83**: 1110–9.

Phadke A, Msall ME, Droste P (2014) Impaired visual fixation at the age of 2 years in children born before the twenty-eighth week of gestation. Antecedents and correlates in the multicenter ELGAN study. *Pediatr Neurol* **51**: 36–42.

Plomin R, Deary IJ (2015) Genetics and intelligence differences: five special findings. *Mol Psychiatry* **20**: 98–108.

Radhakrishnan B, Alwin Prem Anand A (2016) Role of miRNA-9 in brain development. *J Exp Neurosci* **10**: 101–20.

Raff MC, Barres BA, Burne JF, Coles HS, Ishizaki Y, Jacobson MD (1993) Programmed cell death and the control of cell survival: lessons from the nervous system. *Science* **262**: 695–700.

Regev RH, Lusky A, Dolfin T, Litmanovitz I, Arnon S, Reichman B (2003) Excess mortality and morbidity among small-for-gestational-age premature infants: a population-based study. *J Pediatr* **143**: 186–91.

Reiss AL, Kesler SR, Vohr B et al. (2004) Sex differences in cerebral volumes of 8-year-olds born preterm. *J Pediatr* **145**: 242–9.

Reuss ML, Paneth N, Pinto-Martin JA, Lorenz JM, Susser M (1996) The relation of transient hypothyroxinemia in preterm infants to neurologic development at two years of age. *N Engl J Med* **334**: 821–7.

Reuss ML, Paneth N, Susser M (1994) Does the loss of placental hormones contribute to neurodevelopmental disabilities in preterm infants? *Dev Med Child Neurol* **36**: 743–7.

Richardson DK, Corcoran JD, Escobar GJ, Lee SK (2001) SNAP-II and SNAPPE-II: Simplified newborn illness severity and mortality risk scores. *J Pediatr* **138**: 92–100.

Ritchie K, Bora S, Woodward LJ (2015) Social development of children born very preterm: a systematic review. *Dev Med Child Neurol* **57**: 899–918.

Rodriguez A, Miettunen J, Henriksen TB et al. (2008) Maternal adiposity prior to pregnancy is associated with ADHD symptoms in offspring: evidence from three prospective pregnancy cohorts. *Int J Obes (Lond)* **32**: 550–7.

Schuller SS, Kramer BW, Villamor E, Spittler A, Berger A, Levy O (2018) Immunomodulation to prevent or treat neonatal sepsis: past, present, and future. *Front Pediatr* **6**: 199.

Schultz C, Rott C, Temming P, Schlenke P, Moller JC, Bucsky P (2002) Enhanced interleukin-6 and interleukin-8 synthesis in term and preterm infants. *Pediatr Res* **51**: 317–22.

Scott MN, Hunter SJ, Joseph RM et al. (2017) Neurocognitive correlates of attention-deficit hyperactivity disorder symptoms in children born at extremely low gestational age. *J Dev Behav Pediatr* **38**: 249–59.

Seidmann L, Suhan T, Unger R, Gerein V, Kirkpatrick CJ (2013) Imbalance of expression of bFGF and PK1 is associated with defective maturation and antenatal placental insufficiency. *Eur J Obstet Gynecol Reprod Biol* **170**: 352–7.

Sferruzzi-Perri AN, Sandovici I, Constancia M, Fowden AL (2017) Placental phenotype and the insulin-like growth factors: resource allocation to fetal growth. *J Physiol* **595**: 5057–93.

Shen J, Abu-Amer Y, O'Keefe RJ, McAlinden A (2017) Inflammation and epigenetic regulation in osteoarthritis. *Connect Tissue Res* **58**: 49–63.

Singer BH, Newstead MW, Zeng X et al. (2016) Cecal ligation and puncture results in long-term central nervous system myeloid inflammation. *PLoS One* **11**: e0149136.

Sisman J, Logan JW, Westra SJ, Allred EN, Leviton A (2014) Lenticulostriate vasculopathy in extremely low gestational age newborns: inter-rater variability of cranial ultrasound readings, antecedents and postnatal characteristics. *J Pediatr Neurol* **12**: 183–93.

Smyser CD, Wheelock MD, Limbrick DD, Jr, Neil JJ (2019) Neonatal brain injury and aberrant connectivity. *Neuroimage* **185**: 609–23.

Sriram S, Schreiber MD, Msall ME et al. (2018) Cognitive development and quality of life associated with BPD in 10-year-olds born preterm. *Pediatrics* **141**: e20172719.

Srivastav S, Walitza S, Grunblatt E (2018) Emerging role of miRNA in attention deficit hyperactivity disorder: a systematic review. *Atten Defic Hyperact Disord* **10**: 49–63.

Stacy A, McNally L, Darch SE, Brown SP, Whiteley M (2016) The biogeography of polymicrobial infection. *Nat Rev Microbiol* **14**: 93–105.

Streimish IG, Ehrenkranz RA, Allred EN et al. (2012) Birth weight- and fetal weight-growth restriction: impact on neurodevelopment. *Early Hum Dev* **88**: 765–71.

Strunk T, Inder T, Wang X, Burgner D, Mallard C, Levy O (2014) Infection-induced inflammation and cerebral injury in preterm infants. *Lancet Infect Dis* **14**: 751–62.

Theis KR, Romero R, Winters AD et al. (2019) Does the human placenta delivered at term have a microbiota? Results of cultivation, quantitative real-time PCR, 16S rRNA gene sequencing, and metagenomics. *Am J Obstet Gynecol* **220**: 267 e1–267 e39.

Tilley SK, Martin EM, Smeester L et al. (2018) Placental CpG methylation of infants born extremely preterm predicts cognitive impairment later in life. *PLoS One* **13**: e0193271.

Tolsa CB, Zimine S, Warfield SK et al. (2004) Early alteration of structural and functional brain development in premature infants born with intrauterine growth restriction. *Pediatr Res* **56**: 132–8.

Tomlinson MS, Bommarito PA, Martin EM et al. (2017) Microorganisms in the human placenta are associated with altered CpG methylation of immune and inflammation-related genes. *PLoS One* **12**: e0188664.

Tong L, Perez-Polo R (1998) Brain-derived neurotrophic factor (BDNF) protects cultured rat cerebellar granule neurons against glucose deprivation-induced apoptosis. *J Neural Transm* **105**: 905–14.

Ursache A, Merz EC, Melvin S, Meyer J, Noble KG (2017) Socioeconomic status, hair cortisol and internalizing symptoms in parents and children. *Psychoneuroendocrinology* **78**: 142–50.

Van der Burg JW, Allred EN, Kuban K, O'Shea TM, Dammann O, Leviton A (2015) Maternal obesity and development of the preterm newborn at 2 years. *Acta Paediatr* **104**: 900–3.

Van der Burg JW, Allred EN, McElrath TF et al. (2013) Is maternal obesity associated with sustained inflammation in extremely low gestational age newborns? *Early Hum Dev* **89**: 949–55.

Van der Burg JW, Jensen ET, Van de Bor M et al. (2017) Maternal obesity and attention-related symptoms in the preterm offspring. *Early Hum Dev* **115**: 9–15.

Van der Burg JW, O'Shea TM, Kuban K et al. (2018) Are extremely low gestational age newborns born to obese women at increased risk of cerebral palsy at 2 Years? *J Child Neurol* **33**: 216–24.

Van der Burg JW, Sen S, Chomitz VR, Seidell JC, Leviton A, Dammann O (2016) The role of systemic inflammation linking maternal BMI to neurodevelopment in children. *Pediatr Res* **79**: 3–12.

Van Dijk M, Oudejans CB (2011) STOX1: Key player in trophoblast dysfunction underlying early onset preeclampsia with growth retardation. *J Pregnancy* **2011**: 521826.

Van Lieshout RJ, Taylor VH, Boyle MH (2011) Pre-pregnancy and pregnancy obesity and neurodevelopmental outcomes in offspring: a systematic review. *Obes Rev* **12**: e548–59.

Van Well GTJ, Daalderop LA, Wolfs T, Kramer BW (2017) Human perinatal immunity in physiological conditions and during infection. *Mol Cell Pediatr* **4**: 4.

Vanderveen DK, Allred EN, Wallace DK, Leviton A (2016) Strabismus at age 2 years in children born before 28 weeks' gestation: antecedents and correlates. *J Child Neurol* **31**: 451–60.

Volpe JJ (2014) Neonatal neurology – my personal journey and some lessons learned. *Pediatr Neurol* **51**: 753–7.

Voracek M, Haubner T (2008) Twin-singleton differences in intelligence: a meta-analysis. *Psychol Rep* **102**: 951–62.

Wang, Y, Zhang, H, Wang, Z et al. (2018) Therapeutic effect of nerve growth factor on canine cerebral infarction evaluated by MRI. *Oncotarget* **9**: 3741–51.

Whiteley M, Diggle SP, Greenberg EP (2017) Progress in and promise of bacterial quorum sensing research. *Nature* **551**: 313–20.

Wickens RA, Ver Donck L, Mackenzie AB, Bailey SJ (2018) Repeated daily administration of increasing doses of lipopolysaccharide provides a model of sustained inflammation-induced depressive-like behaviour in mice that is independent of the NLRP3 inflammasome. *Behav Brain Res* **352**: 99–108.

Willyard C (2018) Could baby's first bacteria take root before birth? *Nature* **553**: 264–6.

Yang L, Sameshima H, Ikeda T, Ikenoue T (2004) Lipopolysaccharide administration enhances hypoxic-ischemic brain damage in newborn rats. *J Obstet Gynaecol Res* **30**: 142–7.

Yanni D, Korzeniewski S, Allred EN et al. (2017) Both antenatal and postnatal inflammation contribute information about the risk of brain damage in extremely preterm newborns. *Pediatr Res* **82**: 691–6.

Zacchigna S, Lambrechts D, Carmeliet P (2008) Neurovascular signalling defects in neurodegeneration. *Nat Rev Neurosci* **9**: 169–81.

Zagrebelsky M, Korte M (2014) Form follows function: BDNF and its involvement in sculpting the function and structure of synapses. *Neuropharmacology* **76 Pt C**: 628–38.

Glossary

Adhesion molecules: cell-surface molecules that bind to molecules on the surface of other cells. Includes selectins, integrins, and cadherins. Adhesion molecules measured in the ELGAN study include ICAM-1 (CD54), ICAM-3 (CD50), VCAM-1(CD106), and E-SEL (CD62E).

    E-SEL: a selectin cell adhesion molecule expressed only on endothelial cells.

    ICAM: Intercellular adhesion molecule.

    VCAM: Vascular cell adhesion molecule.

Adiposity: increased fat mass.

Ages & Stages Questionnaire (ASQ): developmental screening instrument for infants and young children.

Angiogenic proteins (angio-neurotrophic proteins): proteins that promote the growth of new blood vessels. The angiogenic proteins measured in the ELGAN study include VEGF, VEGF-R1, VEGF-R2, IGF, IGFBP-1, PIGF, ANG-1, ANG-2.

    ANG-1: Angiopoietin 1.

    ANG-2: Angiopoietin 2.

    IGF: Insulin-like growth factor.

    IGFBP-1: insulin-like growth factor-binding protein 1.

    PIGF: Placental growth factor.

    VEGF: vascular endothelial growth factor.

    VEGF-R1: VEGF receptor-1. The ELGAN study measured the soluble form.

    VEGF-R2: VEGF receptor-2. The ELGAN study measured the soluble form.

Asthma: chronic respiratory disease characterized by airway narrowing and inflammation resulting in wheezing, shortness of breath, and cough.

Attention deficit hyperactivity disorder (ADHD): neurodevelopmental disorder characterized by a persistent pattern of inattention and/or hyperactivity and impulsivity.

Autism spectrum disorders: spectrum of neurodevelopmental disorders characterized by impaired social skills, verbal and nonverbal communication, and repetitive behaviors.

Body mass index (BMI): metric for assessing mass relative to height (kilograms/meters^2) and characterizing overweight and obese status.

Brain-derived neurotrophic factor (BDNF): a protein and member of the neurotrophin family of growth factors. BDNF has numerous biologic functions associated with neuroplasticity and neurodevelopmental health.

Bronchopulmonary dysplasia (BPD)/Chronic lung disease (CLD): The ELGAN study considered the child to have BPD/CLD if s/he continued to require supplemental oxygen at 36 weeks post-menstrual age.

Cerebral palsy: a disorder of movement and posture with functional impairment due to a disturbance of the developing brain

> **Leg-predominant symmetric spastic cerebral palsy:** synonymous with diparesis and diplegia; referring to a spastic form of cerebral palsy where the predominant abnormality is found in the legs and both legs are involved.

> **Four-limb symmetric spastic cerebral palsy:** synonymous with quadriparesis and quadriplegia; referring to a spastic form of cerebral palsy where all four limbs are affected.

> **Unilateral spastic cerebral palsy:** synonymous with hemiparesis and hemiplegia; referring to a spastic form of cerebral palsy where the abnormality is found in the arm and leg on the same size of the body.

Chemokines: cytokines that attract cells (leukocytes) to sites of infection/inflammation. Chemokines measured in the ELGAN study include IL-8 (CXCL8), MCP-1 (CCL2), MCP-4 (CCL13), MIP-1ß (CCL4), RANTES (CCL5), I-TAC (CXCL11).

> **I-TAC:** Interferon-inducible T-cell alpha chemoattractant.

> **MCP:** Monocyte chemoattractant protein.

> **MIP:** Macrophage inflammatory proteins.

> **RANTES:** Regulated upon Activation, Normal T cell Expressed and presumably Secreted.

Child Symptom Inventory-4 (CSI-4): a screening inventory of emotional and behavioral symptoms completed separately by parents and teachers.

Chromatin remodeling: regulated alteration of the chromatin structure to transcription (gene expression).

Confounding: Confounding is distortion (inaccuracy) of the estimated measure of association between the primary exposure of interest and the outcome are both associated with a third variable that has not been taken into consideration.

Congenital anomalies: structural or functional defects acquired during fetal development and present, although not necessarily detected, at birth.

Connectome: the complete inventory of white matter tracts. It can be rendered via two different MRI techniques: white matter tractography based on diffusion MRI and white matter fibrography based on qMRI.

C-reactive protein (CRP): protein synthesized by the liver in response to a circulating inflammatory stimulus.

Cytokines: peptides important in cell signaling. Subsumed under the cytokine umbrella are chemokines, interleukins, and tumor necrosis factors. They are neither growth factors nor hormones.

Developmental regulation: orderly changes in cell phenotypes attributed to maturation.

Diffuse astrogliosis: an abundance of (usually hypertrophic) astrocytes often accompanied by (immature) glial fibrils.

DNA methylation: addition of methyl groups to DNA, resulting in alterations to gene transcription (gene expression).

Early and persistent pulmonary dysfunction (EPPD): a pattern of lung disease in the ELGAN cohort characterized by the receipt of mechanical ventilation and high concentrations of oxygen throughout the first two postnatal weeks.

Echolucency: a relative paucity of echoes evident on an ultrasound scan presumed to indicate abnormality of the tissue; synonymous with hypoechoic.

Endotoxin: a toxin produced by, and confined to the outer membrane, of gram-negative bacteria that is released when the bacterial cell disintegrates. Lipopolysaccharides (LPS) are purified endotoxins.

Endodotoxin hypothesis: postnatal: postulates that the cerebral white matter damage associated with postnatal (gam-negative) bacteremia is due, in part, to a circulating product of these organisms, such as endotoxin.

Endodotoxin hypothesis: antenatal: postulates that the cerebral white matter damage associated with maternal urinary tract infection (and perhaps other potentially systemic infections) is due, in part, to a circulating product of infection or inflammation, such as endotoxin.

Epidemiology: study of incidence, prevalence, and determinants of health and disease at the population level.

Epigenetics: literally, above genetics. It refers to mechanisms (e.g. DNA methylation, chromatin remodeling, histone modifications, and non-coding RNA) that modify the influence of the genes we inherit. In essence, these mechanisms turn genes 'on' and 'off'.

Fetal growth restriction (FGR): (also intrauterine growth restriction [IUGR]) is a birthweight below the 10th percentile for gestational age. In the ELGAN study more extreme growth restriction was also defined as a birthweight more than 2 standard deviations below the expected mean (BWZ <−2).

Fetal vascular malperfusion: histologic evidence of an obstruction in the fetal vasculature, typically due to umbilical cord compromise. Features include avascular villi or fibrin deposition in fetal stem vessels.

Gestational diabetes: state of hyperglycemia developing during pregnancy, which increases risk for adverse pregnancy and neonatal outcomes.

Glucose metabolism: metabolism or processing of glucose to release energy to support cellular processes.

Gray matter: regions of the central nervous system consisting mainly of neuronal cell bodies, other supporting cells, and capillaries.

Histologic chorioamnionitis: inflammatory cell infiltration of the placental membranes and umbilical cord.

Hypertrophic astrocytes: plump astrocytes with abundant cytoplasm that stain pink with eosin.

Illness-severity. The concept that information about physiologic disturbances routinely collected in the intensive care unit conveys information about mortality risk. Illness-severity was introduced by health services researchers as a means of comparing mortality risk factors across institutions. The ELGAN study used the Score for Neonatal Acute Physiology (SNAP) (see below) to provide a summary indicator of the severity of physiologic derangements during the first postnatal 12 hours.

Interleukins: proteins that communicate specifically between immune cells (inter- means between and -leukins means leukocytes/white blood cells). These cytokines are typically denoted by IL + number. Interleukins measured in the ELGAN study include IL-1ß, IL-6, IL-6R (the circulating receptor of IL-6), and IL-8 (also listed above as a chemokine).

Interleukin-1alpha (IL-1α): pro-inflammatory cytokine that binds to the interleukin-1 receptor and activates numerous biologic pathways, including acute phase protein synthesis.

Interleukin-1 receptor antagonist (IL-1ra): cytokine that binds to IL-1 receptors and inhibits inflammatory effects of IL-1 proteins (IL-1a and IL-1b).

Interleukin-6 (IL-6): cytokine with both pro- and anti-inflammatory properties, responsible for activating numerous immune-related biological pathways.

Interleukin-8 (IL-8): cytokine functioning as a chemokine to activate neutrophils, promotes cell survival and proliferation in response to hematopoietic cytokines.

Intraventricular hemorrhage: bleeding within the cerebral ventricles.

Lowest temperature: the ELGAN study analyzed the lowest recorded temperature in the first 12 hours after birth. Because mortality risk varied significantly with the lowest recorded temperature in previous validation studies, SNAP-II/SNAPPE-II points were assigned based on the expected contribution of temperature (especially <95°F) to mortality risk.

Magnetic resonance imaging (MRI): collection of techniques using a powerful magnet and radiowaves for taking pictures of the inside of a person. MRI is particularly suited for imaging the soft tissues of the central nervous system: white matter (WM) and gray matter (GM).

> **Diffusion MRI:** special MRI technique that is sensitive to the molecular water motions.

> **MRI pulse sequence:** a specific MRI technique to give a particular image appearance or contrast.

> **Quantitative MRI:** collection of MRI techniques whereby the generated images are direct measures of physico-biological tissue properties.

> **Structural MRI:** image processing techniques geared to partition the brain into tissues types and substructures.

Maternal gestational weight gain: adequacy of the gravida's weight gain during the pregnancy was characterized as insufficient, adequate, or more than adequate according to criteria of the Institute of Medicine, based upon pre-pregnancy BMI status (underweight, overweight, or obese, as defined below).

Maternal obesity: BMI of 30 or greater.

Maternal overweight: BMI of 25–29.9.

Maternal vascular malperfusion: histologic evidence of poor maternal blood flow to the placenta. Features include a small placenta with infarctions or small chorionic villi with syncitiotrophoblastic knots.

Matrix metalloproteinases (MMPs): a group of enzymes that contribute to the degradation of extracellular matrix proteins. The ELGAN study measured MMP-1 and MMP-9.

Maturation-dependent vulnerability: susceptibility to perturbation and the resulting adverse consequences is highest during a specific window of maturation.

MPO: Myeloperoxidase is an enzyme most abundantly expressed in neutrophil granulocytes.

Myelinogenesis: the laying down and maturation of myelin in the developing brain.

National Collaborative Perinatal Project (NCPP): enrolled 55 000 pregnancies (women and their offspring) at 12 sites across the United States from 1959 to 1965 with uniform follow-up assessments for neurological and neurosensory dysfunctions last performed at age 7 years.

Necrotizing enterocolitis: a disorder of the intestines characterized by tissue necrosis (death); nearly all cases occur in newborns in the first months after preterm birth.

Neurotrophins: proteins that promote the survival, development, and function of neurons. Neurotrophins measured in the ELGAN study include neurotrophin 4 (NT4), brain-derived neurotrophic factor (BDNF), and basic fibroblast growth factor (bFGF). Most of the angiogenic proteins measured in this study also have neurotrophic properties.

Oxygen fraction (PO2/FiO2): the oxygen fraction used in calculations of SNAP-II and SNAPPE-II derive from a complex algorithm that identifies the lowest arterial oxygen tension (PO2) and the highest fraction of inspired oxygen (FiO2) in the first 12 hours after birth. Points are assigned to the total SNAP-II or SNAPPE-II score based on the lowest ratio of these recorded measures. In validation studies, SNAP-II and SNAPP-II varied inversely with the PO2/FiO2 ratio, so SNAP-II/SNAPPE-II points were assigned based on three ranges of PO2/FiO2 that correspond, incrementally, to mortality risk.

Preterm birth: occurring before 37 completed weeks of pregnancy. The World Health Organization further categories preterm birth as:

moderate to late preterm (32–37 weeks),

very preterm (28–32 weeks), and

extremely preterm (<28 weeks).

Perivascular amphophilic globules: globules that tend to be located near blood vessels in the developing brain and stain with both acid and basic dyes.

Periventricular leukomalacia: although originally defined by pathologists as histologic evidence of necrosis in the cerebral white matter of newborns, the diagnosis has more recently been applied to cranial ultrasound hypoechoic (echo-poor or echolucent) periventricular images.

pH, serum: in the ELGAN study, pH was measured in serum derived from arterial blood gas samples. The lowest serum pH represented the lowest recorded acidity of the infant's blood (on a logarithmic scale) collected in the first 12 hours after birth. As mortality risk varied significantly with serum pH values, points were assigned based one two ranges of serum pH, and their relative contribution to mortality risk.

Physiologic stability: a term conveying either qualitative or quantitative measures of clinical stability, especially as it pertains to the preservation of organ function or vital signs (e.g. hemodynamic stability, temperature stability, acid-base status).

Polymicrobial: literally, multiple microbes. Many clinicians expect the recovery of only one organism from the site of infection. The recovery of multiple microbes is often interpreted by these people as evidence of contamination. Increasingly, however, the co-occurrence of multiple organisms is seen as biologically important and clinically relevant.

Pulmonary deterioration (PD): a pattern of lung disease in the ELGAN cohort characterized by relatively good lung function in the first postnatal week, followed by need for supplemental oxygen and/or mechanical ventilation in the second week.

Retinopathy of prematurity: a retinal disorder characterized by abnormal blood vessel growth. The ELGAN study used the criteria proposed by the investigators who conducted the Early Treatment for Retinopathy of Prematurity (ET-ROP) study.

SAA: serum amyloid A proteins are mainly secreted by the liver and adipocytes (fat cells) in response to a circulating inflammatory stimulus

Score for Neonatal Physiology (SNAP): an illness severity score based on measures of physiologic dysfunction identified in the first 12 postnatal hours was introduced by Richardson et al. in 1999 to compare mortality risk across institutions and was validated in a population 1621 infants. The score included 34 clinical and physiologic variables associated with mortality risk in term and preterm infants.

Score for Neonatal Acute Physiology – second edition (SNAP-II): SNAP was later simplified and validated. The 34 elements of the original SNAP score were included in a multivariable regression model that identified the best logistic coefficients, creating an additive physiology-based score associated with in-hospital mortality. The elements included in SNAP-II are: lowest recorded serum pH, lowest recorded temperature, lowest recorded mean arterial blood pressure, lowest recorded oxygen fraction (PO2/FiO2) based on arterial blood gas samples and recorded oxygen fractions, the presence of one or more seizures, and urine output, each derived from data collected in the first 12 hours after birth.

Score for Neonatal Acute Physiology *Perinatal Extension* – second edition (SNAPPE-II): SNAPPE-II includes the same physiologic elements included in SNAP-II, but with added points for perinatal risk factors, also associated with mortality. The addition of these three perinatal risk factors (birthweight, low Apgar score, and small for gestational age) significantly enhanced SNAP-II's discrimination for mortality risk. As such, SNAPPE-II includes the six physiologic elements included in SNAP-II, plus three additional perinatal risk factors, for a total of nine elements.

Seizures, multiple: in the ELGAN study, 'multiple seizures' during the first 12 postnatal hours was defined as the presence of more than one seizure that was either highly suspected by at least two clinicians (attending resident, and/or nurse) or confirmed by either a neurologist or an electroencephalogram. A single seizure or suspected seizure did not qualify.

Sepsis: the recovery of bacteria from blood specimens obtained under sterile conditions. This was the definition of documented sepsis or septicemia. Clinical deterioration was not required because most of the infants in the ELGAN study were at one time or another very sick. Presumptive sepsis or septicemia was reported when the clinician considered it prudent to continue antibiotic treatment although blood cultures were negative.

Social and communications dysfunctions: the ELGAN study screened for these dysfunctions using the Social Responsiveness Scale (SRS). It provided an assessment of function in four subdomains of social reciprocity, including social awareness, social cognition, social communication, and social motivation. Dysfunctions were defined as total and component scores ≥65 (i.e., the 96th centile in the general population).

Spasticity: a neurological finding characterized by increased resistance to stretch of a muscle and/or exaggerated deep tendon reflexes

Systemic hypotension: in the ELGAN study, the lowest recorded mean arterial blood pressure (in the first 12 hours after birth) was used to calculate SNAP-II and SNAPPE-II. The ELGAN Study also defined hypotension as (1) the lowest mean arterial pressure (MAP) in the lowest quartile for gestational age, (2) treatment with a vasopressor, and (3) blood pressure lability, defined as the upper quartile of the difference between each infant's lowest and highest MAP.

Tumor necrosis factor- alpha (TNFα): secreted by inflammatory cells, this multifunctional cytokine belongs to a superfamily of type II transmembrane proteins, which distinguishes it from most other cytokines. TNF-R1 and TNF-R2 are circulating receptors of TNFα.

Urine output: in the ELGAN study, urine output was calculated based on the volume of urine collected from the time of birth until the infant was 12 hours of age. In previously published validation studies the contribution to mortality risk was greater for infants with urinary output less than 0.1ml/kg/hour. Therefore, points were assigned based on the relative contribution of urine output (especially <0.1ml/kg/hr) to mortality risk.

Ventriculomegaly: enlargement of the cerebral ventricles, which are fluid-filled cavities in the center of the brain.

Very low birthweight: <1500 grams.

White matter: regions of the central nervous system mainly made up of myelinated axons tracts.

White matter tractography: diffusion based technique with which white matter fibers can be delineated individually or globally thus enabling renditions of the connectome.

Index

NOTE: *f* = figure; *t* = table.

academic achievement 148–9, 197, 199, 203
  reading *vs.* math only 31, 207
  relationship with ADHD 150–1
acidemia 60, 95, 108, 197–8
adhesion molecules 3, 31, 108, 200–1
  definition/types 219
adiposity, maternal 9, 43–9, 205–6
  and cerebral palsy 133
  confounding with other factors 48–9
  consequences for mother 43–4
  developmental outcomes 44–5, 148; potential
    mechanisms 45–8; in term-born 44
  moves to combat 43
  pre-pregnancy *vs.* pregnancy weight gain 45
  prevalence 43, 49
  socioeconomic implications 48
angioneurins 198, 199
APACHE (Acute Physiology And Chronic Health
  Evaluation) 57, 58
APGAR (Appearance, Pulse, Grimace, Activity,
  and Respiration) scores 58
Asperger's syndrome 175
asthma
  not associated with BPD 89, 97
  risk factors 90, 97
ataxia 131
attention deficit hyperactivity disorder (ADHD) 22,
  147–8, 161, 172, 202, 219
  at age 10 174–5, 180–8
  co-morbid 149, 150–1, 175, 207
  comparative study findings 175–6
  complex 206
  gender differences 175
  impact of maternal adiposity 44–5, 45*t*, 46–7,
    206
  prevalence 172, 174
  (problems of) diagnosis 196
Autism Diagnostic Observation Schedule, Second
  Edition (ADOS-2) 151, 157, 196
autism spectrum disorder (ASD) 10, 157–60, 162–6,
  171, 197, 219
  at age 2 132, 157–8, 165–6, 176–80, 196

  at age 10 158–60, 162–3, 175, 196, 207
  antecedents 158–60, 159*t*, 163–5
  and cerebral palsy 132
  co-morbid 151–2
  critical items 158
  impact of bacteremia 77*t*
  impact of maternal adiposity 46–7
  linked to FGR 164, 166, 200
  linked to maternal infection 163–4
  linked to systemic inflammation 164–5, 166, 202
  prevalence 158, 159*f,* 162–3, 166
  screening for 196
Avon Longitudinal Study of Parents and Children xi

bacteremia 73–8, 197, 202, 207
  classification 73
  defined 73
  early *vs.* late 73, 75–6
  future research 78
  means of combating 78
  mechanism/pathophysiology 74–5
  outcomes at 2/10 years 76–8
  pregnancy disorders/neonatal conditions associated
    with 75–6, 76*t*
  prevalence/incidence 73–4, 74*t*
  and ROP 83
Banker, Betty Q. xiii–xiv
basic fibroblast growth factor (bFGF) 199
Bayley Scales of Infant Development II (BSID-II) 17,
  22, 47, 61, 95, 109
  Behavioral Rating Scale (BRS) 146, 171–2
  Mental Development Index (MDI) 76, 112, 132,
    172, 196
  Psychomotor Development Index (PDI) 132, 172,
    196, 200
behavioral development 44, 63, 66, 145, 171–90,
  197, 206
  Age 2 outcomes 146, 171–3, 176–80, 177–9*t*
  Age 10 outcomes 149, 173–5, 180–8, 181–7*t*
  comparative findings 175–88, 177–9*t*
  evaluation 172–3, 173*f*
  future research 189–90

gender differences 146, 175
see also attention deficit hyperactivity disorder;
    social impairment
birthweight(s) 1, 5–6*t*
    relationship with autism 159–60, 200
    relationship with bacteremia 58
    relationship with cerebral palsy 134–5, 138
    relationship with cognitive/behavioral development
        145, 150, 152, 177–9*t*, 181–7*t*
    relationship with illness-severity 58
    and risk of BPD 90, 92
    side effects of medication 96
    very low, defined 224
bleeding, intrauterine 36–7
blood gas derangements 197–8
    and BPD 94–5
    brain-related outcomes 60–1, 61*f*, 108, 197–8
    and cerebral palsy 135
    and illness severity 198
    ultrasound detection 108, 111
    see also specific types
blood pressure, measurement of 197
brain-derived neutrotrophic factor (BDNF) 4, 47–8,
    84, 165, 199, 200, 201, 204, 219
brain dysfunction 10
    impact of maternal adiposity 46–7, 205–6
    indicators 10
brain injury xi, 10, 197
    and blood gas derangements 60–1, 61*f*, 197–8
    correlation with illness-severity 65–6, 198
    high-risk groupings 5
    and hypotension 60, 61*f*
    linked to endodotoxin 2
    'two-hit' model 203
    see also white matter damage
brain structure, periods of 118, 120
British Birth Surveys *see* Avon Longitudinal Study…
bronchopulmonary dysplasia (BPD) xi, 10, 39, 59,
    66, 89–98, 219
    and blood gas values 94–5
    and cerebral palsy 136–7, 138
    definition(s) 89, 137, 219
    and early lung disease 90–2, 91*t*
    future studies 97–8
    genetic factors 97–8
    importance/definitions 89
    linked to FGR 89–90
    linked to gestational age/birthweight 90
    neurodevelopmental outcomes 95–6, 148
    prevalence 136

pulmonary outcomes 96–7
risk factors 89–94
and systemic inflammation 92–4, 93*t*

C-reactive protein (CRP) 47, 93*t*, 94
central nervous system (CNS), relationship with
    immune system 4, 204
cerebral palsy (CP) 2, 3, 9, 17, 22, 44, 60–1, 131–9,
    202
    and bacteremia 76
    and BPD 95, 96
    comorbidities 132, 207
    comparative studies 134–5, 138–9
    defined 220
    degrees of disability 132
    diagnosis, problems of 131
    gender differences 135
    neonatal risk factors 135–9
    and placental lesions 31–2
    prenatal risk factors 133–5, 139
    and protein biomarkers 137–8
    relationship with gestational age 134, 135, 139
    study methods 131–2, 139
    subtypes 22, 96, 110, 131, 132, 136, 139, 220
    ultrasound predictors 109–10, 111–12
    and white matter injury 109–10, 111–12
cervical insufficiency 20, 107
    associated with intrauterine inflammation 35,
        36, 37
Cesarean section, risk of microcephaly 22
chemokines 139, 200–1
    defined 220
    reduced concentration 92
    release of 36
Child Behavioral Checklist (CBC) 22, 109, 163,
    164, 172
    Dysregulation Profile (CBCL-DP) 172, 180
Child Symptom Inventory-4 (CSI-4) 10, 173–4, 220
chorioamnionitis xiii–xiv, 17–18, 172, 221
    impact on brain development 27–8, 31
    prevalence 28*t*, 29–30
    and ROP 84
chorionic plate 201
    infiltration 30
    inflammation 20, 28, 29–30, 29*t*, 133
    thrombi 134–5
    vasculitis 20, 22, 28, 29*t*
cognitive development 10, 145–52, 197
    and ADHD 150–1
    Age 2 outcomes 145–6

Age 10 outcomes 146–9, 207
  and ASD 151–2
  assessment methods 123
  and cerebral palsy 132
  and FGR 200
  genetic factors 49, 205
  impact of bacteremia 75–7, 77t
  impact of BDP/associated factors 95–6, 148
  impact of maternal adiposity 44–5, 45t, 46–7, 206
  impact of pregnancy disorders 39
  and inflammatory protcins 46t
  and SNAP-II scores 62–3, 63t
  socioeconomic factors 204–5
  ultrasound predictions 111
  see also academic achievement
comorbidities 206–7, 208t
confounding 48–9, 220
connectomics 116, 123–4, 125, 220
cytokines 139
  defined 220
  high levels of 39, 200–1
  linked to BPD 92–4
  linked to fetal brain damage 2, 3
  linked to ROP 84
  release of 36–7

Dean Laterality Preference Schedule 196–7
deoxyribonucleic acid (DNA)
  methylation 20, 39, 47, 220
Developmental Epidemiological Network xiii–xiv, 105
developmental regulation 198–9
diabetes, gestational 43, 221
Differential Ability Scales, Second Edition (DAS-II)
  test 47, 77t, 123, 147–8, 150–1, 161, 174, 196
diffuse astrogliosis 2, 220
diffusion tensor imaging (DTI) 116, 119–20
diparesis 22, 96, 110, 131
  relationship with neurodevelopment 136
  specific risk factors 133, 138
dyskinesia 131

early and persistent pulmonary dysfunction
  (EPPD) 220
  linked to BPD 90–1, 93
echolucency 60–1, 105, 202
ELGAN (Extremely Low Gestational Age Newborns)
  study
  achievements/significance 10, 171, 195–209
  comparison of findings with other studies 110–11,
    163, 164, 175–88

data quality 195–7
demographics 5–6t, 7–9, 8t
distributed environment 7–8
ethnic composition 6t, 7–9, 8t
fields/methods of study 5–9
funding 9
future directions 209
genesis xi–xii, xiv, 1–5
objectives 5, 208–9
strengths/weaknesses 189
emotional regulation (ER)
  gender differences 172
  links with extremely preterm birth 171–2
endodotoxin(s) 2, 188, 221
  'endodotoxin hypothesis' 2, 221
  see also lipopolysaccharides
epigenetic age 65
epigenetic modifications 20–1, 39, 204
  and maternal adiposity 47
epigenetics, defined 221
epilepsy 197, 207
  and cerebral palsy 132
epimutations 39
executive dysfunction 147–8, 203
  comorbidities 207
  reduced risk of 199
extremely preterm birth(s)
  defined 1, 223
  demographic characteristics 5–6t, 36
  disorders leading to 35–6
  longterm outcomes xi
  mortality rates 59–60, 59t
  principal morbidities xi
  signal initiators 35–40

fetal growth restriction (FGR) 1, 5, 29, 31, 199,
  200–1
  associated with autism 164, 166
  associated with placental insufficiency 35–6, 37–8
  associated with systemic inflammation 94, 204
  defined 221
  longterm impacts 149
  mortality rates 38
  not associated with CP 133, 135
  as risk factor for BPD 89–90, 91–2, 94
fetal stem vessel thrombosis 31, 39, 172

Generalized Anxiety Disorder 175
Gilles, Floyd 1
Gram-negative organisms 2

gray matter
   changes in biological state 117
   defined 221
   T1/T2 curves 121–2
   volume 118
Gross Motor Function Classification System
   (GMFCS) 132, 146, 149

head circumference *see* microcephaly
'Healthy People' initiative (US) 43
hemiparesis 96, 110, 131
   relationship with neurodevelopment 136
   specific risk factors 138
histologic lesions, placental 27–32, 39
   inflammatory *vs.* abnormal placentation 29,
      31–2, 36
   prevalence 27–8, 28*t*
   relationship with cerebral palsy 133
   relationship with clinical presentation at
      delivery 29
   relationship with recovery of microorganisms
      29–30, 29*t*
   relationship with serum concentrations 30
   value of study 31–2
hypercapnia 60, 94–5, 197–8
hyperechoic lesions, cerebral 107
hyperglycemia 221
hyperoxemia 60, 83, 197–8
hyperoxia
   and lung inflammation 92
   and ROP 81, 84
hypertrophic astrocytes 1–2
hypocapnia 60, 95, 197–8
hypoechoic lesions, cerebral 107, 108
   longterm outcomes 109–10
hypotension, systemic 198
   defined 224
   non-association with CP 135, 139
   relationship with brain injury 60, 61*f*, 108, 197
   treatment 198
hypoxemia 60, 65, 95, 197–8
hypoxia, and cerebral palsy 135
hypoxia-ischemia xiii

illness-severity 57–66, 108
   and blood gas derangements 198
   and brain injury 60–2
   defined 221
   development of scoring system 57
   mortality rates 59–60, 63–4

   need for further studies 66
   neurocognitive outcomes (long-term) 62–3, 63*t*
   relationship with birthweight 58
   relationship with developmental dysfunctions,
      reasons for 65–6
   relationship with early neonatal physiology
      63–6
   short-term outcomes 60
   see also Score for Neonatal Acute Physiology
immune system
   immature, linked to bacteremia 74–5
   relationship with CNS 4, 204
inflammation
   associated with ADHD 172–3, 173*f*,
      174–5, 188
   associated with autism/social impairment 161–2,
      164–5, 166
   associated with FGR 94, 204
   associated with physiologic derangements 66
   associated with ROP 83, 84
   and cerebral palsy 137–9
   epigenetic effects 204
   fetal 2–3
   impaired resolution of 74
   linked to brain injury 74–5, 108–9
   linked to maternal adiposity 46–7, 46*t*, 205–6
   medications 134
   mental health outcomes 188–9
   postnatal 3, 38–9, 200–1
   proteins associated with 3–4, 38, 39, 46*t*, 75*t*,
      84, 92–3, 93*t*, 108, 137–9, 161–2, 162*t*, 165,
      174–5, 203, 204
   (range of) comorbidities 206–7
   range of outcomes 202
   as risk factor for BPD 92–4
   socioeconomic factors 205
   sustained 202–3
   see also intrauterine inflammation; placental
      inflammation
insulin-like growth factors (IGFs) 38, 199
   binding protein (IGFBP-1) 38, 84
   and ROP 84, 85
intelligence quotient (IQ) 149, 150–1, 174, 200
   comorbidities 206, 207
   maternal 148
   and social skills 161
interleukins 47, 93*t*, 137–8, 139, 188, 201, 221
intracranial volume 118
intrauterine growth restriction (IUGR) *see* fetal
   growth restriction

intrauterine inflammation
    combination with other factors 36–7
    neurologic injuries associated with 30–2, 38–9
    pregnancy disorders associated with 36–7,
        39–40, 133
    rates of, in preterm births 36
    and ROP 83
intraventricular hemorrhage (IVH) 59, 221
    and cerebral palsy 136
    isolated *vs.* with white matter injury 109
    longterm outcomes 109, 111
    neuroimaging 105, 106, 107, 110, 111

Lactobacillus sp. 22
language skills, development of 148
    impact of bacteremia 77*t*
    impact of maternal adiposity 45
Larroche, Jeanne Claudie xiii–xiv
laser treatment 82, 85
learning disorders *see* cognitive development
left-handedness 149, 196–7
lipopolysaccharides (LPS)
    defined 221
    impact on developing brain 2, 3, 4, 203, 204
longitudinal magnetization relaxation time (T1) 116,
    121, 123
lung disease 202, 223
    chronic *see* bronchopulmonary dysplasia (BPD)
    early, linked with BPD 90–2

magnesium, administration at delivery 148
magnesium sulfate 134
magnetic resonance imaging (MRI) 10, 222
    development of technology 115
    diffusion (dMRI) 119–20, 120*f,* 124, 125
    methods/pulse sequences 116–17
    metrics 117–18
    structural (sMRI) 117–18
    subject-by-subject processing *vs.* voxel-based
        morphometry 118
    see also multispectral quantitative MRI
mathematical abilities, (delayed) development 31,
    148–9, 207
matrix metalloproteinases (MMPs) 37, 39, 47, 93*t,*
    108, 200–1
    defined 222
Medicaid 195
medications, maternal, association with CP 134
metalloproteinases *see* matrix metalloproteinases
microbiomes 18, 48, 49, 201

microcephaly 46, 60–1, 202
    and cerebral palsy 132, 135
    placental microorganisms and 21–2
    and ROP 85
    ultrasound predictors 109–10
microorganisms, placental 17–22, 201–2
    beneficial 22
    common types 18
    frequency of isolation/log count 18, 19*t*
    methods of investigation 17–19
    relationship with cerebral palsy 22, 133
    relationship with inflammation in newborn 21
    relationship with intrauterine inflammation
        20–1, 39
    relationship with pregnancy complications 20
    relationship with preterm birth 20
    relationship with retinopathy 21–2
    ultrasound detection 107
'minicephaly,' placental microorganisms and 21–2
Modified Checklist for Autism in Toddlers
    (M-CHAT) 132, 157–8, 165, 196
motor development 10, 149
    impact of maternal adiposity 44–5, 45*t*
    ultrasound predictions 111
multiple births 172, 206
multispectral quantitative magnetic resonance imaging
    (MS-qMRI) 115–26
    acquisition protocols 125
    advantages 115
    channels of information 116*f*
    development of techniques 115
    future research 124–5
    image processing 126
    metrics 117
    operating principles 117
    specific parameters 118–22, 119*f* (*see also*
        connectomics; longitudinal magnetization
        relaxation time; proton density; transverse
        magnetization relaxation time; volumetry;
        white matter fibrography/tractography)
    study methods 122–3
    study results 123–4, 125
    theoretical background 116–17
myelin 121–2
    structure 121*f*
myelination 136
myelinogenesis 222

National Collaborative Perinatal Project (NCPP)
    xi, 2, 222

National Institute of Neurological Disorders and
Stroke (NINDS) 9
necrosis, causes of development 1–2
necrotizing enterocolitis (NEC) 59, 66, 135, 138,
197, 222
Neonatal Brain Hemorrhage Study 105, 135, 138
NEPSY-II Auditory Response test 77*t*, 147–8,
150–1, 161, 163, 174, 196
nerve growth factor (NGF) 204
neurotrophins 4, 38, 198–9
definition/types 222
and maternal adiposity 47–8
see also brain-derived neutrotrophic factor
New Jersey Study xiii–xiv
non-steroidal anti-inflammatory drugs (NSAIDs)
134
nutrition, neonatal, and ROP 83

oligodendrocytes 136, 198, 199
Opposition Defiant Disorder 175
Oral and Written Language Scales (OWLS) test 77*t*,
150, 161, 164, 174
organ damage, multiple 203
organ function, immature 64–5
oxygen
fraction, defined 222
low levels/supplementary requirement 90–2,
91*t*
as risk factor for ROP 83

painkillers, association with CP 134
perfusion, cerebral 60
and MRI 121
peripheral retinal ablation 82, 85
periventricular amphophilic globules
bacteriological significance 1–2
and endotoxin hypothesis 2
periventricular hemorrhagic farction 107
periventricular leukomalacia 1–2, 85, 223
neuroimaging 107
pH values 223
physiologic stability, defined 223
Physiologic Stability Index (PSI) 57
placenta
bacteriology 9, 17–22, 195 (*see also*
microorganisms, placental)
biopsies 17–18
epigenetic modifications 20–1
histology 9, 20, 27–32, 195 (*see also*
histologic lesions)

as modulator of inflammatory process/later
outcomes 189–90, 189*f*
polymicrobial infections 201–2
placental abruption 20, 133
associated with intrauterine inflammation 35,
36–7
placental dysfunction 36, 40, 199–200
and ADHD 172
and ROP 83
placental inflammation 31, 35–6, 38, 107
placental insufficiency 199–200, 201
defined 37
impact on pregnancy/newborn 37–8
polymerase chain reaction (PCR) analyses 18–19, 30
polymicrobial placental cultures 201–2
polymorphonuclear cells (PMNs), decrease in 74
postnatal physiologic depression 64
preeclampsia 20, 29, 31, 107, 133, 164, 199
associated with placental insufficiency 35–6, 37–8
correlation with FGR 94
epimutations and 39
mortality rates following 38
relationship with autism 159–60
pregnancy disorders 35–40
developmental correlates 38–40
medication 134
relationship with autism 159–60, 163–4
see also cervical insufficiency; intrauterine
inflammation; placental insufficiency
preterm birth(s)
complications leading to 20, 35–6
defined 223
mortality/morbidity rates 35
spontaneous *vs.* indicated 35, 39
see also extremely preterm birth(s)
preterm labor 20
associated with intrauterine inflammation 35,
36, 37
preterm prelabor rupture of membranes
(pPROM) 20
associated with intrauterine inflammation 35,
36, 37
proteins
angiogenic 38, 199, 204, 219
elevated levels, and ASD 161–2
and reduced risk of dysfunctions 84–5, 199
see also under inflammation
proton density, mapping 118–19, 123
psychiatric dysfunctions 10, 175, 188–9
future research 189–90

pulmonary deterioration (PD) 223
pulmonary surfactant administration xiii

quadriparesis 22, 96, 110, 131, 132
    relationship with neurodevelopment 136
    specific risk factors 133, 138

resuscitation, efforts at 64–5
retinopathy of prematurity (ROP) xi, 10, 39,
    59, 81–5, 207, 223
    classification 81, 82t
    examinations for 82–3
    future research 85
    longterm outcomes 81, 85
    phases of development 81
    placental microorganisms and 21–2
    risk factors 81, 200; in neonatal period 83;
        in pregnancy 83
    treatment 82

Score for Neonatal Acute Physiology (SNAP) 10,
    57–66, 197, 222, 223
    and brain injury 60–2, 65–6
    and cerebral palsy 135
    correlation with mortality 58, 59–60, 59t,
        63–4
    method of calculation 57, 58
    neurocognitive outcomes (long-term) 62–3,
        63t, 197
    Perinatal Extension (SNAP-PE) 58, 197, 223–4
    relationship with gestational age 63–4
    SNAP-II 57, 58–66, 197, 223–4
seizures, multiple 224
sepsis xi, 10, 66, 135, 138
    defined 73, 224
    incidence 73–4
sequential subject-by-subject processing 118
serum concentrations, post-natal 30
smoking (in pregnancy)
    effect on child 148, 172, 180
    effect on pregnancy 36
social impairment (non-autistic) 63, 66, 160–2,
    163–6, 176, 197, 202
    antecedents 163–5
    defined 224
    distinguished from autism 160
    impact of bacteremia 78
    linked to FGR 164, 166
    prevalence 163, 166
    (problems of) definition 157, 160, 224

reduced risk of 84–5
related protein concentrations 161–2, 162t, 165
    and SNAP-II scores 63
    see also autism spectrum disorder
Social Responsiveness Scale (SRS) 77t, 160–2, 163,
    164, 196, 224
socioeconomic status 97, 204–5
    and ADHD 172
    and comorbidities 207
    and maternal adiposity 48
spasticity 131, 136, 224
'sterile womb' hypothesis 18, 201
steroids
    antenatal administration 65, 66, 75, 110–11,
        134
    postnatal administration 95
Stockholm Youth Cohort Study 163, 164
strabismus 85, 197
Streptococcus sp. 39
Susser, Mervyn xiii–xiv
Sweden, extremely preterm studies 134
syncytial knots 28, 35–6, 37–8

thrombosis, placental 39
transverse magnetization relaxation time (T2) 116,
    122, 123, 125
triplets see multiple births
tumor necrosis factor alpha (TNFα)
    defined 224
    levels of 2, 30, 47, 75t, 84, 92
twins see multiple births
'two-hit' studies 203

ultrasound 10, 105–12
    and cerebral palsy 136, 138
    and infant neurodevelopmental outcomes
        109–10, 111
    inter-observer reliability 106–7, 110
    neonatal factors 108–9
    prenatal factors 107
    recommended circumstances 105
    studies, in extremely preterm infants 105–6,
        110–11
umbilical cord vasculitis 22, 29t, 30, 76t
urinary tract infection (maternal), linked to
    developmental impairments 2
urine, output 224

vascular endothelial growth factor (VEGF) 47, 81,
    84, 108, 139, 174–5

vascular malperfusion
    fetal 27, 221
    maternal 27, 28*t*, 29, 222
vasculitis xiii–xiv, 17–18
    chorionic 20, 22, 28, 29*t*
    umbilical 22, 29*t*, 30, 76*t*
ventilation xiii, 91, 136, 202
    risks in later childhood 96
ventriculomegaly 30, 31–2, 60–1, 202, 224
    longterm outcomes 109–10
    neuroimaging 105, 107, 108–9
    reduced risk of 199
Vineland Adaptive Behavior Scales (VABS) 95
visual impairments *see* retinopathy
visual perception tests/impairment 149
volumetry 125
    comparative, results of study 123
    defined 118
voxel-based morphometry 118, 125

Wechsler Individual Achievement Test-III
    (WIAT-III) 47, 77*t*, 148, 150, 151, 174, 198, 207
weight gain, excessive, in pregnancy 45, 206, 222
white matter 224
    changes in biological state 117, 125
    fibrography (WMF) 123–4, 124*f*, 125
    proton density 118–19
    T1/T2 curves 121–2
    tractography (WMT) 116, 119–20, 123, 124, 224
    volume 118
white matter injury 1–2, 60, 95, 134, 199
    and cerebral palsy 136, 138
    and cognitive development 146
    failure to ascertain 138
    longterm outcomes 109–10
    neuroimaging 4–5, 105, 106, 108–9, 110–12
    and reduced brain growth 109
World Health Organization (WHO) 1, 223

Other titles from Mac Keith Press www.mackeith.co.uk

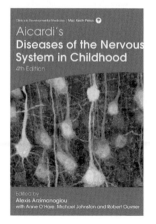

Aicardi's Diseases of the Nervous System in Childhood, 4th Edition
Alexis Arzimanoglou, Anne O'Hare, Michael V Johnston and Robert Ouvrier (Editors)

Clinics in Developmental Medicine
2018 ▪ 1524pp ▪ hardback ▪ 978-1-909962-80-4

This fourth edition retains the patient-focussed, clinical approach of its predecessors. The international team of editors and contributors has honoured the request of the late Jean Aicardi, that his book remain 'resolutely clinical', which distinguishes *Diseases of the Nervous System in Childhood* from other texts in the field. New edition completely updated and revised and now in full colour.

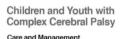
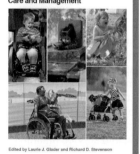

Children and Youth with Complex Cerebral Palsy: Care and Management
Laurie J. Glader and Richard D. Stevenson (Editors)

A Practical Guide from Mac Keith Press
2019 ▪ 404pp ▪ softback ▪ 978-1-909962-98-9

This is the first practical guide to explore management of the many medical comorbidities that children with complex CP face, including orthopaedics, mobility needs, cognition and sensory impairment, difficult behaviours, respiratory complications and nutrition, amongst others. Uniquely, contributors include children and parents, providing applied wisdom for family-centred care. Clinical Care Tools are provided to help guide clinicians and include a Medical Review Supplement, Equipment and Services Checklist and an ICF-Based Care: Goals and Management Form.

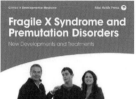
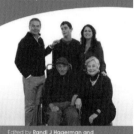

Fragile X Syndrome and Premutation Disorders: New Developments and Treatments
Randi J Hagerman and Paul J Hagerman (Editors)

Clinics in Developmental Medicine
2020 ▪ 192pp ▪ hardback ▪ 978-1-911612-37-7

Fragile X syndrome results from a gene mutation on the X-chromosome, which leads to various intellectual and developmental disabilities. *Fragile X Syndrome and Premutation Disorders* offers clinicians and families a multidisciplinary approach in order to provide the best possible care for patients with Fragile X. Unique features of the book include what to do when an infant or toddler is first diagnosed, the impact on the family and an international perspective on how different cultures perceive the syndrome.

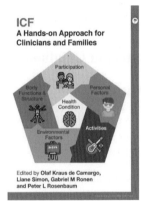

ICF: A Hands-on Approach for Clinicians and Families
Olaf Kraus de Camargo, Liane Simon, Gabriel M. Ronen and Peter L. Rosenbaum (Editors)

A practical guide from Mac Keith Press
2019 ▪ 192pp ▪ softback ▪ 978-1-911612-04-9

This accessible handbook introduces the World Health Organisation's International Classification of Functioning, Disability and Health (ICF) to professionals working with children with disabilities and their families. It contains an overview of the elements of the ICF but focusses on practical applications, including how the ICF framework can be used with children, families and carers to formulate health and management goals.

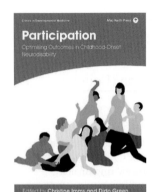

Participation: Optimising Outcomes in Childhood-Onset Neurodisability
Christine Imms and Dido Green (Editors)

Clinics in Developmental Medicine
2020 ▪ 288pp ▪ hardback ▪ 978-1-911612-17-9

This unique book focuses on enabling children and young people with neurodisability to participate in the varied life situations that form their personal, familial and cultural worlds. Chapters provide diverse examples of evidence-based practices and are enriched by scenarios and vignettes to engage and challenge the reader to consider how participation in meaningful activities might be optimised for individuals and their families. The book's practical examples aim to facilitate knowledge transfer, clinical application and service planning for the future.

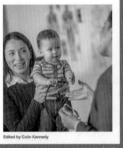

Principles and Practice of Child Neurology in Infancy, 2nd Edition
Colin Kennedy (Editor)

A Practical Guide from Mac Keith Press
2021 ▪ 552pp ▪ softback ▪ 978-1-911612-00-1

Management of neurological disorders presenting in infancy poses many challenges for clinicians. Using a symptom-based approach, and covering a wide range of scenarios, the latest edition of this comprehensive practical guide provides authoritative advice from distinguished experts. It now includes revised coverage of disease prevention, clinical assessment, and promotion of neurodevelopment.

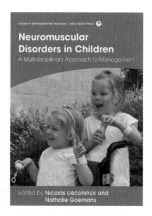

Neuromuscular Disorders in Children: A Multidisciplinary Approach to Management
Nicolas Deconinck and Nathalie Goemans (Editors)

Clinics in Developmental Medicine
2019 ▪ 468pp ▪ hardback ▪ 978-1-911612-09-4

Neuromuscular Disorders in Children: A Multidisciplinary Approach to Management critically reviews current evidence of management approaches in the field of neuromuscular disorders (NMDs) in children. Uniquely, the book focusses on assessment as the cornerstone of management and highlights the importance of a multidisciplinary approach.

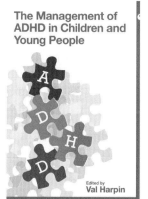

The Management of ADHD in Children and Young People
Val Harpin (Editor)

A Practical Guide from Mac Keith Press
2017 ▪ 292pp ▪ softback ▪ 978-1-909962-72-9

This book is an accessible and practical guide on all aspects of assessment of children and young people with Attention Deficit Hyperactivity Disorder (ADHD) and how they can be managed successfully. The multi-professional team of authors discusses referral, assessment and diagnosis, psychological management, pharmacological management, and co-existing conditions, as well as ADHD in the school setting. New research on girls with ADHD is also featured. Case scenarios are included that bring these topics to life.

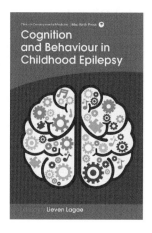

Cognition and Behaviour in Childhood Epilepsy
Lieven Lagae (Editor)

Clinics in Developmental Medicine
2017 ▪ 186pp ▪ hardback ▪ 978-1-909962-87-3

For many parents, cognitive and behavioral comorbidities, such as ADHD, autism and intellectual disability, are the real burden of childhood epilepsy. This title offers concrete guidance and treatment strategies for childhood epilepsy in general, and for the comorbidities associated with each epilepsy syndrome and their pathophysiology. The book is written by experts in the field with an important clinical experience, while chapters by clinical neuropsychologists provide a strong theoretical background.

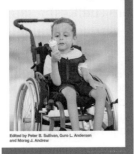

Nutrition and Neurodisability
Peter B. Sullivan, Guro L. Andersen and Morag J. Andrew (Editors)

A Practical Guide from Mac Keith Press
2020 ▪ 208pp ▪ softback ▪ 978-1-911612-26-1

Feeding difficulties are common in children with neurodisability and disorders of the central nervous system can affect the movements required for safe and efficient eating and drinking. This practical guide provides strategies for managing the range of nutritional problems faced by children with neurodevelopmental disability. The easily accessible information on aetiology, assessment and management is informed by a succinct review of current evidence and guidelines to inform best practice.

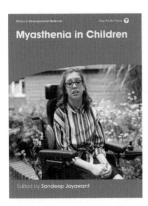

Myasthenia in Children
Sandeep Jayawant (Editor)

Clinics in Developmental Medicine
2019 ▪ 144pp ▪ hardback ▪ 978-1-911612-30-8

Myasthenia is a rare, but underdiagnosed and sometimes life-threatening disorder in children. There are no guidelines for diagnosing and managing these children, especially those with congenital myasthenia, a more recently recognised genetic condition, but there have been significant developments in identification and treatment of myasthenia in recent years. This book will help clinicians and families of children with this rare condition direct management effectively.

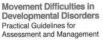
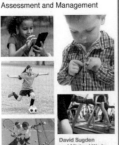

Movement Difficulties in Developmental Disorders
David Sugden and Michael Wade (Authors)

A Practical Guide from Mac Keith Press
2019 ▪ 240pp ▪ softback ▪ 978-1-909962-95-8

This book presents the latest evidence-based approaches to assessing and managing movement disorders in children. Uniquely, children with developmental coordination disorder (DCD) and children with movement difficulties as a co-occurring secondary characteristic of another development disorder, including ADHD, ASD, and Dyslexia, are discussed. It will prove a valuable guide for anybody working with children with movement difficulties, including clinicians, teachers and parents.